EXERCISE IN PREGNANCY

Second Edition

EXERCISE IN PREGNANCY

Second Edition

Editors

Raul Artal Mittelmark, M.D., F.A.C.O.G., F.A.C.S.M.

Professor of Obstetrics, Gynecology and Exercise Sciences
Department of Obstetrics and Gynecology
Division of Maternal-Fetal Medicine
University of Southern California School of Medicine
Los Angeles, California

Robert A. Wiswell, Ph.D.

Associate Professor and Chairman
Department of Exercise Science
Research Associate, Andrews Gerontology Center
University of Southern California
Los Angeles, California

Barbara L. Drinkwater, Ph.D., F.A.C.S.M.

Research Physiologist
Department of Medicine
Pacific Medical Center
Seattle, Washington

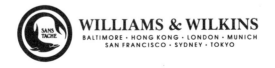

WILLIAMS & WILKINS
BALTIMORE · HONG KONG · LONDON · MUNICH
SAN FRANCISCO · SYDNEY · TOKYO

Editor: Carol-Lynn Brown
Associate Editor: Victoria M. Vaughn
Copy Editors: Shelley Potler, Susan Vaupel
Designer: Wilma E. Rosenberger
Illustration Planner: Ray Lowman
Production Coordinator: Barbara J. Felton
Cover Designer: Wilma E. Rosenberger

RG
558.7
.E94
1991

Copyright © 1991
Williams & Wilkins
428 East Preston Street
Baltimore, Maryland   21202, USA

Accurate indications, adverse reactions, and dosage schedules for
drugs are provided in this book, but it is possible that they may
change. The reader is urged to review the package information
data of the manufacturers of the medications mentioned.

Printed in the United States of America

First Edition 1986

Library of Congress Cataloging-in-Publication Data

Exercise in pregnancy / edited by Raul Artal Mittelmark, Robert A.
  Wiswell, Barbara L. Drinkwater. — 2nd ed.
     p.   cm.
  Includes bibliographical references.
  ISBN 0-683-00258-9
  1. Pregnancy.   2. Exercise for women—Physiological aspects.
I. Artal Mittelmark, Raul.   II. Wiswell, Robert A.   III. Drinkwater,
Barbara L., 1926–
  [DNLM: 1. Exercise—in pregnancy.   2. Pregnancy.   WQ 200 E96]
RG558.7.E94   1990
618.2'4—dc20
DNLM/DLC
for Library of Congress   90-12009
                                                                CIP

90 91 92 93 94
1 2 3 4 5 6 7 8 9 10

*This book is dedicated to our families
for their support and encouragement*

Foreword

The health benefits of exercise are well known and are accompanied by a feeling of well-being. Therefore, an ever-increasing number of women are engaging in some form of regular physical exercise. Exercise programs are initiated while in school and are continued by a substantial number of women after they graduate and begin working in an occupation or at home. When these women become pregnant, most wish to continue their regular forms of exercise but have concerns about possible adverse effects upon the fetus caused by strenuous exercise. Therefore, it is important to obtain information about the effect of different types of exercise, different amounts of exercise, and different intensities of exercise during pregnancy upon both fetal and maternal anatomy and physiology. Dr. Artal and his coeditors and contributors provided much information about this subject in

the first edition of *Exercise in Pregnancy*. Since that volume was published, much new information has been obtained by scientific investigation of the subject. The editors have invited the individuals performing the most important and meaningful studies of various aspects of the effects of exercise during pregnancy to summarize the results and interpretation of the data in the chapters of the second edition of *Exercise in Pregnancy*. This volume will be of great value to all of those in the medical profession who care for or counsel pregnant women.

Daniel R. Mishell, Jr., M.D.
Professor and Chairman
Department of Obstetrics and Gynecology
University of Southern California
School of Medicine
Los Angeles, California

Preface to the Second Edition

Women are continuing an active lifestyle while pregnant and exercise programs are proliferating. The need for updating the information in this rapidly expanding field is essential for health care providers.

In this new expanded edition, we are joined by Dr. Barbara Drinkwater, a prominent exercise physiologist with a career-long interest in exercise in women.

The goal of this second edition of *Exercise in Pregnancy* has been identical to the one set in the first edition: collate all existing significant information to serve as a basis for exercise prescription in pregnancy. In this revised edition, we have given much consideration to the reviews of the first edition as well as to the suggestions advanced by many of our colleagues and associates.

The additions and revisions included in this second edition are numerous and were made possible by the collaboration of new contributors to whom we are most grateful.

The significant advances in the field are reflected in the addition of 13 new chapters.

We intentionally allowed certain overlap of information among chapters to enable most chapters to serve as independent references.

The revised content of the second edition includes a restructured format of three large sections to enable a more logical sequence of information. In addition, we have attempted to provide the physiological background for a variety of physical activities conducted in various environments to include altitude, water, and heat stress.

The data accumulated and published over the past 5 years permit a more accurate determination of normal maternal physiological responses to exercise; and, at the same time, an evaluation of the fetal responses.

We no longer have to claim that there is lack of data to allow safe, moderate exercise prescription in pregnancy. However, some of the data still lack the statistical power to make definitive statements and recommendations regarding strenuous exercise. Valuable information has been accumulated to allow the next step: clinical applications for exercise in pregnancy. One example is the use of exercise as adjunctive therapy in pregnant diabetics.

The editors wish to express their gratitude to the staff of Williams & Wilkins: specifically, Editor, Carol-Lynn Brown; Associate Editor, Victoria Vaughn; Production Coordinator, Barbara Felton; Copy Editor, Shelley Potler; Illustration Planner, Wayne Hubbel; and Designer, Wilma Rosenberger. They have been outstanding in their support and professionalism.

Raul Artal Mittelmark, M.D., F.A.C.O.G., F.A.C.S.M.
Robert A. Wiswell, Ph.D.
Barbara L. Drinkwater, Ph.D., F.A.C.S.M.

Preface to the First Edition

The impetus for writing a book on exercise in pregnancy stemmed from a common interest we shared for the past 5 years. The fascination with and the contemporary attitudes toward physical fitness are frequently carried into pregnancy. Unfortunately, no standards for exercise in pregnancy are available. Pursuing a common interest has allowed invaluable interactions between exercise physiologists and obstetricians. We set out to compile existing information and yet no authoritative source could be identified. The information that we have initially reviewed was rather scarce, anecdotal, and largely related to animal studies.

We see our attempt as a first step toward creating a reference source for exercise prescription in pregnancy. We have included much of our own data; many of the opinions expressed in the book are our own. Some of the opinions may be biased and are based upon long hours of study and observation of pregnant women exercising under laboratory conditions.

We hope this book will generate a stimulus for new research that will help solve the question posed throughout the text: Is exercise beneficial and safe for the mother and her fetus?

Much of the data presented in this text has been the product of collaboration. We would like to express our gratitude to all the contributors who have joined us in this endeavor. We are also very indebted to our research associates whose contribution and input was invaluable: Rao Kammula, Lydia Puglisi, Nazareth Khodiguian, and Fred Dorey. Also, many thanks to the hundreds of volunteers who were willing to accept our curiosity as researchers. Thanks also to our editors Carol-Lynn Brown and Victoria Vaughn for their dedication and for sharing our enthusiasm.

It is our hope that this book will provide a useful resource for all those interested in this topic.

Raul Artal, M.D.
Robert A. Wiswell, Ph.D.

Contributors

Michal Artal, M.D.
Faculty, Los Angeles Psychoanalytical
    Institute
Assistant Clinical Professor of Psychiatry
University of California at Los Angeles
School of Medicine
Los Angeles, California

Samuel P. Bessman, M.D.
Professor and Chairman
Department of Pharmacology and Nutrition
University of Southern California
School of Medicine
Los Angeles, California

Gail Butterfield, Ph.D., R.D., F.A.C.S.M.
Director of Nutrition Studies
Palo Alto Veterans Administration Medical
    Center
Palo Alto, California

Robert C. Cefalo, M.D.
Professor of Obstetrics and Gynecology
Director, Maternal-Fetal Medicine
Department of Obstetrics and Gynecology
School of Medicine
University of North Carolina
Chapel Hill, North Carolina

James F. Clapp III, M.D.
Professor of Obstetrics and Gynecology
Department of Reproductive Biology
Metro Health Medical Center
Case Western Reserve University
Cleveland, Ohio

Denys J. Court, M.B., Ch.B.
Consultant
Department of Obstetrics and Gynecology
National Women's Hospital
Auckland, New Zealand

Val Davajan, M.D.
Professor of Obstetrics and Gynecology
Department of Obstetrics and Gynecology
Division of Endocrinology and Infertility
University of Southern California
School of Medicine
Los Angeles, California

Barbara L. Drinkwater, Ph.D., F.A.C.S.M.
Research Physiologist
Department of Medicine
Pacific Medical Center
Seattle, Washington

Marc J. Friedman, M.D.
Southern California Orthopedic Institute
Van Nuys, California

Elizabeth Gallup, M.D., J.D.
Assistant General Counsel
American Academy of Family Physicians
Kansas City, Missouri
Assistant Clinical Professor
Department of Family Medicine
University of Missouri
Kansas City, Missouri

**Susan Kelemen Gardin, M.S., R.P.T.,
    M.P.H.**
Doctoral Candidate
School of Public Health
Division of Population, Family
    and International Health
University of California
Los Angeles, California

Robert A. Girandola, Ph.D.
Associate Professor of Exercise Science
University of Southern California
Los Angeles, California

Raymond D. Gilbert, Ph.D.
Professor of Physiology, Obstetrics and
   Gynecology
Department of Physiology
Division of Perinatal Biology
Loma Linda University School of Medicine
Loma Linda, California

Jeffrey S. Greenspoon, M.D.
Staff Perinatologist
Director, Perinatal Intensive Care
Cedars-Sinai Medical Center
Los Angeles, California

Ralph Hale, M.D.
Professor and Chairman
Department of Obstetrics and Gynecology
John A. Burns School of Medicine
University of Hawaii
Honolulu, Hawaii

Maureen C. Hatch, Ph.D.
Associate Professor
Department of Epidemiology
Columbia University
New York, New York

Renate Huch, M.D.
Professor of Obstetrics
Department of Obstetrics
Division of Perinatal Physiology
University Hospital
Zurich, Switzerland

Lois Jovanovic-Peterson, M.D.
Senior Scientist
Sansum Medical Research Foundation
Clinical Professor, Department of Medicine
University of Southern California
Los Angeles, California

Ronald P. Karzel, Jr., M.D.
Southern California Orthopedic Institute
Van Nuys, California

Vern L. Katz, M.D.
Assistant Professor
Department of Obstetrics and Gynecology
Division of Maternal-Fetal Medicine
University of North Carolina
School of Medicine
Chapel Hill, North Carolina

Nazareth Khodiguian, Ph.D.
Research Associate
Department of Obstetrics and Gynecology
University of Southern California
School of Medicine
Los Angeles, California

Janet C. King, Ph.D., R.D.
Professor and Chairman
Department of Nutritional Sciences
University of California
Berkeley, California

Thomas H. Kirschbaum, M.D.
Professor of Obstetrics and Gynecology
Division of Maternal-Fetal Medicine
University of Southern California
School of Medicine
Los Angeles, California

Brian J. Koos, M.D., D.Phil.
Associate Professor of Obstetrics and
   Gynecology
Division of Maternal-Fetal Medicine
UCLA School of Medicine
Los Angeles, California

Lawrence D. Longo, M.D.
Professor of Physiology and Obstetrics and
   Gynecology
Division of Maternal-Fetal Medicine
Loma Linda University
School of Medicine
Loma Linda, California

Frederick K. Lotgering, M.D., Ph.D.
Department of Obstetrics and Gynecology
Erasmus University Medical School
Rotterdam, The Netherlands

Damon I. Masaki, M.D.
Assistant Professor
Department of Obstetrics and Gynecology
Division of Maternal-Fetal Medicine
University of Southern California
School of Medicine
Los Angeles, California

Robert G. McMurray, Ph.D.
Associate Professor
Director, Exercise Physiology
Department of Physical Education
University of North Carolina
Chapel Hill, North Carolina

Jill L. McNitt-Gray, Ph.D.
Assistant Professor of Exercise Science
Department of Exercise Sciences
University of Southern California
Los Angeles, California

Raul Artal Mittelmark, M.D., F.A.C.O.G., F.A.C.S.M.
Professor of Obstetrics, Gynecology and Exercise Science
Department of Obstetrics and Gynecology
Division of Maternal-Fetal Medicine
University of Southern California
School of Medicine and Exercise Science
Los Angeles, California

Mark J. Morton, M.D.
Associate Professor of Medicine
Director, Cardiac Catheterization and Heart Research Laboratories
University Hospital
Oregon Health Sciences University
Portland, Oregon

Julian T. Parer, M.D., Ph.D.
Professor of Obstetrics
Associate Staff
Cardiovascular Research Institute
University of California
San Francisco, California

Charles M. Peterson, M.D.
Director of Research
Sansum Medical Research Foundation
Clinical Professor, Department of Medicine
University of Southern California
Los Angeles, California

Marvin D. Posner, M.D.
Chief Perinatologist
Department of Obstetrics and Gynecology
Division of Maternal-Fetal Medicine
Santa Barbara Cottage Hospital
Santa Barbara, California

Gordon G. Power, M.D.
Professor of Physiology and Obstetrics and Gynecology
Department of Physiology
Division of Perinatal Biology
Loma Linda University School of Medicine
Loma Linda, California

Wendy E. St. John Repovich, Ph.D.
Exercise Physiologist
Los Angeles, California

Yitzhak Romem, M.D.
Senior Lecturer
Department of Obstetrics and Gynecology
Director, Genetic Institute
Soroka Medical Center
School of Medicine
Ben-Gurion University of the Negev
Beer-Sheva, Israel

Zena A. Stein, M.D., M.B., B.Ch.
Associate Dean of Research
School of Public Health
Columbia University
Professor of Public Health (Epidemiology)
Co-Director HIV Center for Clinical and Behaviorial Studies
Director, Brain Disorders Department
New York State Psychiatric Institute
New York, New York

Harrison C. Visscher, M.D.
Director of Education
The American College of Obstetricians and Gynecologists
Washington, D.C.

Janet P. Wallace, Ph.D.
Associate Professor
Director of Adult Fitness
Department of Kinesiology
Indiana University
Bloomington, Indiana

Robert A. Wiswell, Ph.D.
Associate Professor and Chairman
Department of Exercise Science
Research Associate
Andrus Gerontology Center
University of Southern California
Los Angeles, California

Itzhak Zaidise, M.D., Ph.D.
Senior Physician
Department of Obstetrics and Gynecology
Diabetes Unit, Endocrinological Institute and
    Diabetes Unit
Rambam Medical Center
Technion Medical School
Haifa, Israel

Contents

Section I/Physiological Adaptations to Pregnancy

Section II/Physiology of Exercise During Pregnancy

Section III/Practical Applications

1

Historical Perspectives

Raul Artal Mittelmark and Susan Kelemen Gardin

In recent years there has been a dramatic increase in the number of women engaging in physical fitness activities. The exercise spirit has enraptured women of all ages, including women in their childbearing years. Confronted suddenly with this revolution, health care providers, obstetricians in particular, are faced with many questions: What are the effects of exercise on the mother and her fetus? What types of exercise are appropriate? How much exercise is safe? Who may exercise in pregnancy? What are the legal and ethical issues involved in recommending prenatal exercise? And, finally, is exercise necessary or desirable in pregnancy? Answers to the previous questions remain indefinite because there is no convincing evidence that exercise in pregnancy is either beneficial or harmful vis-a-vis labor, delivery, and birth outcomes.

Throughout history, recommendations for exercise were based on "common sense" notions of the relationship between maternal physical activity and birth outcomes. In biblical times it was recognized that Hebrew slave women had easier labors than their Egyptian masters: ". . . the Hebrew women are not as the Egyptian women, for they are lively and are delivered ere the midwife come unto them" (Exodus I, 19). One may speculate that Hebrew slave women, while being physically prepared for the demands of childbirth, delivered relatively small infants. Another possible explanation is a higher incidence of premature precipitous deliveries. Conversely, the sedentary life-styles of Egyptian women predisposed them to the delivery of large babies and associated dystocia.

In the 3rd century B.C.E., Aristotle also attributed difficult childbirth to a sedentary maternal life-style (1). Two thousand years later, James Lucas (1788), surgeon at the Leeds General Infirmary in England, strongly advocated maternal exercise in a paper presented to the Medical Society of London. Lucas suggested that maternal exercise could decrease the size of the infant and allow easier passage through the maternal pelvis (2).

The philosophy of the 18th century was to encourage exercise, albeit with strong limitations. In 1781, Alexander Hamilton published his Treatise of Midwifery. In the chapter entitled, "Rules and Cautions for the Conduct of Pregnant Women," he cautioned pregnant women to exercise only in moderation, avoiding "agitation of the body from violent or improper exercise, as jolting in a carriage, riding on horseback, dancing and whatever disturbs the body or mind" (2).

The 19th century was dominated by offensive and patronizing attitudes toward pregnant women. In a popular booklet by Samuel K. Jennings (1808) entitled, "Married Lady's Companion and Poor Man's Friend," exercise was erroneously prescribed to women who could have benefited from rest, and vice versa:

"It is common opinion that breeding women ought to live indolently and feast luxuriously as they are able, lest by exercise they should injure, or by abstinence debilitate the unborn child. . . . Those ladies who are accustomed to idleness and who of course cannot take any considerable degree of exercise without consequent soreness or even fever, ought by no means to indulge in riding on horseback, running or romping, in any stage of pregnancy . . .

The happier class of women, who are in the habit of daily labour and continued exercise, may continue their engagements as before, except only, that it may be

necessary to abate from their common fatigue in a gradual manner, as they advance in pregnancy . . .
If, however, any of the symptoms threatening danger should present themselves, a little blood should be drawn from the arm and repeated as often as necessary" (3).

Although the concept of "moderation" was not based on scientific research, it was consistently maintained up to and including much of the 20th century. Further, it was enforced by moral exhortations regarding the responsibilities of the pregnant woman. In an 1892 book entitled "Advice to Women in the Care of their Health Before, During and After Confinement," the author writes: "When you neglect, risk or injure your own health during pregnancy, you do a direct injustice to, and commit a real crime against your unborn baby" (4).

The 19th century also brought forth the first serious attempts at scientific examination of the relationship between maternal activity and birth outcomes. In 1895, A. Pinard published a study of 1000 births demonstrating a relationship between social class and birth weight. He explained this by differential physical activity in women of heterogenous social classes (5). Letourneur published a similar study in 1896 based on 627 deliveries in Paris, and concluded that physical work at the end of pregnancy was a stronger determinant of birth weight than maternal morphology. He commented that "robust" women engaged in strenuous work (e.g., housemaids) delivered infants of lower birth weight than thinner women involved in less demanding work (e.g., florists) (5). In 1917, Peller published data in Vienna demonstrating that maternal rest resulted in higher birth weights and lower perinatal mortality (5). Naeye and Peters (6) analyzed the outcome of 7722 pregnancies in four different groups of working women defined by: (a) presence or absence of children at home, and (b) home or outside employment. Their results suggest that women who have standing jobs and children at home deliver infants who have significantly lower birth weights (6).

At the turn of the 20th century, there was concern in several countries about the poor health of volunteer recruits for military service. In England, it was estimated that only two-fifths of volunteers were in acceptable health for military service (7). Many British politicians expressed dismay about the "declining quality" of the British population (7). The studies of Pinard, Letourneur, Peller, and others provided a logical plan for improving the quality of the progeny. Legislation was enacted in England, as well as in Holland, Belgium, Portugal, Austria, and Switzerland, prohibiting the employment of pregnant women in factories during the 2–4 weeks preceding childbirth and the 4–6 weeks after childbirth (8). Despite the fact that analogous concerns were voiced in the United States, similar legislation was not adopted (9). Nor was such legislation adopted in Turkey, Russia, Spain, Italy, or France (8).

Moderation in exercise and the need for outdoor air were the two themes of the early 20th century. A handbook for "prospective mothers" published in 1913 contained the following recommendations:

"The amount of exercise which the prospective mother should take cannot be stated precisely, but what can be definitely said is this—she should stop the moment she begins to feel tired . . . Women who have laborious household duties to perform do not require as much exercise as those who lead sedentary lives; but they do require just as much fresh air . . .
Walking is the best kind of exercise . . . Most women who are pregnant find that a two to three mile walk daily is all they enjoy, and very few are inclined to indulge in six miles, which is generally accepted as the upper limit . . .
Very few outdoor sports can be unconditionally recommended to a prospective mother. Because athletic exercise is either too violent or else jolts the body a great deal, it is especially dangerous in the early months of pregnancy . . .
All kinds of violent exertion should be avoided—a rule which at once excludes sweeping, scrubbing, laundry work, lifting anything that is heavy, and going up and down stairs hurriedly or frequently. The use of a sewing machine is also emphatically forbidden" (8).

The expanding list of arbitrary restrictions on activity during pregnancy were derived more from the cultural and social biases of each era than from scientific investigations. A 1935 book entitled "Modern Motherhood" allowed pregnant women to bathe, swim, golf, engage in ballroom dance, while warning against the danger of excessive walking:

"The expectant mother must, of necessity, curtail her usual physical activities because of her extra burden . . . she cannot exercise more than she is accustomed to; she should exercise less. She should not be persuaded to walk a lot because walking is supposed to make birth easier—this superstition is hundreds of years old and still prevalent" (9).

The author also prohibits horseback riding and tennis, but notes that some expectant mothers indulge in these and like activities "with impunity."

Although it is difficult to analyze the impact of various life-styles on pregnancy outcomes, it is clear that this question preoccupies contemporary researchers much as it did ancient and medieval thinkers. One may speculate as to possible differences in the pregnancy impact of pleasurable versus stressful work-related physical activity.

In the late 1920s and early 1930s, the specialized and unique prenatal exercise program came into being. Modern prenatal exercise, attributed to Fairbairn (10, 11) and Randell (12), was directed toward a self-powered successful and natural birth outcome:

"Nothing serves more to improve the chances of a natural outcome than that the prospective mother should have acquired a full understanding of her own part, confidence in her own power to see it through, and the knowledge that there is help behind her should she need it" (10, 11).

During the next decade, these ideas were further developed by several individuals. Between 1933 and 1947, Dick Read developed specific progressive breathing patterns and physical exercises for improving health, muscle-tone, and "sense of well-being," as well as decreasing the pain of childbirth (13). The goal of Read's program was to create a birth experience unhampered by mechanical, pharmacological, and mental factors (13).

The psychoprophylactic method of painless childbirth was developed during this period in Russia by Velvovsky, and was later introduced to the West by Lamaze (14, 15). Lamaze popularized the concept that labor pain is not a disease; therefore, childbirth is not an indication for analgesic drugs.

Margaret Morris (16) promoted maternal exercise from an entirely new slant: She promised improved appearance "in both face and figure" following childbirth as a result of maternity exercises (17).

In England, Kathleen Vaughan advocated improving joint flexibility during pregnancy. The squat position was encouraged with promises of a widened pelvic outlet. Women were urged to adopt tailor-sitting positions and perform pelvic floor exercises in an attempt to prevent tears of the perineum. Women were also encouraged to perform breathing and posture exercises to improve fetal oxygenation and maternal health.

Not surprisingly, the pelvis was and continues to be the focus of proposed change through prenatal exercise programs. Yet, the pelvic floor is a multilayer deep muscle sheet attached to the bony pelvis, and cannot be stretched by tailor sitting. Neither can such sitting increase elasticity to prevent tearing during delivery. As demonstrated by Blankfield (18) bracing the thighs upon the abdomen to resemble the "squat" position is disadvantageous in that it tightens the perineum and does not permit pelvic fixation for good action of the abdominal muscles in bearing down efforts. Pelvic rocking and changes of posture also do not affect the size of the pelvis in labor. However, secondary to hormonal changes, joints and ligaments undergo a rapid process of relaxation in the first trimester of pregnancy and further attempts to "stretch" them are potentially injurious.

Despite their sometimes unsound advice, the new prenatal programs of the 1930s and 1940s were directed toward lofty goals: first, the programs attempted to provide the pregnant woman with a sense that she could develop skills for controlling her experience of childbirth; second, there was a new emphasis on the prospective mother's "non-maternal" interests, both psychological and physical; third, there was a strong emphasis on the positive and active, i.e., what the pregnant woman could accomplish rather than what she was prohibited from attempting. The combined predominant values of these programs were educational and psychological (19).

At the same time these new and "radical" concepts of prenatal activity were being developed, traditional advice regarding moderation and fresh air still retained a primary influence. In a 1942 book entitled "Getting Ready to be a Mother," the following instructions appeared:

"Regular out-of-door exercise promotes digestion, stimulates the activity of the skin and lungs, steadies the nerves, quiets the mind, and promotes sleep. Walking, which is probably the most satisfactory form of exercise, also strengthens some of the muscles that are used during labor . . . The woman who does her own housework may not need additional exercise, but may get her quota of fresh air by resting out of doors each day. Hard work, such as washing, heavy lifting or much running up and down stairs, should not be the lot of the expectant mother. All violent exercise and sports are, of course, to be avoided, particularly swimming, horseback riding and tennis" (20).

Similar guidance appeared in the "Manual for the Conduct of Classes for Expectant Parents," published by the Cleveland Child Health Association in 1942:

"A woman who does her own housework gets plenty of exercise; but she will find she profits by being in the open air for an hour or so each day. Walking is the best exercise (21).

In 1949, the United States Childrens' Bureau issued a publication in which they made standard recommendations for moderation in physical activity:

"A moderate amount of exercise is good for anyone, and this is particularly true for a pregnant woman. Unless you have been ill or unless there is some complication, you can continue your housework, gardening, daily walks and even swim occasionally" (22).

Many books of this era permitted housework, while prohibiting sports, despite the fact that housework is generally more exhausting than sports activities.

Exercise advice of the 1950s and 1960s differed little from earlier advice. Three versions of "Expectant Motherhood" published in 1951, 1957, and 1963, respectively, each contained the identical bland exercise prescription:

"Regular exercise in the open air . . . should form part of your daily routine. For everyone, probably walking is the best type of exercise; for the pregnant woman there can be no question of its superiority . . . For the average woman, a mile or so a day is about the right amount, but it is advisable to divide this into several short walks . . . Light housework . . . is a helpful form of activity and may be stopped short of fatigue, however, in no event should it include lifting of heavy objects.

Violent activity is to be avoided, particularly anything which involves jolting, sudden motion or running. Although physicians vary widely in the forms of exercise they permit in pregnancy, they usually disapprove of horseback riding, tennis and skating. Dancing is harmless, as a rule, if indulged in moderately" (23–25).

Kathleen Vaughan, one of the innovators of the 1930s, published another innovative book in the 1950s entitled "Exercises Before Childbirth." The book contains a forceful attack on the sedentary life of English women:

"The mother who has lived a natural life from her own birth, who was breastfed herself and who has lived on plain, good food, with plenty of free movement in the fresh air when growing, she is the woman who will have an easy confinement when her time comes; while the more luxurious, wrapped-up bottle-fed infant, kept long hours in a perambulator or indoors, with no exercise, and later sitting long hours in school, is very likely to have difficulty in childbearing later on because the natural growth, shape and mobility of the pelvis and its joints have been stunted" (1).

In her book, Vaughan recommends a series of exercises based on the movements of Kashmiri boatwomen at work. A novel approach in Vaughan's book is her recommendation that exercise be performed in group classes for the psychological boost to the prospective mother:

"The advantage of attending a class is that you are stimulated by others also engaged in training for motherhood, with whom you make friends and can compare your babies later on" (1).

During the period of sweeping social change in the 1960s, prenatal exercise established itself as a permanent component of childbirth preparation, and many of the earlier "radical" ideas involving physical and psychological control of childbirth became "de rigeur" in prenatal programs. In a 1977 book entitled "Exercises for Increased Awareness in Education and Counselling in Childbirth," Sheila Kitzinger writes that "exercises should aim at developing poise and a sense of well-being." In discussing pelvic floor exercises she writes:

"There is, therefore, room for exercises, always and flowing, which increase in women a happy consciousness of this part of their body as both good, clean and right, and as under their control" (26).

In the "Exercise Plus Pregnancy Program" (1980), the authors write that:

"Successfully completing an exercise program will give you a greater sense of control over your body. Being in control, while at the same time being relaxed, will give you the confidence and trust you'll need to 'let go' for a smoother labor and delivery" (27).

It is unfortunate that standards for exercise are only recently being developed for pregnant women (see ACOG guidelines, Appendix A). Although the medical community has failed to research and establish prenatal exercise programs systematically based on scientific rationale, social reformers and sports advocates have promoted highly specific programs lacking scientific evaluation or follow-up. Typical programs of the 1970s and 1980s ignore basic physiological changes of pregnancy such as the aortocaval compression syndrome, the increased laxity of joints and ligaments, exaggerated lumbar lordosis and risks of hyperthermia or dehydration. Until recently, few, if any, programs gave any advice on the replenishment of fluids during exercise. These programs generally promote the belief that physical fitness will ease labor and delivery; unfortunately, there is no scientific evidence to date to support this view.

This view has been particularly popularized by the concept of "natural childbirth." Before the origin of modern obstetrics in 1935, fetal and maternal morbidity and mortality were significant, and uncomplicated labor and delivery were regarded as "natural childbirth." Over the years, maternal morbidity and mortality have greatly decreased, and natural childbirth has become synonymous with "painless labor." Many prenatal exercise programs have developed with the latter goal in mind.

Although these programs fulfill an important educational role in instructing women about the process of normal delivery, they also create a childbirth script that results in failure for many participants. Specifically, many programs emphasize verbal analgesia and relaxation activities (e.g., focal point concentration or breathing patterns) to the exclusion of drug therapy. The occurrence of complications in labor is perceived as a personal failure, whereas at other times the blame is shifted to the obstetrician. The psychological impact on patients and physicians is tremendous.

A *Wall Street Journal* article appearing in the August 17, 1984 issue commented on the enormous change in expectations and procedures of childbirth during the last generation. Several statements in the article clearly captured the quandry in which the modern pregnant woman finds herself:

". . . today's middle class mother-to-be is often older and more ambitious than her mother was . . . she approaches childbirth as she does any activity: She studies and prepares and trains as though labor were the bar examination or a sales campaign.

She's so programmed to be in control, however, that if something goes wrong and childbirth doesn't meet her high expectations, she faces a profound sense of guilt and failure. That's the downside risk of the new motherhood.

The variables a mother-to-be can control include diet and exercise. So the conscientious career woman . . . plunges into prenatal exercise classes that strengthen her back, abdomen and pelvic muscles. She also keeps going as long as she can" (28).

It is difficult to determine what proportion of American women exercise regularly throughout their pregnancies. It is estimated that 85 million Americans are involved in some type of fitness programs and 25 million Americans jog regularly (29). Women of reproductive age constitute a significant proportion of this active American public (30). In a 1982 survey published in Morbidity and Mortality Weekly Report, only 10.8% of California women ages 18–34 years admitted to leading sedentary lives (31). In an article published in Newsweek magazine (July 23, 1984), the authors note that ". . . as an outgrowth of the general fitness craze, women are flocking to exercise programs designed to get them in shape for labor and delivery" (32).

Between 1970 and 1973, 42% of all pregnant women worked for some portion of their pregnancy (33). Based on 1977 fertility rates, Kuntz estimates that working American women will constitute over 1 million pregnancies each year (33). Seen in this light, injuries that could result from inappropriate prenatal exercise acquire national economic significance. Estimates of the direct and indirect costs of treating fitness-related injuries in the general population are as high as $40 billion annually.

In the case of pregnant women, one may speculate as to the source of payment for such injuries. According to Sheila Kammerman of Columbia University,

"Unlike 75 other countries, including all other advanced industrialized societies and many among the less developed countries, the United States has no statutory provision that guarantees a woman the right to a leave from employment for a specified period, protects her job while she is on leave, and provides a cash benefit equal to all or a significant portion of her wage while she is not working because of pregnancy and childbirth. Nor does the United States guarantee a working mother the right to health insurance to cover her own medical expenses at the time of pregnancy and childbirth as well as those of her child. Benefits such as these cover most employed women in other countries . . ." (33).

In 1976 the United States Supreme Court ruled in Gilvert v. General Electric Corporation that the exclusion of pregnancy-related disabilities from a company's disability insurance program is not considered sex discrimination, and employers are under no obligation to provide disability insurance benefits to pregnant women (33). The effects of this ruling were essentially reversed with the passage of the 1978 Pregnancy Disability Amendment to Title VII, which requires employers to treat pregnancy and childbirth like other causes of disability insurance or sick leave plans (30). However, only five states (California, Hawaii, New Jersey, New York, and Rhode Island) and Puerto Rico have mandatory state disability laws (33).

Analysis of related legal issues are further discussed in Chapter 27, and recommendations for prenatal activities must be viewed against this background. We have to be aware that certain activities may expose individuals to unwarranted risks (e.g., premature labor) for which unemployment compensation funds may not be available. This may be especially true in cases where an individual requires prolonged periods of hospitalization or confinement at home bed rest.

In view of the current trend toward a more physically active society, the medical community has an obligation to investigate, design, and promote activities that will be safe and maintain the well-being of both mother and fetus. The intensive birthing education of the 1980s provides women with a sense of command, but also leaves them with the fear that some minor dietary error or failure to engage in "prenatal exercises" will result in damage to them or to their unborn children. The emphasis in these programs is on giving the pregnant woman a sense of control over her body, her pregnancy, and her life. By and large, such programs are based on the premise that exercise is an integral part of prenatal care and arguments are often made to push pregnant women into activities they are more prepared to engage in mentally than physically. Pregnancy should not be a state of confinement and women should be encouraged to continue an active life-style, assuming they have no medical or obstetrical complications. Nevertheless, it is irresponsible to promote the notion that prenatal exercise is an absolute requirement for a successful pregnancy. One obligation that we have as health care providers is to reassure women that it is also acceptable to limit exercise in pregnancy. Limiting women to normal daily activities in no way compromises maternal or fetal health.

REFERENCES

1. Vaughn K. Exercises before childbirth. London: Faber and Faber Limited, 1951, pp 11–29.
2. Kerr JMM, Johnstone RW, Phillips MH. Historical review of British obstetrics and gynecology. London: E.S. Livingstone, 1954.
3. Jennings SK. Married lady's companion, or poor man's friend. New York: Lorenzo Dow, 1808, pp 77–80.
4. Stacpoole F. Advice to women on the care of their health before, during and after confinement. London: Cassel, 1892, p 16
5. Briend A. Maternal physical activity: Birth weight and perinatal mortality. Med Hypothesis 1980; 6:1157–1170.
6. Naeye RL, Peters EC: Working during pregnancy: Effects on the fetus. Pediatrics 1982; 69:724–727.
7. Oakley A: The origins and development of antenatal care. In: Enkin M, Chalmers I, eds. Effectiveness and satisfaction in antenatal care. London: Published for Spastics International Medical Publications by Heinemann Medical Books, 1982, pp 1–20.
8. Slemmons JM. The prospective mother: a handbook for women during pregnancy. New York: D. Appleton and Company, 1913, pp 125–135.
9. Enkin M, Chalmers I, eds. Effectiveness and satisfaction in antenatal care. London: Published for Spastics International Medical Publications by Heinemann Medical Books, 1982, pp 266–290.
10. Fairbairn JS. Gynaecology with obstetrics. London: Oxford Medical Publications, 1924.

11. Fairbairn JS. Obstetrics. London: Oxford Medical Publications, 1926.
12. Randell M. Training for childbirth, 3rd ed. London: Churchill, 1945.
13. Read GD. An outline of the conduct of physiological labor. Am J Obstet Gynecol 1947; 54:702.
14. Velvovsky I, Platinor K, Ploticher V, Shugom E. Painless childbirth through psychoprophylaxis. Moscow: Foreign Languages Publishing House, 1960.
15. Lamaze F. Painless Childbirth. London: Burke, 1958.
16. Morris M. Maternity and post-operative exercises. London: Heinemann, 1936.
17. Heaton C. Modern motherhood. New York: Farrar & Rhinehart, 1935, pp 38–40.
18. Blankfield A. The optimum position for childbirth. Med J Austral 1965; 2:666.
19. Burnett C. Value of antenatal exercises. J Obstet Gynaecol Br Emp 1956; 63:40.
20. Van Blarcom C. Getting ready to be a mother. New York: The Macmillan Company, 1942, pp 48–49.
21. Manual for the conduct of classes for expectant parents. Cleveland: Cleveland Child Health Association, 1942.
22. Prenatal Care. Federal Security Agency and Social Security Administration. Children's Bureau Publication No. 4, 1949, pp 25–26.
23. Eastman NJ. Expectant motherhood. Boston: Little, Brown & Co., 1951, pp 74–75.
24. Eastman NJ. Expectant motherhood. Boston: Little, Brown & Co., 1957, pp 73–75.
25. Eastman NJ. Expectant motherhood. Boston: Little, Brown & Co., 1963, pp 79–80.
26. Kitzinger S. Exercises for increased body awareness in education and counselling for childbirth. London: Bailliere-Tindall, 1977, pp 165–171.
27. Cedeno L, Cedeno O, Monroe C. The exercise plus pregnancy program. New York: William Morrow & Company, Inc., 1980.
28. Cox M. Many professional women apply career lessons to job of childbirth. Wall Street Journal, Section 2, August 17, 1984.
29. Medical World News (Psychiatry Edition), July 26, 1984, p 25.
30. Jarrett JC, Spellacy WN. Jogging during pregnancy: An improved outcome? Obstet Gynecol 1983; 63:705–709.
31. MMWR Weekly Report. Annual Summary 1982. 31:128, December 1983.
32. Keerdoja E. Now, the pregnancy workout. Newsweek, July 23, 1984, p 70.
33. Kuntz WD. Pregnant working women: what advice should you give them? Contemp OB/Gyn 1980; 15:69–79.

2

Physiological and Endocrine Adjustments to Pregnancy

Yitzhak Romem, Damon I. Masaki, and Raul Artal Mittelmark

Pregnancy is distinguished by a multitude of physiological and endocrine adjustments directed toward the creation of an optimal environment for the fetus. Every organ system in the expectant mother as well as her personality are intimately involved in this complex process.

The sequence of events is not yet completely elucidated; many times, it is limited to descriptive terms. The changes in the reproductive system must be supported by secondary adjustments of other systems. Because of the complexity of the mechanisms involved, no seemingly ideal adjustment can be achieved. But, by and large, the side effects of the pregnant state do require adjustments and do not constitute a threat to maternal health if properly achieved. Conversely, inadequate adjustment or an imbalance among various body systems results in pathology.

In summarizing the previously mentioned adjustments, our intention is to focus on those systems that can be affected by exercise.

Exercise is a process in which chemical energy is transformed into a movement (or muscular tension in isometric exercise), and inevitably into heat. The human body can be compared to a sophisticated engine, equipped with very sensitive sensors and an immense macroprocessor, that is in continuous need of a mechanism to process fuel (food), dispose of waste products, and dissipate heat. With this somewhat mechanistic view in mind, we divided our description into four sections:

1. Locomotive system (neuromusculoskeletal);
2. Energy-generating system (gastrointestinal, respiratory, cardiovascular);
3. Disposal system (urinary tract, skin); and
4. The endocrine system.

LOCOMOTIVE SYSTEM (NEUROMUSCULOSKELETAL)

The physical fitness of any individual is the result of his or her motor fitness and his or her physical working capacity defined as the maximum level of metabolism (power) of which an individual is capable (1). Listing the elements of motor fitness: strength, speed, agility, endurance, power, coordination, balance, flexibility, and body control, it is clear that these are the results of the performance and integration of the musculoskeletal and neurological systems

Musculoskeletal System

The protruding abdomen, waddling gait, and exaggerated lordosis are familiar features of normal pregnancy. The constantly growing uterus, although a muscular organ not belonging to the musculoskeletal system per se, is the main cause for the changes occurring in the statics and dynamics of the skeleton in the gravida.

From a strictly pelvic organ at 12 weeks, the uterus becomes an abdominal organ displacing the intestines and coming into direct contact with the abdominal wall. Its dimensions increase 150-fold throughout pregnancy and the capacity increases more than 1000-fold (2). Its weight increases up to 20 times at term, not taking into account the weight of the fetus. Altogether, at term, the pregnant uterus with its content contributes an average of 6 kg to the maternal weight gain (3, 4).

The anterior orientation of the uterus expanding into the abdominal cavity displaces the woman's center of gravity, resulting in progressive lumbar lordosis and rotation of the pelvis on the femur. This shifts the center

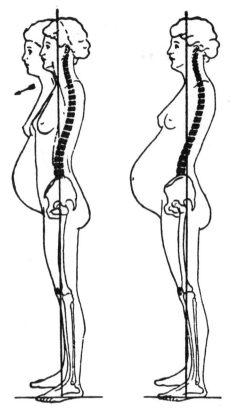

Figure 2.1.   Statics of the nonpregnant or early pregnant woman *(left)* and late pregnant woman *(right)*. (From Greenhill, JP. Obstetrics, ed. 13. Philadelphia: WB Saunders, 1965, p 183.)

of the gravity back over her pelvis preventing a forward fall (Fig. 2.1).

In order to maintain the line of vision and also to compensate for the lumbar lordosis, the gravida increases the anterior flexion of the cervical spine in addition to slumping abduction of the shoulders. Exaggeration of this position can lead to increased paresthesias over the distribution of the ulnar and/or median nerve with increasing motor weakness (the hand syndrome of pregnancy) (5).

In addition, the growing uterus rotates on its long axis, usually to the right. The movement of the uterus is restricted anteriorly by the abdominal wall and posteriorly by the vertebral column. Even in the absence of laxity in an abdominal wall, as in most primigravidas, there is still enough room for displacement. Because the displacement is always in the direction of the inclination, the result is increased instability. The enlarging

breasts (500 g at term), as well, contribute to the change in the center of gravity. As a result of the previously noted changes, the center of gravity in pregnant women is high, rising, and unstable. If those were the characteristics of a ship, there could be a constant threat of capsizing.

A pregnant woman's stability is obtained at the expense of an increased burden upon the muscles and ligaments of the vertebral column. No wonder low back pain is so common in pregnancy.

In addition to its content, the pelvic girdle itself changes profoundly during pregnancy. The bones that compose the pelvis are held together by fibrocartilage with small synovial articular cavities and reinforced with pelvic ligaments: the pubic and sacrosciatic.

Early in pregnancy, secondary to the release of estrogens and/or relaxin, there is increasing relaxation of ligaments. Softening of the cartilage and increase in the synovia and synovial fluid widens the pelvic joints. The result is increased joint mobility and an unstable pelvis reflected in a waddling gait. Changes similar to the one in the pelvis occur in the other joints and muscles.

In the third trimester of pregnancy, the gravida experiences reduced mobility of ankle joints and wrists in spite of increased relaxation of the ligaments. These changes are caused by water retention, mainly in the ground substance of connective tissue, resulting in visible ankle edema in the majority of pregnant women and paraesthesias in the hands, muscular weakness and the carpal tunnel syndrome (6, 7).

It is clear from this description that sports requiring agility, balance, and strength, especially of hands, like skiing, horse riding, gymnastics, and tennis can be more injury producing to the pregnant woman, particularly after the first trimester of pregnancy, whereas swimming is not affected in a similar way.

Neurological System

From the very scanty literature, it appears that the pregnant woman has significant changes in perception senses. In a rather old report (1930), but still the most comprehensive, J. P. Johns (8) describes the definite concentric contraction of form and color fields and also enlargement of the blind spot during pregnancy with a return to normal about 10 days postpartum.

The corneal sensitivity as well as the corneal topography change, most probably secondarily to edema. That is the rationale for not prescribing new optical corrections until some weeks after delivery (9, 10).

It is common knowledge, although not validated in strictly scientific terms, that heightening or dulling of the senses of taste and smell may account for the cravings and aversions toward certain food during pregnancy (11, 12).

Reaction time and upper extremity strength, especially when rapid movement and shift in balance are required, may be affected during pregnancy (13). This has safety implications for both work and exercise.

There is a paucity of data about other senses and their adaptations during pregnancy.

There is evidence that even the most sophisticated activities controlled by the central nervous system, namely, the emotional and cognitive processes, may be altered in pregnancy with a tendency toward insomnia, lability of mood, anxiety, as well as slightly impaired cognitive functions (14).

ENERGY-GENERATING SYSTEMS

The energy utilized by the body is chemical and released in the process of oxygenation. The oxygen serves as an oxidant, via the pulmonary tract. The distribution system for the above is the cardiovascular system.

The energetic cost of pregnancy is estimated at about 80,000 kcal or 300 kcal/day (15). This is required to cover the growth and development of the fetus, buildup of maternal tissue such as the uterus, breasts, fat, and to compensate for the increased metabolism due to increased activtiy of the cardiovascular, respiratory, and urinary systems, and the addition of the fetal metabolism (Table 2.1). The demand is unevenly distributed, being at maximum during the two middle quarters of pregnancy, an extra need of about 390 kcal/day. It is mainly caused by fat storage during that period. The last quarter of pregnancy is less demanding, only an additional 250 kcal/day is needed for the growing fetus, while the fat storage ceases (Table 2.2; Fig. 2.2).

There are two ways to meet this energetic cost of pregnancy, either by increased intake or reduced expenditure of energy. Both ways are utilized during pregnancy. The average pregnant woman eating an unrestricted diet probably increases her total daily energy con-

Table 2.1. The Extra Components of Oxygen Consumption in Pregnancy[a]

Source of Extra Energy Output	Increment at Weeks of Pregnancy				Estimated Cost (ml O₂/min)	Increment of O₂ Consumption (ml/min) Weeks of Gestation			
	10	20	30	40		10	20	30	40
Cardiac output (liters/min)	1.0	1.5	1.5	1.5	About 20 at 4.5 liters/min; increase pro rata	4.5	6.8	6.8	6.8
Respiration (liters/min)	0.75	1.50	2.25	3.00	1.0/liter ventilation	0.8	1.5	2.3	3.0
Uterine muscle (g)	140	320	600	970	3.7/kg	0.5	1.2	2.2	3.6
Placenta (g)									
Wet	20	170	430	650	3.3/100 g dry weight	0	0.5	2.2	3.7
Dry	2	17	65	110					
Fetus (g)	5	300	1500	3400	3.65/kg	0	1.1	5.5	12.4
Breasts (g)	45	180	360	410	3.3/kg	0.1	0.6	1.2	1.4
Kidneys (mEq Na reabsorbed)	7	7	7	7	1.0/mEq	7	7	7	7
					Total ml/min	12.9	18.7	27.2	37.9

[a]From Hytten FE. Nutrition. In Hytten FE, Chamberlain G, eds. Clinical Physiology in Obstetrics. Oxford: Blackwell, 1980, p 167.

Table 2.2.   Cumulative Energy Cost of Pregnancy Computed for the Energy Equivalents of Protein and Fat Increments and the Energy Cost of Maintaining the Fetus and Added Maternal Tissues[a,b]

| | Equivalent (kcal/day) per Weeks of Pregnancy: | | | | Cumulative Total (kcal)[c] |
	0–10	10–20	20–30	30–40	
Protein	3.6	10.3	26.7	34.2	5,186
Fat	55.6	235.6	207.6	31.3	36,329
Oxygen consumption	44.8	99.0	148.2	227.2	35,717
Total net energy	104.0	344.9	382.5	292.7	77,234
Metabolizable energy (total net energy + 10%)	114	379	421	322	84,957

[a]The total is derived from oxygen consumption figures (Table 2.1) and assumes an RQ of 0.90. Note: for the first 10-week period total increment is divided by 56 since pregnancy is dated from the last menstrual period.
[b]From Hytten FE, Nutrition. In Hytten FE, Chamberlain G, eds. Clinical Physiology in Obstetrics. Oxford: Blackwell, 1980, p. 165.
[c]Taken as 5.6 kcal/g for protein and 9.5 kcal/g for fat.

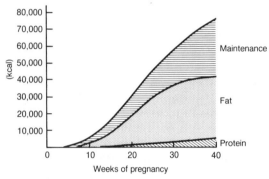

Figure 2.2.   The cumulative energy cost of pregnancy and its components. (From Hytten FE. Nutrition. In Hytten FE, Chamberlain G, eds. Clinical Physiology in Obstetrics. Oxford: Blackwell, 1980, p 166.)

sumption by approximately 150–300 kcal due to increased appetite (16). Conversely, it is common for pregnant women to reduce their physical activity, not only because of the demands imposed by the growing fetus, and the mechanical instability and laxity of joints, but also because of the feeling of lassitude and somnolence caused by the surge in hormones, mainly progesterone (17, 18).

If dietary intake is inadequate to meet the caloric and nutrient needs of the expectant mother, protein will be catabolized. Since pregnancy is, in essence, an anabolic state with positive nitrogen balance throughout, increased breakdown of proteins to combat the inadequate energy supply will reduce the availability of amino acids for maternal buildup and fetal growth, with adverse results (19). Similar adverse effects on the fetus will most probably occur with a diet restricted in pro-

teins in spite of adequate caloric intake. This issue is compounded because of the close relationship between optimal protein use and the adequacy of the energy sources (20).

Adequate weight gain is the most practical indicator of caloric intake. It is estimated that a healthy primigravida, eating without restriction, will gain an average of 27.5 lb (12.5 kg) (21). This estimation served as a baseline for the compilation of the Recommended Daily Dietary Allowance (RDAs) for Pregnancy. Yet, it is important to keep in mind that the RDAs

Table 2.3.   Recommended Daily Dietary Allowance (RDAs) for Pregnancy[a]

Energy (kcal)	2,400 (2,300)[b]
Protein (g)	78 (76)[b]
Vitamin A (IU)	5,000
Vitamin D (IU)	400
Vitamin E activity (IU)	15
Ascorbic acid (mg)	60
Folic acid (mg)	800
Niacin (mg)	16
Riboflavin (mg)	1.7
Thiamine (mg)	1.4
Vitamin B_6 (mg)	2.5
Vitamin B_{12} (μg)	4.0
Calcium (mg)	1,200
Phosphorus (mg)	1,200
Iodine (μg)	125
Iron (mg)	18[c]
Magnesium (mg)	450
Zinc (mg)	20

[a]Source: Committee on Maternal Nutrition, Food and Nutrition Board, National Research Council: *Recommended Dietary Allowances*, ed 9, publication 2216. Washington, D.C., National Academy of Sciences, 1980.
[b]Recommended for gravidas more than 23 years old.
[c]Recommended for gravidas more than 19 years old. The increased requirement cannot be met by the diet; supplemental iron is recommended.

published by the Committee on Maternal Nutrition, Food and Nutrition Board, National Research Council (Table 2.3) are intended as guidelines for average population, not individuals. Additional information on these topics can be found in Chapter 9.

More recently, the average maternal weight gain is 33.7 lb (15.3 kg) (22). Maternal weight was determined to be an important factor in subsequent fetal birth weight in nonobese women (<135% of ideal body weight) and therefore, at least a 24-lb (11-kg) weight gain is recommended. Low prepregnancy weight (<90% of ideal body weight) conversely was associated with lower fetal birth weights (23). In contrast, maternal fat accretion was not found to correlate with subsequent birth weights (23, 24).

Gastrointestinal System

It is rather controversial whether the anatomic and physiological changes in the gastrointestinal tract encourage the efficiency of the food intake or the increased caloric intake occurs in spite of it.

The main change in the function of the gastrointestinal tract in pregnancy is its decline in activity. The esophageal peristalsis has a slower wave speed and lower amplitude. The lower esophageal sphincter responses to hormonal pharmacological and physiological stimuli are reduced. In addition, the intraesophageal pressure is reduced while the intragastric pressure is slightly elevated compared to the nonpregnant state, lowering the barrier pressure (25, 26).

As pregnancy progresses, the growing uterus displaces the stomach and the intestines. The relatively common displacement of the lower esophageal sphincter upward into the negative pressure region of the thorax contributes to its reduced compliance (27). In all, these changes favor gastroesophageal reflux and result in frequent indigestion and regurgitation.

There is a decrease in the tone and motility of the gastrointestinal tract that results in prolongation of the gastric emptying time (28) and delayed intestinal passage (29). As a result of the reduced intestinal motility and the slow passage of the food through the large bowel, with increased absorbtion of water, the feces are dry, hard, and difficult to expel; constipation is a common complaint (30).

In pregnancy, the oropharynx is affected by excessive salivation and hyperemia with softening of the gums, which are easily traumatized and bleed. The gallbladder is usually hypotonic and distended with thick and tarry bile, emptying slower in pregnancy (31, 32).

Respiratory System

The changes in the respiratory system are extensive, including anatomic and functional alterations. These changes occur very early due to hormonal influence, mainly progesterone, even before the growing uterus mechanically impairs ventilation. Actually, in spite of the space occupied by the uterus, the total lung capacity (TLC) shows relatively little change (reduction of 300 ml) in pregnancy (33–35). The rise of the diaphragm by about 4 cm caused by flaring of the lower ribs, as is seen observing the progressively increasing subcostal angle from about 68° in early pregnancy to 103° in late pregnancy, is compensated for by increasing the transverse

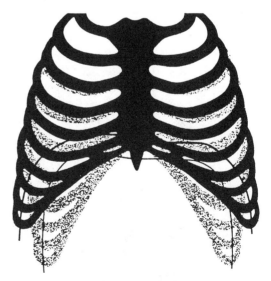

Figure 2.3.   The ribcage in pregnancy *(black),* and the nonpregnant state *(stippled)* showing the increased subcostal angle, the increased transverse diameter, and the raised diaphragm in pregnancy. (From deSwiet M. The respiratory system. In Hytten FE, Chamberlain G, eds. Clinical Physiology in Obstetrics. Oxford: Blackwell, 1980, p 86.)

diameter of the chest (Fig. 2.3) (36). The net result is that the thoracic cavity is not reduced. More than that, the diaphragmatic excursion is increased with breathing (37).

Significant respiratory functional changes are observed in pregnancy. The respiratory center has a reduced threshold for Pco_2 and increased sensitivity to any increase in Pco_2. For a given increase in Pco_2, the induced increase in pulmonary ventilation rate is about 4 times greater during pregnancy (38). The increased ventilation is achieved by breathing more deeply and not more frequently.

There is a gradual increase up to 40% in tidal volume (V_T), from 500 ml in the non-pregnant state to about 700 ml in late pregnancy (39). Because the vital capacity is changed very little during pregnancy (increase of about 100 ml), the change in V_T must come at the expense of other functional lung volumes, namely the expiratory reserve volume (ERV), as illustrated in Figure 2.4. The ERV decreases by about 200 ml while residual volume (RV) decreases by 300 ml, reducing the functional reserve capacity (RV + ERV) by 500 ml. It means that, at the end of quiet expiration, there is a smaller

oxygen reserve in the lung (40) and, thus, a reduced ability to withstand periods of apnea, a factor that should be taken into account when considering participation in sports like diving or short sprints. The cause for the reduction in the residual volume is unclear and the answer may lie with the increased central blood volume (CBV), which includes the lung, heart, and great vessels. The CBV rises by 20% or 260 ml and is illustrated on chest radiographs by the increased prominence of the pulmonary vasculature (41, 42).

The increased minute ventilation, which is directly related to the increased V_T and rises, as expected, by 40% from 7.5 liters/min to 10.5 liters/min, results in a significant decrease in Pco_2 from about 39 mm Hg in the nonpregnant state to 31 mm Hg during pregnancy (43, 44). The changes in respiration occur as early as the 7th week of pregnancy with a 24% increase in minute ventilation and 10% increase in O_2 consumption (40).

Obviously, the increased minute ventilation increases the oxygen supply by at least 40% and even more, up to 50% because the alveolar ventilation increases proportionally more than expected with increased pulmonary ventilation as expressed by the minute volume. One additional explanation is that the fixed respiratory dead space caused by the increased V_T, as the sole promoting factor for increased minute volume, involves a relatively smaller dilutional effect of the unventilated air trapped in the dead space.

The adaptation of the respiratory system should be viewed from two different perspectives: Does it meet the increased oxygen demand of pregnancy? And what portion of the inborn functional reserve is utilized in the adaptation process?

The basal oxygen consumption increases through pregnancy by about 40 ml/min (44, 46); the main consumers being the heart and the kidney, in addition to the fetus and the placenta (Fig. 2.5).

The approximately 20% increase in oxygen consumption is facilitated by the 40–50% increase in ventilation.

The increase in ventilation may be the cause of the common subjective feeling of dyspnea in pregnancy in spite of the increased oxygen

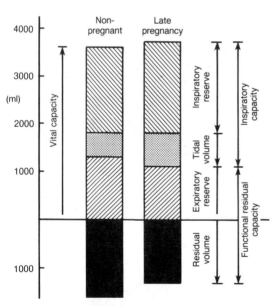

Figure 2.4. Subdivisions of lung volume and their alterations in pregnancy. (From deSwiet M. The respiratory system. In Hytten FE, Chamberlain G, eds. Clinical Physiology in Obstetrics. Oxford: Blackwell, 1980, p 81.)

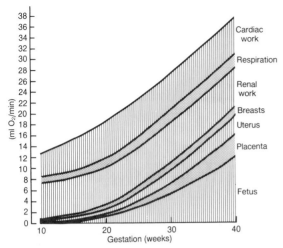

Figure 2.5. Partition of the increased oxygen consumption in pregnancy among the organs concerned. (From deSwiet M. The respiratory system. In Hytten FE, Chamberlain G, eds. Clinical Physiology in Obstetrics. Oxford: Blackwell, 1980, p 91.)

supply. The usual explanations for dyspnea, i.e., mechanical restriction or airways resistance were not validated in pregnancy (47).

Additional stress, like the one caused by exercise, is easily compensated within the respiratory system with the capacity to increase 10-fold (48). (See Chapter 15 for additional information.)

Cardiovascular System

The goal of the adaptation of the cardiovascular system, teleologically speaking, is to provide increased amounts of oxygen and fuel to all the organs with increased activity. The cardiovascular performance augments

more than physiologically needed as reflected by the increased oxygen consumption. In addition, whereas the cardiac output increases about 40%, there is an increase of only 13% in body mass to be supplied by maternal blood. The major increase in cardiac output occurs early in pregnancy at the end of the first trimester (49) during which period the oxygen consumption only starts to rise (Fig. 2.5). Furthermore, the arterial-venous (A-V) oxygen difference is reduced remarkably at the beginning of pregnancy and reaches prepregnant levels only at term (49–51).

The aforementioned facts defy the teleological explanations for the increased cardiovascular performance. A more plausible hypothesis is that the increase in cardiac output follows the increase in blood volume either in time or magnitude; both rise as early as 6–8 weeks of gestation, reaching the peak toward the end of the second trimester. Cardiac output and blood volume both increase in the range of 40–50% (Fig. 2.6).

The increase in the blood volume is a result of an increase in plasma volume up to 50% and red cell volume up to 20% (52, 53). This discrepancy between the increase in plasma volume and the red cell volume has a dilutional effect causing a drop in hematocrit from about 40% in the nonpregnant state to 35% at term. Therefore, the term "physiological anemia" is a misnomer, implying only negative connotations. Actually, the relative reduction in red cell mass does not interfere with oxygen distribution to the various organs as evidenced by decreased A-V differ-

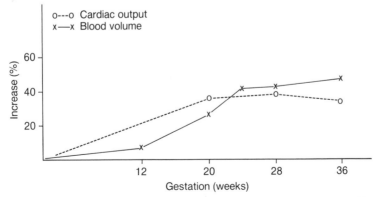

Figure 2.6. Changes in cardiac output and blood volume throughout pregnancy. Based on data from Pyorala (54) and Lund and Donovan (53).

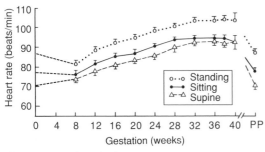

Figure 2.7. Serial changes in heart rate during pregnancy. (From Wilson M, et al. Am J Med 1980;68:97.)

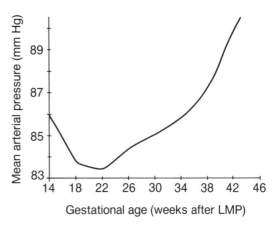

Figure 2.8. Mean arterial pressure by gestational age for single, white, term live births (nulliparas, 25–34 years of age). (From Page EW, Christianson R. Am J Obstet Gynecol 1976;125:740.

ence, which shows that more oxygen is carried to the tissues than is necessary.

Both components of cardiac output, the stroke volume and the heart rate, contribute to this increase. The latter contributes more during early pregnancy. The stroke volume increases at midpregnancy, up to 30% declining toward term (49, 54, 55). The resting heart rate starts to rise as early as 8 weeks of gestation by 8 beats per minute (bpm) (51). The resting heart rate rises through pregnancy reaching a plateau by 32 weeks, about 20 bpm higher than in the nonpregnant state (Fig. 2.7) (57).

The increased cardiac output is achieved at the expense of the enlargement of the heart. The mean end-diastolic volume of the heart increases between 70 and 80 ml during pregnancy due to increased diastolic filling and, most probably, also by muscle hypertrophy (58, 59). The contractility of the myocardium is changed in pregnancy, whether it is increased or decreased is still a matter of controversy (60–62). The increased excitability of the heart leads to more frequent atrial and ventricular extrasystoles (63). Such individuals must be closely supervised during exercise.

The 40% increase in cardiac output of about 1.5 liters/min is similar in percentage to the increase in pulmonary function, but it represents a much higher proportion in the cardiac function reserve. Taking into consideration that the maximum cardiac output can be increased no more than 3-fold (64) in comparison to 10-fold increase in pulmonary function, the cardiovascular performance is therefore lagging and constitutes a limiting factor in work capability.

There are some other very specific phenomena concerning the cardiovascular system in pregnant women:

As stated, the cardiac output rises significantly in pregnancy while, at the same time, the mean arterial pressure (MAP) drops. The decrease in MAP occurs as early as the first trimester, being lowest at midpregnancy and rising toward the nonpregnant state values at term (Fig. 2.8). The systolic blood pressure changes are relatively insignificant (65). As a result, pregnant women have an increased pulse pressure with a throbbing pulse. The inevitable conclusion from the rising cardiac output concomitantly with the drop in blood pressure is that the peripheral resistance of the circulation in pregnancy must be significantly reduced. Indeed, it was found that peripheral resistance in midpregnancy of 979 dyne·sec/cm^5 rose to 1200–1300 toward term gestation, compared to over 1200 for the nonpregnant state (51, 54).

The cardiovascular clinical state as we find it in pregnancy: throbbing, rapid pulse, increased cardiac output, increased oxygen consumption, and decreased peripheral resistance, is that of a hyperkinetic state similar to hyperthyroidism.

An important factor that should be taken into consideration when advising physical activity to pregnant women is the change in cardiac output and arterial blood pressure that may occur with changes in posture. Because of uterine mobility, change in posture changes its axis. In an upright position, the uterus falls forward, while supine, it falls backward and rests upon the vertebral column, often compressing the inferior vena cava and the abdominal aorta. The result is reduced cardiac output and supine hypotension (54, 66–68).

DISPOSAL SYSTEMS

By-products of increased metabolism in pregnancy result in increased heat and waste production, which need to be disposed. Changes occurring in pregnancy in skin and kidneys facilitate these functions.

The mechanism for heat dissipation has particular relevance in the gravida who engages in physical activities. There are three ways to dissipate heat: radiation, conduction, and evaporation. Heat is produced mainly in the core of the body and must be conducted to the outer layer, the skin, in order to be effectively dissipated. We have to keep in mind that the subcutaneous tissue abundant in fat is a very efficient insulator, therefore, direct conduction is impaired (69).

It is the capillary network of the skin that serves as a radiator for the body, with the blood serving as a coolant. The abundant sweat glands are instrumental in exploiting the mechanism of evaporation to lose heat.

The significant increase of blood flow to the skin starts at the beginning of the 2nd trimester, reaching the highest level at about 30 weeks of gestation when it levels off until delivery (70, 71). It is accomplished via peripheral vasodilatation (72), which is also evident in congestion of the nasal mucous membranes (73, 74), leading to occasional nose bleeding or snoring.

Along with increased hyperemia of the skin, there is an increase in the activity of the sebaceous and sweat glands that causes increased sweating.

The mechanism of radiation and conduction are effective only under conditions where the temperature of the surroundings is less than that of the skin. Otherwise, the only means by which the body can rid itself of the heat is by evaporation. Any disruption in proper functioning of the protective mechanisms described, as in the case of dehydration with arrest of perspiration or exercising in high humidity areas, has immediate repercussions on the fetus. The fetus depends totally on the mother for his or her heat dissipation. Any increase in maternal core temperature is immediately reflected in elevated fetal body temperature. It has been suggested by experimental teratology and retrospective studies that hyperthermia is teratogenic and may lead to neural tube defects in the offspring. These reports have to be viewed very cautiously because they linked such effects to maternal temperatures in excess of 38.9°C. These temperatures are reached fairly easily during exercise activities (75, 76).

The kidneys have an intrinsically large functional capacity as exemplified by the fact that an indiviudal may lose 50% function (unilateral nephrectomy) and yet maintain normal creatinine values. Furthermore, within 1–2 weeks of the nephrectomy, the remaining kidney attains a compensatory increase in function only slightly below the preoperative value for both kidneys (77).

It seems, therefore, that the expectant mother is well equipped to deal with the burden of having to clear additional waste products of fetal metabolism added to her own. Changes imposed by pregnancy are in direct proportion to the increase in the kidney's functional capability. Anatomically, the urinary system enlarges during pregnancy. The kidneys increase in weight and size, but the main change is seen in the collecting system, with dilatation of calyces, renal pelvis, and ureters (78).

The functional equivalent of the anatomical changes is the 30–50% increase in glomerular filtration rate (GRF) as expressed by creatinine clearance (79). The increase in GRF facilitates not only the filtration of waste products, but also in the process, other vital elements are lost. The most significant of those is the sodium. It is the increased tubular reabsorption of sodium, which is responsible for a considerable proportion of the specific metabolic cost of pregnancy, that prevents the critical process of sodium depletion (80).

Still, there are other important constituents of plasma that are filtered and lost because of the increased GFR: the glucose, amino acids, and water-soluble vitamins.

In pregnancy the tubular reabsorption of glucose, amino acids, and water-soluble vitamins (nicotinic acid, ascorbic acid, and folate) is less than optimal, with greater excretion in the urine compared to the nonpregnant state. The loss of amino acids may reach 2 g/day (81, 82). Although a regular, well-balanced diet provides an ample substitute for the urinary loss, in cases of increased demand, as in exercise, this particular point should be taken into account. (For additional information, see Chapters 5 and 16).

ENDOCRINE SYSTEM

The endocrine system is involved in significant changes in pregnancy. These changes are modulated, in part, by the ovaries and the fetoplacental unit and by the maternal endocrine glands.

The main source for pregnancy-sustaining hormones during the first 6–8 weeks of gestation is the ovarian corpus luteum. From the very beginning, most probably from the day of conception, the trophoblast produces the human chorionic gonadotropin (hCG) that prevents the corpus luteum from involution (83).

At a gestational age of 6–8 weeks, the placenta becomes the main source for hormone production (84).

Contrary to the common belief, the corpus luteum activity persists until term (85). Two kinds of hormones are produced by the corpus luteum: the steroids, and a unique polypeptide, relaxin. The ovaries appear to be the only source for production of relaxin during pregnancy. Relaxin is a 6500 low molecular weight peptide, structurally similar, in part, to the insulin molecule. By present assay techniques, it is detectable only in pregnancy. Plasma levels are highest at the end of the 1st trimester and maintained somewhat lower throughout pregnancy (86). The function of relaxin is still unclear, but as the name suggests, its main functions are thought to be relaxation of ligaments, softening and stretching of fibrocartilage by collagenolytic

activity in preparation for delivery. Such functions have been demonstrated in animals (87).

Among the steroids secreted by the corpus luteum, progesterone is the most essential and vital for the maintenance of pregnancy. Throughout pregnancy, the bulk, about 90%, originates from the placenta. But during the first 6–8 weeks of gestation, the corpus luteum is the principal source for progesterone (84).

The production of steroids by the corpus luteum reaches its peak 3–4 weeks after ovulation and then decreases, but does not entirely stop until the end of pregnancy. This pattern of production can be detected by monitoring the production of 17-hydroxyprogesterone, a metabolite of progesterone secreted almost exclusively by the ovarian tissue until late midpregnancy (Fig. 2.9) (88).

Two other groups of steroids secreted by the corpus luteum are the estrogens and androgens. Of the estrogens, only estradiol and estrone are secreted by the corpus luteum in significant amounts. Estriol, the estrogen most commonly associated with pregnancy, is produced almost exclusively by the fetoplacental unit (89).

The androgen production by the corpus

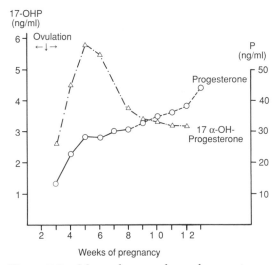

Figure 2.9.   Mean plasma values of progesterone *(P)*, and 17 α-hydroxyprogesterone *(17-OHP)* of 10 normal patients followed weekly from the 3rd to 13th week of pregnancy. ↓ indicates the presumed time of ovulation. (From Tulchinsky D, Hobel CJ. Am J Obstet Gynecol 1973;117:884.

luteum is noticeable only when in excess, as in the case of pregnancy luteoma, causing virilization of the expectant mother (90). It is conceivable that androstenedione, dehydroepiandrosterone (DHEA), and testosterone significantly add to the anabolic changes of pregnancy, yet the pregnant woman is relatively protected from excessive influence of androgens, whatever their source, by an increased level of sex-binding globulins generated by high levels of estrogens. The high efficiency of the placenta to convert androgens into estrogens acts as a protective barrier for the fetus against virilization by androgens originating from the mother (91).

Placenta

The placenta can be seen as the major endocrine organ of pregnancy. Either alone or in conjunction with the fetus, it modulates the physiological homeostasis of the mother and fetus.

The protein hormones of the placenta are closely related in their structure and function to the pituitary hormones. The human placental lactogen (hPL) and hCG share a common unit with the luteinizing hormone (LH), human growth hormone and thyrotropic stimulating hormone (TSH); thus, the similarities in biological function of LH and hCG. The same can be stated for the hPL, prolactin, and hGH.

hCG functions and regulation are enigmatic; they rise rapidly in the early stages of pregnancy, reaching a peak between 8 and 10 weeks of gestational age. Following, there is a relatively rapid decline up to 18 weeks, and, thereafter, the levels remain constant with a slight increase toward term. This type of pattern is in total contrast to those of other protein hormones of the placenta and does not simulate placental growth (Fig. 2.10).

Undoubtedly, hCG has a key role in the maintenance of the corpus luteum of pregnancy, but its function after 8 weeks of gestation is poorly understood. It is speculated that hCG has a role in fetal development like induction of fetal testosterone secretion from the Leydig cells of the testis, or some regulatory function for the adrenal fetal zone (92, 93).

In pathological conditions (trophoblastic diseases, hyperemesis gravidarium), the high levels of hCG highlight thyrotropic properties and increase the body metabolic rates (94). One common complication of early pregnancy, "morning sickness," is attributed to the high hCG levels (95).

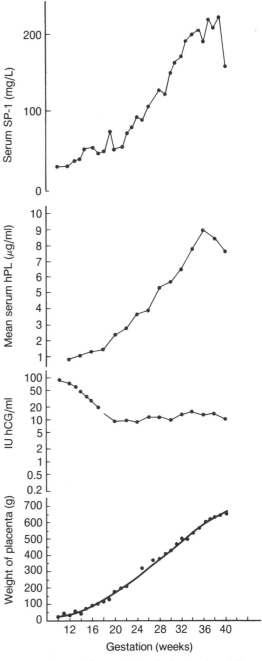

Figure 2.10.   Relationship of placental weight to plasma concentration of hormones through pregnancy.

hPL follows a more predictable pattern, with concentrations in direct proportion to the growth of the placenta (Fig. 2.10). Being closely related to hGH, the hPL activities involve lypolysis, nitrogen retention, hyperinsulinism, and peripheral resistance to insulin in pregnancy, all known to have diabetogenic effects (96). The pregnant woman, even when not affected by diabetes mellitus, is more prone to develop metabolic acidosis and hypoglycemia in the event of relative starvation or increased energy consumption not supported by appropriate caloric intake (97) as is likely to occur in diet-minded pregnant joggers.

Placental proteins currently studied are the schwangerschaftsprotein I (SP1), the pregnancy-associated plasma protein A (PAPP-A), the pregnancy-associated plasma protein B (PAPP-B), and the placental protein 5 (PP5). The distribution of these proteins throughout pregnancy resembles that of the hPLs, however, their function is as yet unknown (98) (Fig. 2.10).

Placental Steroids

ESTROGENS

Three estrogens, among the many hormones known to be produced by the placenta, have been the target of attention for both researchers and clinicians: the estradiol, estriol, and estetrol. Estriol is produced in large quantities by the fetoplacental unit and secreted via maternal circulation; therefore, it has been used as a predictor of fetal well-being (99).

The concentration of estrogens in plasma rises constantly, reaching levels up to and in excess of 15 ng/ml, increasing 2- to 5-fold throughout pregnancy (Fig. 2.11).

PROGESTAGENS

There are three biologically active progestagens produced in the placenta, the major one, progesterone, is the most abundant and biologically active. The other two are the 20-alpha (α)- and 20-beta (β)-hydroxylated derivatives of progesterone and are much less active and produced in small amounts. Unlike estrogens, their production is indepen-

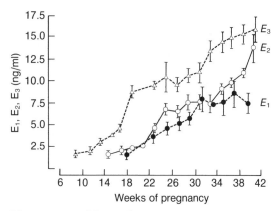

Figure 2.11. Mean plasma concentrations of estrogens during pregnancy. E_1 = estrone; E_2 = estradiol; E_3 = estradiol. The *bars* represent the standard error of the means. (From Tulchinsky D, et al. Am J Obstet Gynecol 1972;112:1095.

dent of the fetus. Progesterone levels increase from 40 ng/ml during the 1st trimester of pregnancy to 160 ng/ml during the 3rd trimester (Fig. 2.12).

The effects of the steroidal hormones can be divided into two groups: those promoting growth and those having mixed effects, mainly metabolic.

The primary target cells for the steroids that promote growth are the reproductive organs: the uterus and the breasts.

Under estrogenic and progestative influence, the uterus alters in size from $7.5 \times 5 \times 2.5$ cm with a capacity of 4 ml to $28 \times 24 \times 21$ cm and capacity of about 4000 ml at term. The

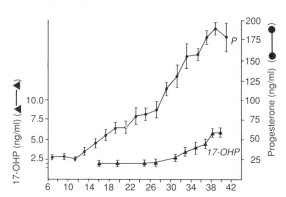

Figure 2.12. Progesterone *(P)* and 17-hydroxyprogesterone *(17-OHP)* mean plasma levels during human pregnancy. (From Tulchinsky D, et al. Am J Obstet Gynecol 1972;112:1095; and MacNaughton MC in Klopper A. Plasma Hormone Assays in Evaluation of Fetal Well-being. Edinburgh: Churchill Livingstone, 1976.)

weight increases from 30–60 g before pregnancy to 750–1000 g at term (2).

The increase of the uterine mass is accompanied by significant vascular changes. The arteries and the veins increase both in diameter and length. The net result is that, at term, the uterus and the associated blood vessels contain one-sixth or more of the total maternal blood volume. The uterine blood flow increases from about 50 ml/min at 10 weeks of gestation to a maximum of 500–700 ml/min at term (100,101). This change could be seen as equivalent to implanting an additional kidney (renal plasma flow equals 700–800 ml/min).

The estrogens also change the functional properties of the uterine muscle, increasing the elastic properties and the contractility, while the progesterone has a quiescent effect keeping the uterus in a nonactive state (102).

The breasts, another specific target organ for estrogens and progesterone, enlarge through the process of hypertrophy and hyperplasia of the gland and, at the same time, increase the fat content and vascularity. The estrogens influence the ductal growth, whereas the progesterone influences the alveolar growth (103). The nipples which progressively enlarge become more pigmented and erectile, while the breast seems to be less sensitive to tactile stimulation (104).

Progesterone generates an overall systemic smooth muscle relaxation effect in pregnancy and is the principal cause for venous dilatation, and atony of the bowel (105).

Progesterone also has a profound effect on the hypothalamic control centers. Progesterone resets the respiratory center, lowering the threshold for Pco_2 as a consequence, causing hyperventilation and a decrease in Pco_2. The insignificant increase in pH is due to compensatory and concomitant decrease in bicarbonate (38, 106). Resetting of the "lipolytic center" involves fat deposition, mainly during 1st and 2nd trimesters of pregnancy.

There is change in the appetite-satiety center toward increased ingestion of food, a contributing factor to the weight gain, while there is some evidence that progesterone engenders a feeling of lassitude, acting as an additional factor for energy saving (17, 18, 107).

An additional important effect of progesterone is resetting of the thermoregulatory control center with an elevation of at least 0.5°F (108) in addition to the increase in body temperature because of a higher metabolic rate.

Changes in ground substance of the connective tissue that may underlie the increased laxity of the joints, or water retention in the interstitial space, are thought to be caused by direct estrogenic activity (109).

The indirect influences of steroidal hormones are transmitted by changes exerted on the maternal endocrine system as described later in this chapter.

Pituitary

High levels of estrogens have various effects on the anterior pituitary. The production of follicular stimulating hormones (FSH) and LH declines in pregnancy to luteal phase levels of the menstrual cycle causing an anovulatory state (110, 111). The suppression of FSH and LH production is potentiated by the inhibitory influence of high levels of the placental analog for those hormones, the hCG (112).

In spite of the stimulatory effect of estrogens on hGH levels in the nonpregnant state, in pregnancy hGH levels are lower than in the nonpregnant state, because of the prevailing inhibitory effect of placental lactogen (113).

Conversely, prolactin levels, in spite of the inhibitory effect of high levels of its placental analog, the hPL, rise in pregnancy and are 10-20 times higher at term than in the nonpregnant state (114). There is a well-recognized function for prolactin to prepare the breast for lactation. The remainder of functions remains to be elucidated. There are animal studies to support the concept that osmoregulation in the fetus is modulated by prolactin (115). In addition, it also appears that prolactin has a role in the maternal metabolism of calcium by enhancing the transformation of 25-hydroxycholecalciferol to its most active form the 1,25-dihydroxycholecalciferol (116).

The actions of corticotrophin (ACTH) and thyrotropin (TSH), two other hormones originating in the anterior pituitary, do not appear to change during pregnancy.

Thyroid

Tachycardia, up to 100 bpm, elevated basal metabolic rate, intolerance to heat and, very often, emotional lability are common features of the pregnant state. Falsely, it can be deduced that these are results of a hyperactive thyroid, but measurements of free T_3 and T_4 levels that modulate the metabolic state, reveal no change from the nonpregnant state (117). The elevation of total T_3 and T_4 is caused by increases in thyroxin-binding globulin (TBG), a known effect of estrogenic hormones (118). The elevated BMR is actually normal if we take into account in the equation the increased metabolic activity of the mother secondary to the enlarged uterus, increased work of lung and heart, and the metabolism of the products of conception (119).

Parathyroid and Calcium Metabolism

The parathyroid gland is the source of two hormones involved in the regulation of calcium metabolism: the parathyroid hormone (PTH) and calcitonin (CT). In addition, the regulatory mechanism involves vitamin D and its metabolites, phosphorous and magnesium. From a teleological point of view, there is a sound rationale for a complex regulatory system, because of the multiple inflow and outflow sources for calcium in plasma. Absorption of calcium (Ca) is accomplished through the gastrointestinal tract and bone reabsorption, and is lost in urine, feces, and bone deposition.

Certain changes occurring in pregnancy, such as an increase in maternal extracellular fluid volume, maternal glomerular filtration, and Ca transfer across the placenta in the amount of about 30 g throughout pregnancy (120), result in a progressive reduction in serum Ca as pregnancy advances. The total serum Ca concentration in pregnant women reflects the significant decline in Ca that is bound to plasma protein, primarily albumin (Fig. 2.13). The ionic Ca, the functional fraction, does not change, except for a slight decline in the 3rd trimester. Concurrently, in

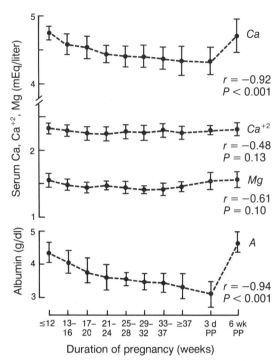

Figure 2.13. Mean ($\pm$ SD) levels of Ca, Ca^{+2}, Mg, and A during pregnancy and the puerperium. (From Pitkin RM, et al. Am J Obstet Gynecol 1979;133:781.

the 3rd trimester, the fetus incorporates Ca at the maximal rate of 200-300 mg/day (121).

The increase in demand is met by: increased digestive tract absorption, reduction in urinary loss, increased bone mobilization, or any combination of the above.

The homeostasis of Ca in pregnancy is maintained mainly by increased levels of PTH (Fig. 2.14). The PTH affects the increased production in the kidneys of the most active vitamin D derivative, the 1,25-hyrdoxycholecalciferol, whose role is to enhance intestinal absorption and reduce renal excretion.

Contrary to the common belief, the positive Ca balance in pregnancy does not result in marked maternal bone tissue loss. Selective blocking of PTH activity on bone tissue prevents the resorption activated by the hormone.

Protection of the maternal skeleton is achieved, most probably, through the effects of high levels of estrogen and progesterone that inhibit PTH activity and promote bone deposition. CT levels in pregnancy tend to decline (122).

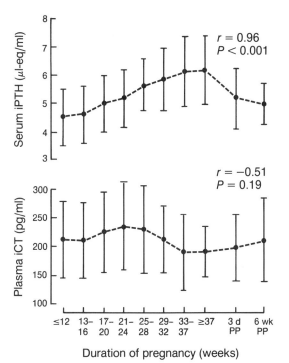

Figure 2.14. Mean (±SD) levels of inhibitory parathyroid hormone *(iPTH)* and calcitonin *(iCT)* during pregnancy and the puerperium. (From Pitkin RM, et al. Am J Obstet Gynecol 1979;133:181.

Although the RDA for Ca is 1200 mg, the ideal minimal dose is 400–600 mg (123). That amount is easily acquired by regular diet. In cases of starvation, when maternal diet is lacking calcium or vitamin D and there is lack of exposure to sun and/or renal disease, the fetal Ca demands will be met by demineralization of the maternal skeleton. Phosphorus (P) and magnesium (Mg) metabolism are intimately related to the metabolism of Ca.

P and Ca are both regulated by the same intestinal, renal, and skeletal factors; PTH modulates their activity in a similar fashion mobilizing effects on bone tissue for both. The mechanism of intestinal absorption is similar with the exception that vitamin D is not essential for P absorption.

The kidney is the regulatory organ for P plasma levels. The kidney has a P transport maximum (T_m), which means that, under certain levels in plasma, all filtrated P will be reabsorbed. This particular mechanism is influenced by PTH, CT, estrogens, and adrenal steroids resulting in an increased urinary loss of P.

The GH and, most probably, hPL due to its GH-like effect, increase the T_m, reducing the P urinary loss. The net result of these various activities in pregnancy is a tendency toward decline in P levels during the first two-thirds of pregnancy with a nadir at about 30 weeks of gestational age, and thereafter a slight rise (122).

An important aspect is that an increase in P blood levels promotes the Ca incorporation into the bone tissue (124), lowering the plasma Ca level.

Because of a very efficient intestinal absorption and renal recovery, and abundant amounts of P found in any food, there is no P deficiency recognized in pregnancy, and it is believed that high levels of P are the cause for leg cramps (122).

Little is known about Mg homeostasis. By and large, it is influenced by the same factors as Ca and P, including PTH.

Adrenal Gland and Water Metabolism

Despite increased concentrations of hormones originating in the adrenal, no anatomic enlargement is found in pregnancy (125). Specific binding proteins, like sex hormones, globulins, or transcortin increase in pregnancy secondary to high levels of estrogens.

It is believed that steroids play a crucial role in the homeostasis of pregnancy by modulating the activity of other hormones and by their own direct action. The adrenal estrogen production is negligible compared to the large amount produced in the fetoplacental unit or the ovary. Testosterone is found in higher concentrations during pregnancy, but is less active because of the diminished free fraction and reduced peripheral conversion to dihydrotestosterone, the more potent derivative (126).

DHEA and its sulfate derivative, the most abundant of androgens, are produced almost exclusively by the adrenals, are very efficiently metabolized by the placenta, and are aromatized to estradiol and estrone (91).

Circulating catecholamines, epinephrine and norepinephrine, are not changed in pregnancy compared to the nonpregnant state, but they increase significantly during labor and delivery (127).

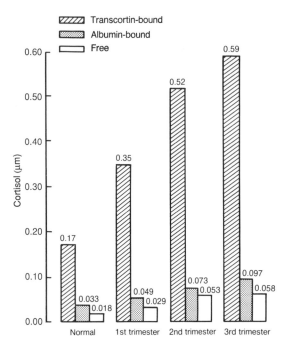

Figure 2.15.   Distribution of bound and unbound cortisol in pregnancy plasma. (From Rosenthal HE, et al. J Clin Endocrinol Metabol 1969;29:352.

The plasma levels of cortisol are elevated in the 1st trimester and rise thereafter until delivery. This elevation is caused largely by the estrogen-mediated increase in transcortin. More significantly, there is also an increase in the free fraction that is the active part of the hormone (Fig. 2.15). The free cortisol concentration in plasma, during pregnancy, reaches levels encountered in pathological states such as Cushing's syndrome (128, 129). The reason for this rise is only partially understood. The increase in free cortisol appears not to be related to pituitary ACTH, which levels, although rising, are within the normal range during pregnancy (130), but subject to other sources of stimulating hormones. There is some evidence that the placenta is capable of producing ACTH-like hormone (131). Indirect evidence for the extrapituitary source of the stimulating hormone is the inability to suppress cortisol production after stimulation with corticosteroids (132).

The additional mechanism responsible for elevated cortisol levels is reduced elimination with a half-life that is double compared to the nonpregnant state (133). It is not clear why, despite high levels of cortisol, there is no clinical, Cushing-like manifestation. The reason could be attributed to the competitive actions of other hormones, particularly progesterone, that has a high affinity to cytosol receptors for cortisol (134).

Mineralocorticoids and Water Metabolism

The two potent mineralocorticoids produced by the zona glomerulosa of the adrenal cortex, aldosterone and 11-deoxycorticosterone (DOC) are elevated during pregnancy, and a clear distinction can be made between the two. Plasma levels of aldosterone increase significantly at about 12 weeks of gestation, and reach a plateau at 30 weeks of gestation, 3- to 5-fold higher than in the nonpregnant state (Fig. 2.16). Increased levels of sodium suppress aldosterone production whereas ACTH increases it (135). Conversely, plasma levels of DOC rise progressively, mainly during the 3rd trimester of pregnancy, increasing at term 10- to 15-fold from the nonpregnant state (Fig. 2.16). DOC levels are unresponsive to changes in salt intake or ACTH (136, 137). A significant portion of DOC originates during the 3rd trimester from peripheral extra-adrenal 21-hydroxylation of maternal progesterone and the fetus (138, 139).

Aldosterone production is modulated by various systems; the renin angiotensin, which responds to changes in mean arterial pressure, sodium and potassium levels, and by direct stimulation of ACTH. As previously maintained, ACTH levels do not change significantly during pregnancy. The sodium and potassium levels are the result rather than the cause of aldosterone changes.

High estrogen levels stimulate liver production of angiotensinogen, the substrate for renin to product angiotensin II. Angiotensin II, in turn, stimulates aldoesterone production.

Reduced MAP in pregnancy is a trigger for the increased release of renin. The cumulative effect of this phenomenon is sodium retention expressed as fluid retention and intravascular fluid expansion. It happens in spite of increased GFR and reduction in colloid osmotic pressure (140, 141).

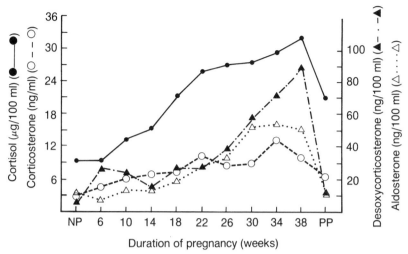

Figure 2.16. Mean steroid levels in 11 women throughout pregnancy and postpartum *(PP)* compared to levels in nonpregnant *(NP)* women. (Data from Wintour EM, et al. Clin Exp Pharmacol Physiol 1978;5:399.

Theoretically, the changes described in elevated aldosterone and angiotensin II levels should have harmful effects: i.e., depletion of potassium, excessive retention of sodium, and hypertension. The fact is that usually neither depletion of potassium with excessive sodium retention nor hypertension occur in pregnancy. The counteractive action is believed to be secondary to progesterone, which guards for stable potassium concentration and prevents excess of sodium retention (142). The hypertensive effects of angiotensin II are counteracted by reduced responsiveness of the renal and systems vasculature under the influence of high levels of prostaglandins, and by high estrogen activity (143).

Toward the end of pregnancy, the expectant mother accumulates an excess of 8.5 liters of water. Up to 30 weeks of gestation, the measured gain is close to the expected one from added maternal blood, tissue, and products of conception. However, at term, only part of the total extracellular fluid gain (6.5 liters) can be recovered by computation of the volume added in the known sites (4.0 liters) (144). The excess 2.5 liters are most probably distributed in the ground substance of the connective tissue, visible as pitting ankle edema in about 40–50% of otherwise normal pregnant women.

Atrial natriuretic peptide (ANP), isolated in 1981, has natriuretic and vasoactive prop-

erties and is thought to be an important determinant in volume homeostasis. The highest levels have been found in volume-expanded conditions in the nonpregnant individual such as in a patient with congestive heart failure. ANP levels during pregnancy would predictably be elevated but this is presently controversial. An early study reported an elevated ANP level during pregnancy that correlated with weight gain (145). An increase in mean ANP level but without diurnal variation, as seen with aldosterone, was subsequently reported in pregnancy (146). Other studies showed either no increase in ANP in pregnancy (147) or an increase during the immediate puerperium (148). ANP's role during volume-depleted states, such as may occur with exercise, has not been reported.

As a whole, the adaptive anatomical and physiological changes in pregnancy have a significant impact on the ability of the pregnant woman to maintain physical fitness or to participate in certain sports activities. It is important to recognize those limiting factors whenever attempting to prescribe exercise programs in pregnancy.

REFERENCES

1. DeVries HA. Physiology of Exercise, ed. 3. Dubuque, Iowa: William C. Brown, 1980, p 246.
2. Davey AD. Normal pregnancy: physiology and management. In Dewhurst J, ed. Integrated Ob-

stetrics and Gynecology for Postgraduates, 3rd ed. Oxford: Blackwell, 1981, p 105.

3. Hytten FE, Cheyne GA. The size and composition of the human pregnant uterus. J. Obstet Gynaecol Br Commonw 1969; 76:400.

4. Hytten FE. Weight gain in pregnancy. In Hytten FE, Chamberlain G, eds. Clinical Physiology in Obstetrics. Oxford: Blackwell, 1980, pp 208–209.

5. Crisp WE, DeFrancesco S. The hand syndrome of pregnancy. Obstet Gynecol 1964; 23:433.

6. Tobin SM. Carpal tunnel syndrome in pregnancy. Am J Obstet Gynecol 1967; 23:493.

7. Voitk AJ, Mueller JC, Farlinger DE, Johnson RU. Carpal tunnel syndrome in pregnancy. Can Med Assoc J 1983; 128:277.

8. Johns JP. The influence of pregnancy on the visual field. Am J Ophthalmol 1930; 13:956.

9. Millodot M. The influence of pregnancy on the sensitivity of the cornea. Br J Ophthalmol 1977; 61:646.

10. Weinreb RN, Lu A, Key T. Maternal ocular adaptations during pregnancy. Obstet Gynecol Surv 1987; 42:471–483.

11. Jacobs WH, Janowitz HD. The digestive tract. In Rovinsky JJ, Guttmacher AF, eds. Medical, Surgical and Gynecologic Complications of Pregnancy. Baltimore: Williams & Wilkins, 1965, p 177.

12. Hansen R, Langer W. Über geschmacks Veränderung in der Schwangershaft. Klin Wochenschr 1935; 14:1173.

13. Masten WY, et al. Reaction time and strength in pregnant and nonpregnant employed women. J Occup Med 1988; 30:451–456.

14. Jarrahi-Zadeh A, Kane Jr FJ, Van de Castlf RL, Lachenbruch PA, Ewing JA. Emotional and cognitive changes in pregnancy and early puerperium. Br J Psychiatry 1969; 115:797.

15. Hytten FE. Nutrition. In Hytten FE, Chamberlain G, eds. Clinical Physiology in Obstetrics. Oxford: Blackwell, 1980, p 165.

16. Bruce NH. Gestational adaptation: major systems. In Iffy L, Kaminetzky HA, eds. Principles and Practice of Obstetrics and Perinatology. New York: John Wiley & Sons, 1981, p 688.

17. Merryman M, Borman R, Barnes L, Rothchild I. Progesterone "anasthesia" in human subjects. J Clin Endocrinol Metab 1954; 14:1567.

18. Selye HJ. Studies concerning anesthetic action of steroid hormones. J Pharmacol Exp Ther 1941; 73:127.

19. Kaminetzky HA, Baker H. Nutritional needs in pregnancy. In Iffy L, Kaminetzky HA, eds. Principles and Practice of Obstetrics and Perinatology. New York, John Wiley & Sons, 1981, p 665.

20. Pitkin RM: Nutritional support in obstetrics and gynecology. Clin Obstet Gynecol 1976; 19:489.

21. Thompson AM, Billewicz WZ: Clinical significance of weight trends during pregnancy. Br Med J 1957; 1:243.

22. Abrams BF, Laros RK. Prepregnancy weight, weight gain, and birth weight. Am J Obstet Gynecol 1986; 154:503–509.

23. Langhoff-Ross J, Lindmark G, Kylberg E, Gebre-Medhin M. Energy intake and physical activity during pregnancy in relation to maternal fat accretion and infant birthweight. Br J Obstet Gynaecol 1987; 94:1178–1185.

24. Langhoff-Ross J, Lindmark G, Gebre-Medhin M. Maternal fat stores and fat accretion during preg-

nancy in relation to infant birthweight. Br J Obstet Gynaecol 1987; 94:1170–1177.

25. Ulmsten U, Sundström G. Esophageal manometry in pregnant and non-pregnant women. Am J Obstet Gynecol 1978; 132:260.

26. Fisher RS, Roberts GS, Grabowski CJ, Cohen S: Altered lower esophageal sphincter function during early pregnancy. Gastroenterology 1978; 74:1233.

27. Bassey OO. Pregnancy heartburn in Nigerians and Caucasians with theories about aetiology based on manometric recordings from oesophagus and stomach. Br J Obstet Gynaecol 1977; 84:439.

28. Davison JS, Davison MC, Hay DM. Gastric emptying time in late pregnancy and labour. J Obstet Gynaecol Br Commonw 1970; 77:37.

29. Parry E, Shields R, Turnbull AC. Transit time in the small intestine in pregnancy. J Obstet Gynaecol Br Commonw 1970; 77:900.

30. Parry E, Shields R, Turnbull AC. The effect of pregnancy on the colonic absorption of sodium potassium and water. J Obstet Gynaecol Br Commonw 1970; 77:616.

31. Gerdes MM, Boyden EA. The rate of emptying of the human gallbladder in pregnancy. Surg Gynecol Obstet 1938; 66:145.

32. Potter MG. Observations of the gallbladder and bile during pregnancy at term. JAMA 1936; 106:1070.

33. Gazioglu K, Kaltreider NL, Rosen M, Yu PN. Pulmonary function during pregnancy in normal women and in patients with cardiopulmonary disease. Thorax 1970; 25:445.

34. Alaily AB, Carrol KB. Pulmonary ventilation in pregnancy. Br J Obstet Gynaecol 1978; 85:518.

35. Knuttgen HG, Emerson K. Physiological response to pregnancy at rest and during exercise. J Appl Physiol 1974; 36:549.

36. Thomson KJ, Cohen ME. Studies on the circulation in pregnancy; II. Vital capacity observations in normal pregnant women. Surg Gynecol Obstet 1938; 66:591.

37. McGinty AP. The comparative effects of pregnancy and phrenic nerve interruption on the diaphragm and their relation to pulmonary tuberculosis. Am J Obstet Gynecol 1938; 35:237.

38. Prowse CM, Gaensler EA. Respiratory and acid-base changes during pregnancy. Anaesthesiology 1965; 26:381.

39. Lehmann V, Fabel H. Lungen funktionsuntersuchungen an schwangeren feil; II. Ventilation, Atemmechanik und Diffisionkapazitat. Z Geburtshilfe Perinatol 1973; 177:397.

40. Archer GW, Marx GF. Arterial oxygen tension during apnoea in parturient women. Br J Anaesth 1974; 46:358.

41. Adams JQ. Cardiovascular physiology in normal pregnancy: Studies with the dye-dilution technique. Am J Obstet Gynecol 1954; 67:741.

42. Rovinsky JJ, Jaffin H. Cardiovascular hemodynamics in pregnancy; III. Cardiac rate, stroke volume, total peripheral resistance, and antral blood volume in multiple pregnancy. Synthesis of results. Am J Obstet Gynecol 1966; 95:787.

43. Bouterline-Young H, Bouterline-Young E. Alveolar carbon dioxide levels in pregnant parturient and lactating subjects. J Obstet Gynaecol Br Emp 1956; 63:509.

44. Pernoll ML, Metcalfe J, Schlenker TT, Welch JE,

Matsumoto JA. Oxygen consumption at rest and during exercise in pregnancy. Respir Physiol 1975; 25:285.

45. Clapp III JF, Seaward BL, Sleamaker RH, Hiser J. Maternal physiologic adaptations to early human pregnancy. Am J Obstet Gynecol 1988; 159:1456–60.
46. Knuttgen HG, Emerson K. Physiological response to pregnancy at rest and during exercise. J Appl Physiol 1974; 36:549.
47. Campbell EJM, Howell JBL. The sensation of breathlessness. Br Med Bull 1963; 19:36.
48. Comroe J, Forster RE, Dubois AB, Briscoe WA, Carlsen E. The Lung: Clinical Physiology and Pulmonary Function Tests. Chicago: Year Book, 1962.
49. Walters WAW, MacGregor WG, Hills M. Cardiac output at rest during pregnancy and the puerperium. Clin Sci 1966; 30:1.
50. Lees MM, Taylor SH, Scott DB, Kerr MG. A study of cardiac output at rest throughout pregnancy. J Obstet Gynaecol Br Commonw 1967; 74:319.
51. Bader RA, Bader ME, Rose PJ, Braunwald E. Haemodynamics at rest and during exercise in normal pregnancy as studied by cardiac catheterization. J Clin Invest 1955; 34:1524.
52. Pirani BBK, Campbell DM. Plasma volume in normal first pregnancy. J Obstet Gynaecol Br Commonw 1973; 80:884.
53. Lund CJ, Donovan JC. Blood volume during pregnancy. Am J Obstet Gynecol 1967; 98:393.
54. Pyorala T. Cardiovascular response to the upright position during pregnancy. Acta Obstet Gynecol Scand 1966; 45(suppl):5.
55. Ueland K, Novy MJ, Peterson EN, Metcalfe J. Maternal cardiovascular dynamics; IV. The influence of gestational age on the maternal cardiovascular response to posture and exercise. Am J Obstet Gynecol 1969; 104:856.
56. Clapp III JF. Maternal heart rate in pregnancy. Am J Obstet Gynecol 1985; 152:659–660.
57. Wilson M, Morganti AG, Zervoudakis I, Letcher RL, Romney BM, Von Oeyon P, Papera S, Sealey JE, Laragh JH. Blood pressure, the unine-aldosterone system and sex steroids throughout normal pregnancy. Am J Med 1980; 68:97.
58. Gemzell CA, Robbe H, Strom G. Total amount of haemoglobin and physical working capacity in normal pregnancy and the puerperium. Acta Obstet Gynaecol Scand 1957; 36:93.
59. Ihrman K. A clinical and physiological study of pregnancy in material from northern Sweden; VII. The heart volume during and after pregnancy. Acta Soc Med Upsala 1960; 65:326.
60. Rubler S, Schneebaum R, Hammer N. Systolic time intervals in pregnancy and the post-partum period. Am Heart J 1973; 86:182.
61. Burg JR, Dodek A, Kloster FE, Metcalfe J. Alterations of systolic time intervals during pregnancy. Circulation 1974; 49:560.
62. Liebson PR, Mann LI, Evans MI, Duchin S, Arditi L. Cardiac performance during pregnancy: serial evaluation using external systolic time intervals. Am J Obstet Gynecol 1975; 122:1.
63. Szekely P, Snaith L. Heart Disease and Pregnancy. Edinburgh: Churchill Livingstone, 1974.
64. Ueland K, Novy MJ, Metcalfe S. Hemodynamic responses of patients with heart disease to pregnancy and exercise. Am J Obstet Gynecol 1972; 113:47.

65. MacGillivray I, Rose GA, Rowe B. Blood pressure survey in pregnancy. Clin Sci 1969; 37:395.
66. Voyrs N, Ullery JC, Hanusek GE. The cardiac output changes in various positions in pregnancy. Am J Obstet Gynecol 1961; 82:1312.
67. Kerr MG, Scott DB, Samuel E. Studies of the inferior vena cava in late pregnancy. Br Med J 1964; 1:532.
68. Bieniarz J, Crottongini JJ, Curuchet E, Romero-Salinas G, Yoshida T, Poseiro JJ, Caldeyro-Barcia R. Aortocaval compression by the uterus in late human pregnancy. An angiographic study. Am J Obstet Gynecol 1968; 100:203.
69. Guyton AC. Medical Physiology, ed. 6. Philadelphia: WB Saunders, 1981, p 887.
70. Spetz S, Jansson I. Forearm blood flow during normal pregnancy studied by venous occlusion plethysmography and 133-xenon muscle clearance. Acta Obstet Gynaecol Scand 1966; 48:285.
71. Katz M, Sokal MM. Skin perfusion in pregnancy. Am J Obstet Gynecol 1980; 137:30.
72. Melbard SM. Valeur diagnostique de la capillaroscopie dans la grossesse et dans la sepsie puerperale. Gynecol Obstet 1938; 37:100.
73. Scott JH. Heat-regulating function of the nasal mucose membrane. J Laryngol Otol 1954; 65:308.
74. Fabricant ND. Sexual functions and the nose. Am J Med Sci 1960; 239:498.
75. Miller P, Smith DW, Shepard TH. Maternal hyperthermia as a possible cause of anencephaly. Lancet 1978; 1:519.
76. Pleet HB, Graham JM, Harvey MA. Patterns of malformations resulting from the teratogenic effects of trimester hyperthermia. Pediatr Res 1980; 14:587.
77. Davison JM. The urinary system. In Hytten FE, Chamberlain G, eds. Clinical Physiology in Obstetrics. Oxford: Blackwell, 1980, p 302.
78. Marchant DJ. Alterations in anatomy and function of the urinary tract during pregnancy. Clin Obstet Gynecol 1978; 21:855.
79. Davison JM, Hytten FE. Glomerular filtration during and after pregnancy. J Obstet Gynaecol Br Commonw 1975; 8:583.
80. Lindheimer MD, Katz AI, Nolten WE, Oparil S, Ehrlich EN. Sodium and mineralocorticoids in normal and abnormal pregnancy. Arch Nephrol 1977; 7:33.
81. Davison JM. Renal nutrient excretion with emphasis on glucose. Clin Obstet Gynecol 1975; 2:365.
82. Hytten FE, Cheyne GA. The aminoaciduria of pregnancy. J Obstet Gynaecol Br Commonw 1972; 63:509.
83. Mishell Jr DR, Nakamura RM, Barberia JM, Thorneycroft IH. Initial detection of human chorionic gonadotropin in serum in normal human gestation. Am J Obstet Gynecol 1974; 118:990.
84. Csapo AI, Pulkkinen M. Indispensability of the human corpus luteum in maintenance of early pregnancy. Lute-ectomy evidence. Obstet Gynecol Surv 1978; 33:69.
85. Mikhail G, Allen WM. Ovarian function in human pregnancy. Am J Obstet Gynecol 1967; 99:308.
86. Quagliarello J, Szlachter N, Steinetz BG, Goldsmith LT, Weiss MD. Serial relaxin concentrations in human pregnancy. Am J Obstet Gynecol 1979; 135:43.
87. Porter DG, Amoroso EC. The endocrine functions of the placenta. In Philipp E, Barnes J, Newton M, eds. Scientific Foundation of Obstetrics and Gynaecology. Chicago: Year Book, 1977, p 700.

88. MacNaughton MC. Hormone assays in early pregnancy. In Klopper A, ed. Plasma Hormone Assays in Evaluation of Fetal Well-Being. Edinburgh: Churchill Livingstone, 1976, p 42.

89. Lauritzen C, Klopper A. Estrogens and androgens. In Fuchs F, Klopper A, eds. Endocrinology of Pregnancy, ed. 3. Philadelphia: Harper & Row, 1983, p 80.

90. Garcia-Bunuel R, Berek JS, Woodruff JD. Luteomas of pregnancy. Obstet Gynecol 1975; 45:407.

91. Bolte E, Mancuso S, Eriksson G, Wigust N, Diczfalusy E. Studies on the aromatization of neutral steroids in pregnant women; 3. Overall aromatization of dehydroepiandrosterone sulphate circulating in the fetal and maternal compartments. Acta Endocrinol 1964; 45:576.

92. Wilson JD, Griffith JE, George FW, Leshin M. The role of gonadal steroids in sexual differentiation. Recent Prog Horm Res 1981; 37:1.

93. Lauritzen C, Lehman WD. Levels of chorionic gonadotropin in the newborn infant and their relationship to adrenal dehydroepiandrosterone. Acta Endocrinol (suppl) Kbh 1965; 100:112.

94. Nisula BC, Morgan FJ, Caufield RE. Evidence that chorionic gonadotropin has intrinsic thyrotropic activity. Biochem Biophys Res Commun 1974; 59:86.

95. Fairweather DVI. Nausea and vomiting in pregnancy. Am J Obstet Gynecol 1968; 102:135.

96. Osathanondh R, Tulchinsky D. Placental polypeptide hormones. In Tulchinsky D, Ryan KJ, eds. Maternal-Fetal Endocrinology. Philadelphia: WB Saunders, 1980, p 29.

97. Felig P, Lynch V. Starvation in human pregnancy: hypoglycemia, hypoinsulinemia and hyperketonemia. Science 1970; 170:990.

98. Klopper A. The new placental proteins. Biol Med 1979; 1:89.

99. Curet LB, Olson RW. Oxytocin challenge tests and urinary estriols in the management of high risk pregnancies. Obstet Gynecol 1980; 55:196.

100. Assali NS, Rauramo L, Peltonen T. Uterine and fetal blood flow and oxygen consumption in early human pregnancy. Am J Obstet Gynecol 1960; 79:86.

101. Metcalfe J, Romney SL, Ramsey LH, Burwell CS. Estimation of uterine blood flow in normal human pregnancy at term. J Clin Invest 1955; 34:1632.

102. Klopper A. The ovary. In Hytten FE, Chamberlain G, eds. Clinical Physiology in Obstetrics. Oxford: Blackwell, 1980, p 434.

103. Guyton AC. Textbook of Medical Physiology, ed. 6. Philadelphia: WB Saunders, 1981, p 1033.

104. Robinson JE, Short RV. Changes in breast sensitivity at puberty, during the menstrual cycle and at parturition. Br Med J 1977; 1:1188.

105. Kumar D. In vitro inhibitory effect of progesterone on extrauterine human smooth muscle. AM J Obstet Gynecol 1962; 84:1300.

106. Lyons HA, Antonio R. The sensitivity of the respiratory center in pregnancy and after the administration of progesterone. Trans Assoc Am Physicians 1959; 72:173.

107. Harvey GR. Regulation of energy balance. Nature 1969; 222:629.

108. Moghissi KS, Syner FN, Evans TN. A composite picture of the menstrual cycle. Am J Obstet Gynecol 1972; 114:405.

109. Langgard H, Hvidberg E. The composition of oedema fluid provoked by estradiol and of acute inflammatory oedema. J Reprod Fertil 1969; 9(suppl):37.

110. Faiman C, Ryan RJ, Jarrck SJ, Rubin ME. Serum FSH and hCG during human pregnancy and puerperium. J Clin Endocrinol Metab 1968; 28:1323.

111. Jeppsson S, Rannevik G, Thorell JI. Pituitary gonadotropin secretion during first weeks of pregnancy. Acta Endocrinol 1977; 85:177.

112. Miyake A, Tanizawa O, Aono T, Yasuda M, Kurachi K. Suppression of luteinizing hormone in castrated women by the administration of human chorionic gonadotropin. J Clin Endocrinol Metab 1976; 43:928.

113. Mochizuki M, Morikawa H, Kawaguchi K, Tojo S. Growth hormone, prolactin and chorionic somatomammotropin in normal and molar pregnancy. J Clin Endocrinol Metab 1976; 43:614.

114. Rigg LA, Lein A, Yen SSC. The pattern of decrease in circulating prolactin levels during human gestation. Am J Obstet Gynecol 1977; 129:454.

115. Tyson JE. The evolutionary role of prolactin in mammalian osmoregulation: effects on fetoplacental hydromineral transport. Semin Perinatol 1982; 6:216.

116. Spanos E, Pike JW, Haussler MR, Colston KW, Evans IMA, Goldner AM, McCain TA, MacIntyre I. Circulating 1-alpha-25-dihydroxy vitamin D in the chicken: enhancement by injection of prolactin and during egg laying. Life Sci 1976; 19:1751.

117. Souma JA, Niejadlik DC, Cottrell S, Rankel S. Comparison of thyroid function in each trimester of pregnancy with the use of triiodothyronine uptake, thyroxine iodine, free thyroxine, and free thyroxine index. Am J Obstet Gynecol 1973; 116:905.

118. Dowling JT, Freinkel N, Ingbar SH. The effect of oestrogens upon peripheral metabolism of thyroxine. J Clin Invest 1960; 39:1119.

119. Sandiford I, Wheeler T. Basal metabolism before, during and after pregnancy. J Biol Chem 1924; 62:329.

120. Pitkin RM. Calcium metabolism in pregnancy: a review. Am J Obstet Gynecol 1975; 121:724.

121. Irwin MI, Kienholtz WW. A conspectus of research on calcium requirements of man. J Nutr 1973; 103:1019.

122. Pitkin RM, Reynolds WA, Williams GA, Hargis GG. Calcium metabolism in normal pregnancy: A longitudinal study. Am J Obstet Gynecol 1979; 133:781.

123. Reeve J. Calcium metabolism. In Hytten FE, Chamberlain G, eds. Clinical Physiology in Obstetrics. Oxford: Blackwell, 1980, p 263.

124. Slatopolsky E, Rutherford E, Hruska K, Martin K, Klahr S. How important is phosphate in the pathogenesis of renal osteodystrophy: Arch Intern Med 1978; 138:848.

125. Whiteley JH, Stoner HB. The effect of pregnancy on the human adrenal cortex. J Endocrinol 1957; 14:325.

126. Saez JM, Forest MG, Morera AM, Bertrand J. Metabolic clearance rate and blood production rate of testosterone and dehydrotestosterone in normal subjects during pregnancy and in hyperthyroidism. J Clin Invest 1972; 51:1226.

127. Lederman RP, Lederman E, Work Jr, BA, McCann PS. The relationship of maternal anxiety, plasma catecholamines and plasma cortisol to progress in labor. Am J Obstet Gynecol 1978; 132:495.

128. Burke CW, Roulet F. Increased exposure of tissues to cortisol in late pregnancy. Br Med J 1970; 1:657.

129. Rosenthal HE, Slaunwhite WRJ, Sandberg AA. Transcortin: a corticosteroid-binding protein of plasma; X. Cortisol and progesterone interplay and unbound levels of these steroids in pregnancy. J Clin Endocrinol Metab 1969; 19:352.

130. Carr BR, Parker Jr, CR, Madden JD, MacDonald PC, Porter JC. Maternal plasma adrenocorticotroph and cortisol relationships throughout human pregnancy. Am J Obstet Gynecol 1981; 139:416.

131. Genazzani AR, Fraioli F, Hurlimann J, Fioretti P, Felber JP. Immunoreactive ACTH and cortisol plasma levels during pregnancy. Detection and partial purification of corticotropin-like placental hormone: The human chorionic corticotropin (hCC). Clin Endocrinol 1975; 4:1.

132. Nolten WE, Rueckert PA. Elevated free cortisol index in pregnancy: Possible regulatory mechanisms. Am J Obstet Gynecol 1981; 138:492.

133. Cohen M, Stiefel M, Reddy WJ, Saidlaw JC. The secretion and disposition of cortisol during pregnancy. J Clin Endocrinol Metab 1958; 18:1076.

134. Nolten WE, McKenna MV, Rueckert PA, Ehrlich EN. Inhibition of 3H-dexamethasone binding to lymphocytes in vitro; relevance to the apparent development of refractoriness to cortison in pregnancy. Clin Res 1980; 28:7624.

135. Erlichs EN, Lindheimer MD. Effect of administered mineralocorticoid or ACTH in pregnant women: Attenuation of kaliuretic influence of mineralcorticoids during pregnancy. J Clin Invest 1972; 51: 1301.

136. Ehrlich EN, Nolten WE, Oparil S, Lindheimer MD. Mineralocorticoids in normal pregnancy. In Lindheimer MD, Katz AI, Zuspan FP, eds. Hypertension in Normal Pregnancy. New York: John Wiley & Sons, 1976, p 1989.

137. Nolten WE, Lindheimer MD, Opard S, Erlich EN. Desoxycortisterone in normal pregnancy; 1. Sequential studies of the secretory patterns of desoxycarbiosterone, aldosterone and cortisol. Am J Obstet Gynecol 1978; 132:414.

138. Winkel CA, Milewich L, Gant NF, Parker Jr CK, Gant NF, Simpson ER, MacDonald PC. Conversion of plasma progesterone to deoxycorticosterone in men, nonpregnant and pregnant women and adrenalectomized subjects. Evidence for steroid II-hydroxylase activity in nonadrenal tissues. J Clin Invest 1980; 66:803.

139. Nolten WE, Holt LH, Rueckert PA. Desoxycorticosterone in normal pregnancy; III. Evidence of a fetal source of desoxycorticosterone. Am J Obstet Gynecol 1981; 139:477.

140. Davison JM, Hytten FE. Glomerular filtration during and after pregnancy. J Obstet Gynaecol Br Commonw 1975; 81:583.

141. Robertson EG. Increased erythrocyte fragility in association with osmotic changes in pregnancy serum. J Reprod Fertil 1968; 16:323.

142. Landau RL, Lugibihl K. Inhibition of the sodium retaining influence of aldosterone by progesterone. J Clin Endocrinol Metab 1958; 18:1237.

143. Everett RB, Worley RJ, MacDonald PC, Gant NF. Effect of prostaglandin synthetase inhibitors on pressor response to angiotensin II in human pregnancy. J Clin Endocrinol Metab 1978; 46:1007.

144. Hytten FE. Weight gain in pregnancy. In Clinical Physiology in Obstetrics. Oxford: Blackwell, 1980, p 216.

145. Cusson JR, Gutkowska J, Rey E, Michon N, Boucher M, Larochelle P. Plasma concentration of atrial natriuretic factor in normal pregnancy. N Engl J Med (Letter) 1985; 313:1230–1231.

146. Miyamoto S, Shimokawa H, Sumioki H, Touno A, Nakano H. Circadian rhythm of plasma atrial natriuretic peptide, aldosterone, and blood pressure during the third trimester in normal and preeclamptic pregnancies. Am J Obstet Gynecol 1988; 158:393–399.

147. Bond AL, August P, Druzin ML, Atlas SA, Sealey JE, Laragh JH. Atrial natriuretic factor in normal and hypertensive pregnancy. Am J Obstet Gynecol 1989; 160:1112–1116.

148. Rutherford AJ, Anderson JV, Elder MG, Bloom SR. Release of atrial natriuretic peptide during pregnancy and immediate puerperium. Lancet (Letter) 1987; 1:928–929.

3

Fuel Metabolism in Pregnancy— Theoretical Aspects

Itzhak Zaidise, Raul Artal Mittelmark, and Samuel P. Bessman

There is no other period in adult life in which such major physiological changes occur as in pregnancy. All available resources are channeled to the fetus without harming the mother. These functions are regulated by a variety of hormones, including the specific gestational placental hormones.

Fats, proteins, and carbohydrates are recognized as fuels because they are capable of supplying energy requirements. They are also the major building blocks of the body. Their demand during pregnancy is increased to supply these functions.

FUEL COMPONENTS AND STORAGE

All of the three major components, proteins, carbohydrates, and fats, can be utilized as fuels because they are oxidized for energy (ATP) production. The utilization rate varies and depends on the specific need of each organ. The most selective organ is the brain that, under normal conditions, uses exclusively glucose.

Fuel supply is derived from either external sources, namely diet, or from internal stores. Of the three possible fuels, only fat is stored in significant amounts in the adipose tissues. A nonpregnant 60-kg woman stores about 18 kg of fat, which can generate 160,000 kcal. Carbohydrates stored as glycogen are very limited, estimated as 800–1000 kcal, about half stored in the liver and the other half stored in skeletal muscles. Only liver glycogen is readily available for immediate utilization. In 24 hours of continuous fasting, the liver is virtually depleted of glycogen, but the muscles still possess about 80% of their glycogen.

Proteins are not stored in the body in the usual sense because every known protein has a specific physiological role (enzymes, functional proteins as actin or myosin, structural as collagen and bone proteins). Every protein broken down and utilized for energy may affect some important physiological function. The major body proteins are collagen (25%) and actomyosin (20%) that, under conditions of increased demand, undergo degradation. Such degradation is more pronounced in myosin than in collagen. Loss of more than 10% of body proteins is known to cause major impairments of physiological functions, while a 30–50% loss is lethal.

Fat is a readily stored substrate. Not only does it have twice the caloric value of carbohydrates and proteins, but it is also unhydrated while the other two fuels are hydrated with about four times their weight of water. Therefore, 1 kg of fat yields the same amount of energy as about 10 kg of carbohydrates or proteins. Thus, storage of fat has a clearly evolutionary advantage over carbohydrates. Fat cannot supply the entire energy needed for the organism because the brain and other tissues (red blood cells and the renal cortex) cannot utilize it. Such needs are supplied by glycogen.

The average weight gain during pregnancy is about 12 kg, with the conceptus accounting for 4.950 kg (fetus, 3.5 kg; placenta, 0.65 kg; amniotic fluid, 0.8 kg). Maternal tissues directly affected by pregnancy (uterus and breasts) along with fluid gain account for about 4.3 kg for a total of 9.250 kg (1). The rest, 2.75 kg, is believed to be the net fuel storage increase. In the human, these stores are assumed to be mainly fat (2) (Fig. 3.1). Weight gain during gestation is inversely related to maternal weight before pregnancy. Obese patients gain less than lean ones (3). In the rat, total body weight increases during gestation by about 30%, fat is increased 50%, while proteins are increased 20% (4). The proteins accumulated are well distributed

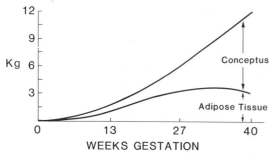

Figure 3.1. Constituents of maternal weight gain during pregnancy. Fat content is established from measurement of total body water. The conceptus consists of the fetus, placenta, uterus, amniotic fluid, and membranes. The conceptus plus fat could account for all maternal weight gain during pregnancy. (From Hytten FE, Leitch I. The physiology of human pregnancy, ed. 2. Oxford: Blackwell, 1971, p 333–369.)

among the various organs (liver, 35%; heart, 30%; kidneys, 28%; gastrointestinal tract, 40–50%) (5). Protein metabolism in the rat appears to be biphasic, anabolic in the early stage of pregnancy and catabolic later on (6).

It is not clear what changes in total body protein occur in human pregnancy. Johnstone et al. (7) performed a 12-day nitrogen balance test in 68 normal pregnant women in late gestation (30–34 weeks); no nitrogen retention or loss could be demonstrated. A total gain of about 1 kg protein equivalent to 5 kg lean body mass in human pregnancy was calculated by Hytten and Leitch (8); almost all of it has been related to the fetus, placenta, and uterus. The remainder of protein accumulation occurs early in pregnancy

and is generated to accommodate the increased metabolic needs, but not for storage. Proteins are utilized as fuel in cases of fuel shortage as in starvation or when excess proteins are ingested.

INTERCONVERSION OF FUELS

The most essential fuel is glucose, which must be continuously available, yet it is stored in relatively small amounts. In the rat, placental transfer of fat is poor, and the fetus mobilizes its energy and synthesizes fat from glucose and amino acids (9). In other animals and humans, there is a limited transfer of fatty acids, but primarily amino acids and glucose cross the placenta.

Some interconversion of fuels does exist. Glucose can be converted to fat through acetyl coenzyme A, the main pathway for excess carbohydrates and amino acids. The reverse pathway, fatty acids to glucose, is trivial. About 5% of the triglyceride (TG) carbons, the glycerol moiety, can be converted to glucose. Glucose can also be utilized to form the carbon skeleton of almost all the nonessential amino acids. Also, proteins can be converted to glucose, approximately 60 g of glucose for every 100 g of protein (Fig. 3.2).

CONTROLLED STRESS CONCEPT

Bessman and his group have proposed the "controlled stress" hypothesis to explain the biochemical effects caused by the interplay among the catabolic stress hormones and anabolic insulin (10). They postulated that all

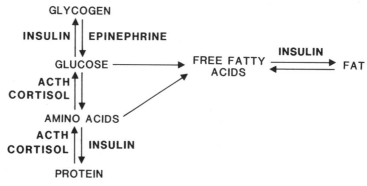

Figure 3.2. Interconversion of fuel elements. Note that there is no conversion from fatty acids to glucose. Epinephrine stimulates the breakdown of glycogen and fat. ACTH and cortisol stimulate breakdown of protein to amino acids and the transformation of these into glucose (gluconeogenesis). Insulin reverses the epinephrine and ACTH-cortisol effects.

types of stress, including trauma, infection, and psychological stress, constitute an emergency survival mechanism in which the organism is rapidly supplied with large amounts of fuels, glucose for the brain and free fatty acids (FFA) for the muscles, to enable them to cope with the "fight and flight" requirements.

Epinephrine, the most primitive stress hormone (11), is responsible for the primary stress reaction. Its mechanism of action is a rapid activation of pre-existing inactive enzymes through cAMP-adenyl cyclase system (12, 13). Both glycogenolysis and lipolysis are markedly increased. By and large, the epinephrine effect is uncontrolled and results in excess supply of these fuels, exceeding the capacity of the cell to metabolize. This results in hyperglycemia, hyperlipidemia, ketonemia, and lactic acidemia from incomplete oxidation of FFA and glucose. The acids cause a decrease in blood bicarbonate and pH (Table 3.1). All these changes can be observed clinically in diabetic ketoacidosis. Epinephrine effect causes excessive expenditure of the limited glycogen depots. This is phase I of stress.

Insulin is known to elicit anabolic reactions and, as such, can be regarded as the true growth hormone (14). Insulin counteracts the action of epinephrine (Table 3.2) by its stimulation of protein, fat, and glycogen synthesis. Insulin limits the supply of all fuels by reference to the blood glucose level. It is secreted when the glucose level rises higher than 100 mg/dl, the optimal concentration for brain metabolism. It acts by increasing the resynthesis of fat and glycogen without affecting their breakdown rate.

If stress continues for several hours, the effects of cortisol, ACTH, and growth hormone (GH) (phase II of stress) become man-

Table 3.1. Epinephrine Effects on Blood Chemistry

1. Glucose	↑	
2. Free fatty acids	↑	
3. Lactate	↑	
4. Ketone acids	↑	
5. Bicarbonate	↓	
6. pH	↓	

Table 3.2. Insulin Effects

Metabolism		Blood	
Glycogen synthesis	↑	Glucose	↓
Protein synthesis	↑	Amino acids	↓
Glucose transport	↑	Glucose	↓
Fatty acid synthesis	↑	Ketones	↓
Fat synthesis	↑	Free fatty acids	↓

ifested (Table 3.3). They are secreted along with epinephrine, but because their mechanism of action is slow, their effects are delayed (e.g., induction of enzymes). Phase II hormones increase protein breakdown to amino acids, thereby stimulating gluconeogenesis, so that an adequate supply of glucose for the brain continues even after liver glycogen reserves are exhausted. Insulin controls phase II by increasing the opposite reaction, protein synthesis from amino acids, therefore depriving gluconeogenesis of substrate when the glucose blood level exceeds the optimum of 100 mg/100 ml. Protein breakdown is not affected by insulin (15). Because the fuel to be conserved is glucose, it represents the signal for pancreatic β-cell secretion of insulin.

When the stress is over, both epinephrine and the phase II hormones are no longer secreted. Epinephrine effects cease immediately, while phase II effects continue for hours or even days because their decline depends on the half-life of the newly synthesized enzymes evoked by phase II hormones (cortisol, ACTH, GH) (Fig. 3.3).

Pregnancy appeared late in evolution. It exists only in vertebrates, mainly, mammals. Gestation-related hormones, estrogen, pro-

Table 3.3. Steroid-Peptide Hormone Effects

Metabolism		Blood	
Protease	↑	Amino acids, ketones and lactate	↑
Glucose-6-phos- phatase Fructose-1,6-di- phosphatase Pyruvate carboxylase Phosphoenolpyruvate carboxykinase		Glucose	↑

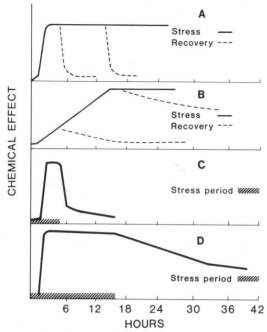

Figure 3.3. Schematic relationship between chemical effects of stress hormones of phase I and II stress and duration of actual stress. *A*, Phase I of stress—epinephrine. *B*, Phase II of stress—steroid-peptide hormones. *C*, Actual manifestations of short-term stress—combined effect of phase I and II hormones. *D*, Actual manifestation of long-term stress—combined effect of phase I and II hormones. (From Zaidise I, Bessman SP. The diabetic syndrome—uncontrolled stress. In Belfiore F, Galton DJ, Reaven GM, eds. Frontiers in Diabetes. Basel: Karger, 1984; vol 4, p 77–92.)

gesterone, human placental lactogen, and prolactin, play a secondary role, as modifiers, in the main scheme of fuel metabolism previously discussed. Their major metabolic role is to ensure adequate substrate supply to the fetus through catabolism of maternal stores. They are secreted independently of the day-to-day metabolic variations so that the fine-tuning of fuel metabolism is regulated by the major stress hormones and insulin.

HORMONES AFFECTING FUEL SUPPLY IN PREGNANCY

In nonstressful conditions, epinephrine levels do not change in pregnancy (16).

ACTH and cortisol do increase during pregnancy (17, 18). Progressively increasing cortisol levels are accompanied by higher circulating cortisone-binding globulin (19, 20).

ACTH levels rise in late pregnancy. It was postulated (20) that the hypothalamus demonstrates a reduced sensitivity to cortisol due to high maternal concentrations of cortisone antagonists such as progesterone and 17-hydroxyprogesterone (21). A direct positive effect of estrogen on ACTH secretion was also suggested (6). The placenta probably secretes a significant part of the maternal ACTH (22) because the placental content of the hormone is higher than can be explained by the blood distribution of the hormone. This explains also the resistance of cortisol production to dexamethasone inhibition. The pregnant woman, therefore, can be considered to be continually in phase II of stress augmented by the catabolic effect of those hormones particularly associated with pregnancy.

Fasting growth hormone (hGH) is essentially unchanged throughout pregnancy. Pituitary hGH secretion in response to stimuli (as hypoglycemia) is increased during the first 24 weeks and depressed thereafter.

In reviewing the current literature, it appears that glucagon plays only a minor role in modifying the pregnancy-related changes of fuel metabolism (3).

Estrogen secretion rises from below 100 μg/day to 33 mg/day near term gestation (23). This hormone increases lipolysis and gluconeogenesis via protein breakdown, the latter effect is assumed to be facilitated by ACTH secretion. Conversely, natural estrogen improves glucose tolerance, both in laboratory animals and in human subjects (24), probably through a positive effect on insulin secretion, for it also causes hypertrophy of the pancreatic islets, which has been shown to occur in pregnancy (25). This process may explain the increased basal levels of insulin in late pregnancy in spite of lower fasting blood glucose.

Progesterone has a limited effect, in the human, on glucose tolerance, but it does increase basal plasma insulin (26, 27). Progesterone was also found to diminish insulin receptor response (28). Its secretion rises progressively, reaching a level of 250 mg/day at term.

hPL is a single chain, placenta-secreted polypeptide. Immunologically, it is closely related to hGH. hPL causes mobilization of FFA from maternal depots. The lipid, lipoprotein, and apolipoprotein levels increase during pregnancy are positively correlated with changes in estradiol, progesterone, and hPL (29). It has a diabetogenic effect and its administration provokes glucose intolerance in women who have had impaired glucose tolerance tests in previous pregnancies (30). The increase of insulin-like growth factors (IGF) that occur in pregnancy are probably related to the GH-like activity of hPL. Blood levels at term are 5–8 μg/ml (31). It has been suggested that hPL is modulated by glucose and/or FFA (32).

Prolactin has actions similar to those of hGH. Its levels in pregnancy are steadily increasing (33, 34). Prolactin is secreted by the maternal pituitary, myometrium, and endometrium. Uterine prolactin secretion is mediated by estrogen, progesterone, and relaxin (35). The "anti-insulin effect" of prolactin is well established. Its administration causes an elevation of blood FFA level in the human (36), and a delayed increase (5 hours) of blood glucose and glucose turnover in the dog (37). In hyperprolactinemic nonpregnant women, the glucose tolerance curve, basal insulin levels, and postchallenge plasma insulin responses are significantly higher than in normal women, mimicking the metabolic responses of late gestation (38). These phenomena can be explained through the "controlled stress" concept, because prolactin increases gluconeogenesis that could appear clinically as diminution of insulin sensitivity. The delayed changes in glucose metabolism are similar to those seen in phase II stress, reflecting stimulated catabolic enzyme synthesis.

METABOLIC ADAPTATION TO PREGNANCY

Fat accumulation and increased protein synthesis start early in pregnancy. These changes are partly explained by enhanced maternal appetite. Pregnancy is characterized by increased levels of circulating insulin and insulin resistance (39, 40). This leads to higher insulin requirements in diabetic patients (41). Early in pregnancy, hPL, prolactin, and cortisone levels are low so that the glucose tol-

erance test results are generally unaltered and may even improve in the diabetic patient (42), probably due to enhanced insulin secretion.

A major metabolic change occurs in the second half of pregnancy. Fat accumulation ceases; in many cases, there is actual decline in fat depots. Some investigators report a reduction in lean body mass in laboratory animals. During this period, cortisol, GH, and insulin levels continue to rise. Fasting blood levels of glucose, amino acids, FFA, and ketones do not significantly alter throughout pregnancy (Fig. 3.4*A*). A further fast of 4–6 hours results in lower blood glucose and amino acids while FFA and ketones hike markedly (Fig. 3.5) (43, 44).

The metabolic changes mimic those seen in prolonged starvation and, indeed, Freinkel termed them as a state of "accelerated starvation" (45). The above metabolic shift is partly allied to the fetal requirements. The fetus triples its weight during the last trimester. Although the fetus' metabolic expenditure per kg body weight, expressed in calories, is not much different from that of the mother, the composition of the substrates used is dissimilar. Because very limited amounts of fatty acids cross the placenta, fat and protein synthesis are derived mostly from glucose and amino acids.

The continuous transplacental drainage of glucose and amino acids does not affect maternal blood levels of these nutrients during daytime. However, after an overnight fast, plasma glucose and amino acids are depressed in late pregnancy. With exhaustion of liver glycogen depositories, protein becomes the only source for glucose and amino acids. Under these conditions, lipolysis occur. However, because glucose is drained, the maternal organism does not respond with insulin secretion (46) to control the excess TG breakdown as in the normal compensated stress reaction. If starvation persists, FFA formation exceeds its complete oxidation rate, resulting in generation of ketones (Fig. 3.4*B*). This simulates the sequence of events occurring during starvation in the nonpregnant individual, but much faster because the catabolic hormones are initially higher in preg-

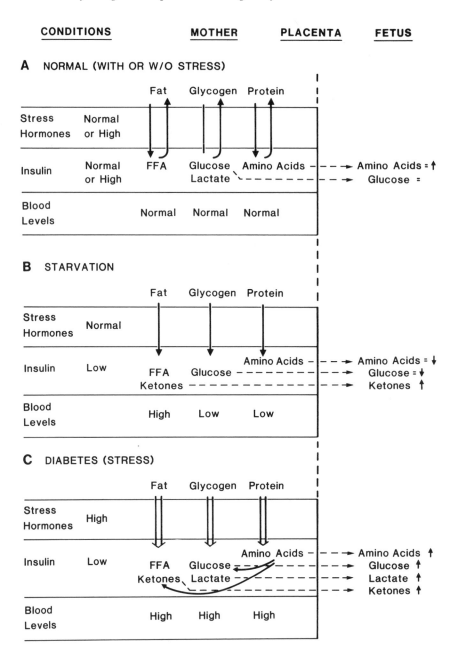

Figure 3.4.   Hormonal effects on fuel supply and availability in pregnancy. *A, Normal:* A balance exists between breakdown and synthesis of fuels due to the mutual effects of stress hormones and insulin. Blood levels of fuels and their products are normal. No change is observed during stress because insulin secretion increases to counteract stress hormone activity. *B, Starvation:* Due to glucose drainage from the maternal system, insulin activity is low. As fat breakdown continues without activation of fat synthesis by insulin, FFA and ketones rise, resulting in ketonemia in the mother and fetus. *C, Diabetes with stress:* Both phase I and II of stress are activated and are not controlled by insulin. PFA, ketones, glucose, lactate, and amino acids are elevated in maternal blood (diabetic ketoacidosis). All of them except FFA are elevated also in the fetus. The fetus reacts with hyperinsulinemia and transforms these substrates to fat and proteins, resulting in the typical macrosomic baby seen in diabetic pregnancies.

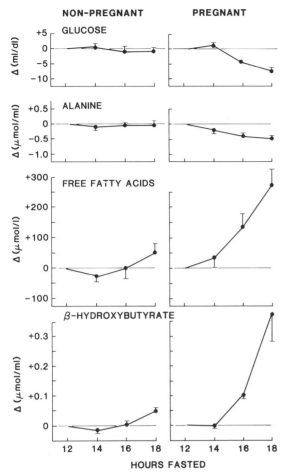

NON-PREGNANT   PREGNANT

Figure 3.5. Changes in plasma concentrations of glucose, alanine, free fatty acids, and β-hydroxy-butyrate in nonpregnant and pregnant women between 12 and 18 hours' fast. Values are shown as absolute increments or decrements from base values. (Modified from Metzger BE, Ravnikar V, Vileisis RA, Freinkel N. "Accelerated starvation" and the skipped breakfast in late normal pregnancy. Lancet 1982;1:588–592.

nancy and glucose utilization is enhanced. An elevated lipolytic activity was found in vitro in the fat tissues of pregnant animals (47) exposed to cortisol and hPL.

The decreased glucose tolerance observed in late pregnancy is interpreted by this mechanism. During a glucose load, insulin has to counteract the increased gluconeogenesis effects of pregnancy hormones and cortisone by diverting glucose to fat and glycogen. Some other hypotheses have been advanced to explain glucose intolerance in pregnancy

despite higher insulin secretion: reduced binding affinity of insulin receptor (48); post-receptor defect; faster removal of insulin from the circulation (49) by special receptor proteins (inactive receptor or enhanced insulin catabolism by higher insulinase activity and/ or concentration). The rat and human both have placental insulinase activity, but there is no increase in insulin clearance in the human (50). The combined effect of these processes was termed "insulin insensitivity." Insulin sensitivity in pregnancy is about one-fifth of that found in the nonpregnant woman (51).

The factors determining insulin sensitivity are not clear, e.g., hormone-, enzyme-, or receptor-related. In general, the insulin insensitivity components themselves can be explained by the controlled stress mechanism. Puavilai and coworkers (52) found, in late pregnancy, during glucose load, increased insulin binding to peripheral monocytes together with a high plasma glucose to insulin ratio. They suggested a "postreceptor" defect in insulin action. These same data can be interpreted as intact insulin action in the face of high gluconeogenesis rate caused by ACTH, cortisol, and hPL, which are elevated during late gestation without need to postulate unknown postreceptor effects.

Maternal insulin does not cross the placental barrier. In the fetus, insulin can be detected already at 12–15 weeks and its concentration increases rapidly thereafter. A simple monophasic insulin response to glucose is observed early in the 2nd trimester. The physiological biphasic response develops only in the postnatal period (53).

Transplacental passage of fatty acids in the nondiabetic human is small, but may reach a large proportion in other species (54, 55). Essential fatty acids, such as linoleate, cannot be synthesized by the fetus and must be transported across the placenta. On the basis of fetal linoleate content, it has been estimated that up to 50% of total fetal lipids is contributed by the mother (55). On the other hand, Koren and Shafrir (9) found in the rat that only 1–2% of intravenously injected palmitate cross the placenta over 16–18 hours. Small maternal contribution over long time periods may, therefore, add to a large total amount of fatty acids.

The human placenta has a lipoprotein lipase activity (56). Therefore it may uptake TG as well as FFA although the rate is by far higher for the latter. The placenta stores some FFA but mostly reesterifies them to TG. All fats are liberated into the fetal circulation as FFA.

Placental transfer of FFA is regulated mainly by their transplacental gradient (57). All components of plasma lipids are elevated in pregnancy (58). Further increase of FFA and TG are seen in maternal diabetes. Other important factors affecting FFA transfer are: placental blood flow, umbilical blood flow, maternal and fetal albumin concentrations, and intratrophoblastic fatty acid-binding protein (59).

CONSEQUENCES OF GESTATIONAL KETOSIS

As discussed previously, gestational ketosis is common and should probably be regarded as a physiological rather than a pathological state. Unlike fatty acids, ketones readily cross the placenta (60), and their levels in fetal circulation equal that of the mother (61). Whether this poses risks for the fetus is still under debate. Gestational ketosis in normal women is often considered to have the same pathological significance as diabetic ketoacidosis. The latter is a totally different metabolic situation, where ketosis is accompanied by metabolic acidosis and glucose levels are usually highly elevated. Metabolic acidosis per se may harm the fetus by decreasing uterine blood flow (62).

The Collaborative Perinatal Project of the National Institute of Neurological Disorders and Stroke consists of an 8-year prospective follow-up of 53,518 pregnancies in 12 United States hospitals between 1959 and 1966 (63). Some studies were based upon the diabetic mothers' subgroup of this database. Churchill et al. (64) found lower IQ scores (mean of 83) in infants of diabetic mothers who had had episodes of ketonuria within 24 hours of delivery as compared with those who had not had such episodes (mean 101) or of those of normal nondiabetic mothers (mean 102). Analyzing the same data, Naeye (65) found

no difference among any of these groups in the IQ scores. Stehbens and co-workers (66) followed, prospectively, 80 children of diabetic mothers. By the age of 5 years, they found a lower IQ score among those children whose mothers had had ketonuric episodes during pregnancy.

In these studies, the exact occurrence of ketoacidosis vs. ketosis only is unknown. The results, therefore, cannot be extrapolated to normal women with physiological ketosis of pregnancy. Naeye and Chez (67), analyzing the Collaborative Perinatal Project database, did not find any psychoneurological impairment among children of normal mothers who had had ketosis during starvation. In certain conditions, the fetus can even benefit from ketones because it can utilize them for energy (68) and for cerebral lipid synthesis (69).

Nevertheless, ketosis should be avoided by frequent meals and snacks especially before night sleep. Skipping breakfast is another unwanted habit because it prolongs the overnight fast to 16–18 hours (44). Some food is also recommended before exercise.

METABOLIC FATE OF GLUCOSE

On the average, pregnant women who do not limit their food intake consume approximately 2300–2800 kcal (70). Because very little net maternal weight gain (excluding pregnancy products and fluids) is observed during late gestation, all fuels are used for maternal and fetal energy needs and fetal growth. Assuming an average daily intake of 2500 kcal with 40% carbohydrates, the available glucose amounts to 1000 kcal or 250 g. Maternal inflexible requirements are about 150 g/day (120 g for the brain and 30 g for other glucose-dependent tissues).

Fetal oxygen consumption near term is about 5 ml/kg/hour (71). Based on the assumption that the primary fuel for the fetus is glucose, Widdowson (5) calculated that the fetal energy requirement per kg of body weight is the same as that of the mother. Fetal and maternal inflexible needs at that time add up to 215 g (72), leaving only 35 g of glucose for other metabolic needs. It has been found experimentally that uterine glucose utilization (mainly the conceptus) represent 30–50% of overall glucose utilization by the mother (73). The previously mentioned data are consistent with the common belief that, in late pregnancy, glucose is "reserved" for fetal needs. Glucose utilization is also dependent on its maternal plasma concentration. In the ovine fetus glucose satisfies about 50% of the energy requirements in the fed state, but only 15% in the starved condition. Insulin-induced hypoglycemia has a similar effect (74).

In early pregnancy, fetal metabolic needs are practically nil. Glucose disappears from the blood after meals faster than it can be oxidized. When 50 g glucose are injected intravenously, blood glucose will return to the preload level within 1 hour. At the same time, only about 70 kcal are exploited for energy. Even if all the energy were produced from glucose (which is probably an overestimation), it accounts for only 35% of the administered glucose. Therefore, most of the glucose is diverted into fat and a smaller amount into glycogen. Each molecule of glucose transformed into fat is lost for the maternal glucose-dependent tissues and for the fetus later in pregnancy.

Glucose utilization by the resting muscle is insulin dependent. Glucose uptake by the tissue is increased in the presence of higher circulating glucose levels even in the absence of insulin (75). Glucose utilization for energy is higher in the absorptive period because both glucose and insulin are elevated at that time, while significantly diminished thereafter. In late pregnancy, muscle glucose oxidation is relatively higher because the absorptive period is prolonged (reduced glucose tolerance) and basal insulin levels are higher.

Exercising muscle utilizes glucose independently of insulin. In the diabetic patient, exercise lowers blood glucose, an insulin-like effect. It has been shown by Artal et al. (76) that, during exercise in pregnancy, glucose is reduced similarly in the healthy and diabetic patients. The mechanism of this phenomenon was worked out by Bessman and his group (77–80). They suggested a creatine-phosphocreatine shuttle for energy transfer from the mitochondria to the myofibrils. When the muscle is exercised, more phosphocreatine is consumed by the myofibrils. The free creatine liberated diffuses to the mitochondrial membrane where phosphocreatine is regenerated. The latter reaction is ATP dependent and the net effect, in the mitochondrial compartment, is the depletion of ATP and an increased adenosine diphosphate (ADP). Because ADP controls energy generation, its greater availability results in a higher rate of energy production.

METABOLIC CONSIDERATIONS ON DIABETES IN PREGNANCY

Viewing insulin as the only antistress hormone, diabetes can be considered as a disease of "uncontrolled stress." The organism is fully capable of producing the epinephrine and peptide hormones phases of stress, but unable to modulate them with pancreatic insulin and prevent the ill effects of the full blown stress reaction. In practice, a diabetic patient balanced with a certain dose of insulin can cope with normal life quite well. However, as soon as any kind of stress intervenes: infection, surgery, or emotional stress, the diabetic patient is driven out of balance and goes into an excessive catabolic state that requires a higher dose of insulin.

Pregnancy may be considered a state of chronic stress; not only the original stress phase II hormones are elevated, but also some pregnancy-related stress hormones, i.e., hPL and prolactin, are elevated. Glucose levels fluctuate in normal late gestation more than in any other period, and with them, insulin demands also change. Metzger and Freinkel (81) concluded that the effect of pregnancy on maternal fuel metabolism is to amplify the magnitude of the oscillation during transitions between the fed and fasted states (Fig. 3.6). Insulin oscillates in parallel with glucose.

The pregnant diabetic is incapable of secreting the required amount of insulin in response to glucose stimulation. The blood levels of the fuels will oscillate even wider than in normal pregnancy. The experimental data support these considerations. Glucose is elevated in the fed state, although it does not return to normal in the fasted state due

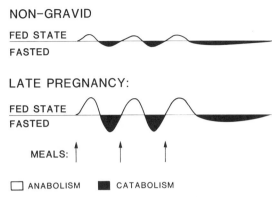

Figure 3.6. Effect of pregnancy on metabolic fuels. (From Metzger BE, Freinkel N. Effects of diabetes mellitus in the endocrinologic and the metabolic adaptation of gestation. Semin Perinatol 1978;2:309–318.)

to increased gluconeogenesis (82). The same is observed for amino acids (81). Circulating FFA and ketones are higher in pregnant diabetic patients than in normal pregnant women, both in the fed and the fasted states (83). The increase is most pronounced after an overnight fast (84).

In insulin-dependent diabetes, the physician and the patient assume the role of the pancreas in monitoring the metabolic state and controlling stress. The better the control, the closer the patient is to normal. Any metabolic study of diabetes reflects only the success or failure of a certain treatment scheme in a certain group of patients (85). Normally, insulin secretion is adjusted many times a day to control the correct supply and storage of the main fuels as reflected by glucose blood levels. A diabetic patient given two to four doses of insulin daily may get his or her average requirement of the hormone, but certainly not his or her immediate needs. Most of the time, the diabetic patient has either too much or too little circulating insulin. The organism oscillates enormously between anabolic and catabolic states. This constant shift between synthesis and breakdown, especially of proteins, may be responsible for the late complications of the disease. For the short run, the body can accommodate such fluctuations unless a rapid increase in insulin levels is needed as in the case of severe stress.

Pregnancy is a period of rapid metabolic

changes requiring a better adjustment of insulin administration. Moreover, for reasons beyond the scope of this chapter, fetal outcome appear best when maternal glucose levels are constantly stabilized around 80–100 mg/100 ml (85–89). Accomplishing better control necessitates strict dietary (90, 91) and activity control as well as regular monitoring of blood glucose (85, 92), a better distribution of insulin dosage and avoidance of prolonged fasting, and any possible stress.

Several open-loop insulin pumps have been introduced (93, 94). They administer insulin continuously and may take into account the changes in insulin requirements during meals, and be programmable for activity and overnight fasting. However, because they are preprogrammed, strict dietary and activity control must be retained, and no factor that cannot be predetermined is taken into account. The periods of increased insulin requirement due to stress are, we believe, most destructive.

The optimal solution is a closed-loop system that will monitor blood glucose and deliver the exact amount of insulin needed as

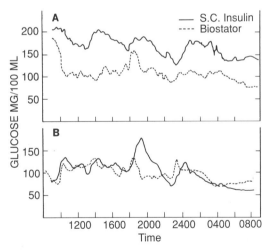

Figure 3.7. Blood glucose levels obtained with a closed-loop insulin delivery system (Biostator, Miles Laboratories, Elkhart, IN) and optimal conventional therapy with diet and multiple injections of subcutaneous insulin. A, Juvenile diabetes. B, Mature onset diabetes. The closed-loop system not only brings mean blood glucose down to a predetermined level, but also reduces the catabolic and anabolic fluctuations represented by glucose levels.

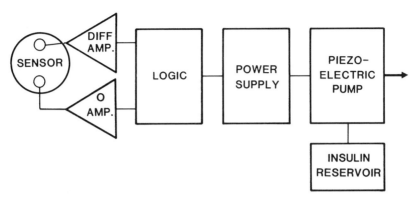

Figure 3.8.   Schematic representation of the implantable artifical β cell. The glucose oxidase electrode senses *tissue* glucose and activates the piezoelectric pump when glucose levels are above predetermined value. Insulin is delivered either subcutaneously or intraperitoneally. Note that the vascular system is not involved to avoid coagulation problems.

does the normal pancreas. A large, relatively immobile unit is available and has proved efficient for short-term treatment such as delivery, cesarean section, or ketoacidotic events (Fig. 3.7) (95, 96). An implantable long-term device was developed by Bessman and his group. This "artificial pancreas" is based on a glucose oxidase sensor measuring directly tissue glucose and activating a piezoelectric pump to deliver minute amounts of insulin as needed (Fig. 3.8). Experimental models have been tested (97–99). Such systems may prove to be essential for insulin-dependent diabetics who wish to engage in regular physical activity.

One of the known complications in infants of diabetic mothers is macrosomia. Its etiology was thought to be maternal hyperglycemia and fetal hyperinsulinism. Normalization of maternal blood glucose did not eliminate the problem. It was shown that the concentrations of maternal amino acids and FFA play a major role in determining fetal birth weight. These findings may also explain the high incidence of macrosomia in infants of obese, nondiabetic women (24). Conversely, low placental uptake of amino acids was found in small for gestational age infants (100).

REFERENCES

1. Jacobson NH. Nutrition and pregnancy. In Wallace H, Gold EM, Lis EF, eds. Maternal and child health practices. Springfield, IL: Charles C Thomas, 1973.

2. Hytten FE, Thompson AM, Taggart N. Total body water in normal pregnancy. Obstet Gynaecol Br Commonw 1966; 73:553–561.

3. Knopp RH, Montes A, Childs M, Job RL, Hirushi M. Metabolic adjustments in normal and diabetic pregnancy. Clin Obstet 1981; 24:21–49.

4. Spray CM. A study of some aspects of reproduction by means of chemical analysis. Br J Nutr 1950; 4:354–360.

5. Widdowson EM. The demands of the fetal and maternal tissues for nutrients, and the bearing of these on the need of the mother to "eat for two". In Dobbing J, ed. Maternal nutrition in pregnancy—eating for two? London: Academic Press, 1981; p 1–17.

6. Naismith DJ. The fetus as a parasite. Proc Nutr Soc 1969; 28:25–31.

7. Johnstone FD, Campbell DM, MacGillivaray I. Nitrogen balance studies in human pregnancy. J Nutr 1981; 111:1884–1893.

8. Hytten FE, Leitch I. The physiology of human pregnancy, ed 2. Oxford: Blackwell, 1971; p 333–369.

9. Koren Z, Shafrir E: Placental transfer of free fatty acids in the pregnant rat. Proc Soc Exp Biol Med 1964; 116:411–414.

10. Zaidise I, Bessman SP. The diabetic syndrome—uncontrolled stress. In Belfiore F, Galton DJ, Reaven GM, eds. Frontiers in diabetes. Basel: Karger, 1984; vol 4, p 77–92.

11. Falkmar S, Wilson S. Comparative aspects of the immunology and biology of insulin. Diabetologia 1967; 3:519–528.

12. Rall TW, Sutherland EW. Formation of cyclic adenine ribonucleotide by tissue particles. J Biol Chem 1985; 232:1065–1076.

13. Sutherland EW, Rall TW. The relation of adenosin 3', 5'-phosphate and phosphorylase to the action of catecholamines and other hormones. Pharmacol Rev 1960; 12:265–299.

14. Bessman SP. Diabetes mellitus. Observations, theoretical and practical. J Pediatr 1960; 56:191–203.

15. Mohan C, Bessman SP. In vitro protein degradation measured by differential loss in methionine and 3-methylhistidine: The effect of insulin. Anal Biochem 1981; 118:11–22.

16. Zuspan SP. Urinary excretion of epinephrine and

norepinephrine during pregnancy. J Clin Endocrinol 1970; 30:357–360.

17. Kalkhoff RH, Kissebah AH, Kim HG. Carbohydrates metabolism in pregnancy: relationship to gestational hormone action. Semin Perinatol 1978; 2:291–307.

18. Cousins L, Yen SSC, Meis P, Halberg F, Brink G. Circadian rhythm and diurnal excursion of plasma cortisol in diabetic pregnant women. Am J Obstet Gynecol 1986; 155:1176–1181.

19. Burke CW, Roulet F. Increased exposure of tissues to cortisol in late pregnancy. Br Med J 1970; 1:657–659.

20. Demey-Ponsart E, Foidart JM, Sulon J, Sodoyez JC. Serum CBG, free and total cortisol and circadian patterns of adrenal function in normal pregnancy. J Steroid Biochem 1982; 16:165–169.

21. Burden J, Harrison DJ, Hillhouse EW, Ironmonger MR, Jones MT. Effect of chlorpromazine, pentabarbitone, vasopressin, angiotensin II, bradykinin and ACTH on secretion of CRF from hypothalamus in vitro. J Endocrinol 1975; 67:45.

22. Rees LH, Buarke CW, Chard T, Evans SW, Letchorth AT. Possible placental origin of ACTH in normal pregnancy. Nature 1975; 256:620–622.

23. Oakey RE. The progressive increase in estrogen production in human pregnancy: an appraisal of factors responsible. Vitam Horm 1970; 28:1–36.

24. Kalkhoff RK, Kandaraki E, Morrow PG, Mitchell TH, Kelber S, Borkowf HI. Relationship between neonatal birthweight and maternal plasma amino acid profiles in lean and obese nondiabetic women and in type I diabetic pregnant women. Metabolism 1988; 37:234–239.

25. Aerts L, Van Asshe FA. Ultrastructural changes of the endocrine pancreas in pregnant rats. Diabetologia 1975; 11:285–289.

26. Costrini NV, Kalkhoff RK. Relative effects of pregnancy estradiol and progestrone on plasma insulin and pancreatic islet insulin secretion. J Clin Invest 1971; 50:992–999.

27. Kalkhoff RK, Jacobson M, Lember D. Progesterone pregnancy and the augmented plasma insulin response. J Clin Endocrinol Metab 1970; 31:24–28.

28. Krauth MC, Schillinger E. Changes in insulin receptor concentration in rat fat cells following treatment with the gestagens clomegestone acetate and cyproterone acetate. Acta Endocrinol (Copenh) 1977; 86:667–672.

29. Desoye G, Schweditsch MO, Pfeiffer KP, Zechner R, Kostner GM. Correlation of hormones with lipid and lipoprotein levels during normal pregnancy and postpartum. J Clin Endocrinol Metab 1987; 64:704–912.

30. Goebelsmann U. Protein and steroid hormones in pregnancy. J Reprod Med 1979; 23:166–177.

31. Genazani AR, Pocolar F, Neri P, Fioretti P. Human chorionic somatomammotropin (HCS): plasma levels of normal and pathological pregnancies and their correlation with placental function. Acta Endocrinol 1972; 167(suppl):1–39.

32. Tyson JE, Austin K, Farinholt J, Fiedler J. Endocrine-metabolic response to acute starvation in human gestation. Am J Obstet Gynecol 1976; 125:1073–1084.

33. Jacobs LS, Daughaday WH. Physiologic regulation of prolactin secretion in man. In Josimovich JB, Reynolds M, Cobo E, eds. Lactogenic hormones, fetal nutrition, and lactation. New York: John Wiley & Sons, 1974; p 351–377.

34. Rigg LA, Lein A, Yen SSC. Pattern of increase in circulating prolactin levels during human gestation. Am J Obstet Gynecol 1977; 129:454–456.

35. Huang JR, Tseng L, Bischof P, Janne OA. Regulation of prolactin production by progestin, estrogen and relaxin in human endometrial stromal cells. Endocrinology 1987; 121:2011–2017.

36. Berle P, Finsterwalder E, Apostolakis M. Comparative studies on the effect of human growth hormone, human prolactin and human placental lactogen on lipid metabolism. Horm Metab Res 1974; 6:847–850.

37. Rathgeb I, Winkler B, Steel R, Alszuler N. Effect of ovine prolactin administration on glucose metabolism and insulin levels in the dog. Endocrinology 1971; 88:718–722.

38. Gustafson AB, Banasiak MF, Kalkhoff RK, Hagen TC, Kim HK. Correlation of hyperprolactinemia with altered insulin and glucagon: similarity of effects of late human pregnancy. J Clin Endocrinol Metab 1980; 51:242–246.

39. Lind T, Billewicz WZ, Browh G. A serial study of changes occurring in the oral glucose tolerance test in pregnancy. J Obstet Gynaecol Br Commonw 1973; 80:1033–1039.

40. Spellacy WN, Goetz FC. Plasma insulin in normal late pregnancy. N Engl J Med 1963; 268:988–991.

41. Langer O, Anyaegbunam A, Brustman L, Guidetti D, Levy J. Mazze R. Pregestational diabetes: insulin requirements throughout pregnancy. Am J Obstet Gynecol 1988; 159:616–621.

42. Silverstone FA, Solomon E, Rubricius J. The rapid intravenous glucose tolerance test in pregnancy. J Clin Invest 1961; 140:2180–2189.

43. McDonald-Gibson RG, Young M, Hytten FE. Changes in plasma nonesterified fatty acids and serum glycerol in pregnancy. Br J Obstet Gynaecol 1975; 82:460–466.

44. Metzger BE, Ravnikar V, Vileisis RA, Freinkel N. "Accelerated starvation" and the skipped breakfast in late normal pregnancy. Lancet 1982; 1:588–592.

45. Freinkel N, Metzger BE, Nitzan M, Daniel R. Surmaczynska BZ, Nagel TC. Facilitated anabolism in late pregnancy: some novel maternal compensation for accelerated starvation. In Malaisse WJ, Pirart J, eds. Proceedings of the Eight Congress of the International Diabetes Federation. Amsterdam, Excerpta Medica, 1975.

46. Felig P, Lynch V. Starvation in human pregnancy: Hypoglycemia, hypoinsulinemia and hyperketonuria. Science 1970; 170:990–992.

47. Knopp RH, Herrera E, Freinkel N. Carbohydrate metabolism in pregnancy; VIII. Metabolism of adipose tissue isolated from fed and fasted pregnant rats during late gestation. J Clin Invest 1970; 49:1438–1446.

48. Pagano G, Cassoder M, Massobri M, Bozzon C, Tossare GF, Menato G, Lenti G. Insulin binding in human adipocytes during late pregnancy in healthy, obese and diabetic states. Horm Metab Res 1980; 12:177–181.

49. Goodner CJ, Freinkel N. Carbohydrate metabolism in pregnancy: The turnover of I^{131}-insulin in the pregnant rat. Endocrinology 1960; 67:862–872.

50. Bellman O, Hartmann E. Influence of pregnancy on the kinetics of insulin. Am J Obstet Gynecol 1975; 122:829–833.

51. Fisher PM, Sutherland HW, Bewsher PD. The in-

sulin response to glucose infusion in gestational diabetes. Diabetologia 1980; 19:15–20.

52. Puavilai G, Drobny EC, Domont LA, Baumann G. Insulin receptors and insulin resistance in human pregnancy: evidence for a post receptor defect in insulin action. J Clin Endocrinol Metab 1982; 54:247–253.

53. Otonkoski T, Andersson S, Knip M, Simell O. Maturation of insulin response to glucose during human fetal and neonatal development. Studies with perifusion of pancreatic islet like cell clusters. Diabetes 1988; 37:286–91.

54. Shafrir E, Barash V. Placental function in maternal-fetal fat transport in diabetes. Biol Neonate 1987; 51:102–112.

55. Hull D, Elphick MC. Evidence for fatty acid transfer across the human placenta. In Pregnancy metabolism, diabetes and the fetus. Ciba Foundation Symposium No. 63, Amsterdam: Excerpta Medica, 1979; p 75–86.

56. Elphick MC, Hull D. Rabbit placenta clearing factor lipase and transfer to the foetus of fatty acids derived from triglycerides injected into the mother. J Physiol (London) 1977; 273:475–487.

57. Shafrir E, Khasis S. Maternal fetal fat transport versus new fat synthesis in the pregnant diabetic rat. Diabetologia 1982; 22:111–117.

58. Knopp RH, Warth MR, Charles D. Childs M, Li JR, Mabuchi H, Van Allen MI. Lipoprotein metabolism in pregnancy, fat transport to the fetus, and the effects of diabetes. Biol Neonate 1986; 50:297–317.

59. Thomas CR. Placental transfer of non-esterified fatty acids in normal and diabetic pregnancy. Biol Neonate 1987; 51:94–101.

60. Schade DS, Perkins RP, Drumm DA. Interpreting ketosis warning in pregnancy. Contemp Obstet Gynecol 1983; 21:91–109.

61. Herrera E, Gomez-Coronado D, Lasuncion MA. Lipid metabolism in pregnancy. Biol Neonate 1987; 51:70–77.

62. Blechner JN, Stenger VG, Prystowski H. Blood flow to the human uterus during maternal metabolic acidosis. Am J Obstet Gynecol 1975; 121:789–794.

63. The Collaborative Study on Cerebral Palsy: Mental retardation and other neurological and sensory disorders of infancy and childhood manual. Bethesda, MD: U.S. Department of Health, Education and Welfare, 1966.

64. Churchill JA, Berendes HW, Nemore J. Neuropsychological deficits in children of diabetic mothers. A report from the collaborative study of cerebral palsy. Am J Obstet Gynecol 1969; 105:257–268.

65. Naeye RL. The outcome of diabetic pregnancies: A prospective study. Ciba Foundation Symposium No. 63. Amsterdam: Excerpta Medica, 1979; p 227–241.

66. Stehbens JA, Baker GL, Kitchell M. Outcome at age 1, 3 and 5 years of age of children born to diabetic women. Am J Obstet Gynecol 1977; 127:408–413.

67. Naeye RL, Chez RA. Effects of maternal acetonuria and low pregnancy weight gain on children's psychomotor development. Am J Obstet Gynecol 1981; 139:189–193.

68. Hawkins RA, Williamson DH, Krebs HA. Ketone body utilization by adult and suckling rat brain in vivo. Biochem J 1971; 122:13–18.

69. Webber RJ, Edmond M. The in vivo utilization of acetoacetate, D-(-)-3-hydroxybutyrate, and glucose for lipid synthesis in brain of 18-day-old rat. Evi-

dence for an acetyl-CoA bypass to sterol synthesis. J Biol Chem 1979; 254:3912–3920.

70. King JC. Protein metabolism during pregnancy. Clin Perinatol 1975; 2:243–254.

71. Sinclair JC: Metabolic rate and temperature control. In Smith CA, Nelson NM, eds. The physiology of the human infant, ed 4. Springfield, IL: Charles C Thomas, 1976; p 354.

72. Zaidise I, Artal R, Bessman SP. Fuel metabolism in pregnancy. In Artal R, Wiswell RA. Exercise in pregnancy, I edition. Los Angeles, Williams & Wilkins, 1986; p 83–97.

73. Kalhan SC, D'Angelo LJ, Savin SM, Adam PAJ. Glucose production in pregnant women at term gestation. Sources of glucose for human fetus. J Clin Invest 1979; 63:388–394.

74. Herrera E, Palacin M, Martin A, Lasuncion MA. Relationship between maternal and fetal fuels and placental glucose transfer in rats with maternal diabetes of varying severity. Diabetes 1985; 34(suppl 2):42–46.

75. Soskin S. The endocrines in diabetes. Springfield, IL: Charles C Thomas, 1948.

76. Artal R, Wiswell R, Romem Y, Kammula RK, Sperling M. Hormonal responses to exercise in pregnant diabetic and non-diabetic patients. In Proceedings of the Society for Gynecologic Investigation 1983; 225.

77. Bessman SP. Interrelations of various food materials. In Ghadim H, ed. Total parenteral nutrition. New York: John Wiley & Sons, 1975; 335–342.

78. Bessman SP, Fonio A. The possible role of the mitochondria bound creatine kinase in regulation of mitochondrial respiration. Biochem Biophys Res Commun 1966; 22:597–602.

79. Bessman SP, Geiger PG. Transport of energy in muscle: the phosphorylcreatine shuttle. Science 1981; 211:448–452.

80. Yang WCT, Geiger PJ, Bessman SP, Borrebaek B. Formation of creatine phosphate from creatine and ^{32}P-labeled ATP by isolated rabbit heart mitochondria. Biochem Biophys Res Commun 1977; 76:882–887.

81. Metzger BE, Freinkel N. Effects of diabetes mellitus in the endocrinologic and the metabolic adaptation of gestation. Semin Perinatol 1978; 2:309–318.

82. Gillmer MDG, Persson B. Metabolism during normal and diabetic pregnancy and its effect on neonatal outcome. In Pregnancy metabolism, diabetes and the fetus. Ciba Foundation Symposium No. 63, Amsterdam: Excerpta Medica, 1979; p 93–121.

83. Persson B, Lunell NO. Metabolic control in diabetic pregnancy. Am J Obstet Gynecol 1975; 122:737–745.

84. Gillmer MDG, Beard RW, Oakley NW, Brooke FM, Elphick MC, Hall D: Diurnal plasma free fatty acid profile in normal and diabetic pregnancies. Br Med J 1977; 2:670–673.

85. Artal R, Golde SH, Dorey F, McClellan SN, Gratacos J, Lirette T, Montoro M, Wu PYK, Anderson B, Mestman J. The effect of plasma glucose variability on neonatal outcome in the pregnant diabetic. Am J Obstet Gynecol 1983; 147:537–541.

86. Farrag OA. Prospective study of 3 metabolic regimens in pregnant diabetics. Aust NZ J Obstet Gynaecol 1987; 27:6–9.

87. Karlsson K, Kjellmer I. The outcome of diabetic pregnancies in relation to the mother's blood sugar level. Am J Obstet Gynecol 1972; 112:213–220.

88. Landon MB, Gabbe SG, Piana R, Mennuti MT, Main EK. Neonatal morbidity in pregnancy complicated by diabetes mellitus: predictive value of maternal glycemic profiles. Am J Obstet Gynecol 1987; 156:1089–1095.

89. Tevaarwerk GJM, Harding PGR, Milne KJ, Jaco NT, Rodger NW, Hurst C. Pregnancy in diabetic women: Outcome with a program aimed to normal glycemia before meals. Can Med Assoc J 1982; 125:435–441.

90. Schulman PK, Gyves MT, Merkatz IR. Role of nutrition in the management of the pregnant diabetic patient. In Merkatz IR, Adams PAJ, eds. The diabetic pregnancy: a perinatal perspective. New York: Grune & Stratton, 1979; p 35–44.

91. Seeds AE, Knowles HC. Metabolic control of diabetic pregnancy. Clin Obstet Gynecol 1981; 24:51–62.

92. Sonksen PH. Home monitoring of blood glucose by diabetic patients. Acta Endocrinol 1980; 94(238):145–155.

93. Potter JM, Reckless JPD, Cullen Dr. The effect of continuous subcutaneous insulin infusion and conventional insulin regimes on 24-hour variations of glucose and intermediary metabolites in the third trimester of pregnancy. Diabetologia 1981; 21:534–539.

94. Rudolf MCJ, Coustan DR, Sherwin RS, Bates SE, Felig P. Efficacy of insulin pump in the home treatment of pregnant diabetics. Diabetes 1981; 30:891–895.

95. Nattras M, Alberti KGMM, Dennis KJ, Gillibrand PN, Letchworth AT, Buckle ALJ. A glucose-controlled insulin infusion system for diabetic women during labour. Br Med J 1978; 2:599–601.

96. Santiago JV, Clarke WL, Arias F. Studies with a pancreatic beta cell simulator in the third trimester of pregnancy complicated by diabetes. Am J Obstet Gynecol 1978; 132:455–463.

97. Bessman SP, Layne EC, Thomas LJ, Zaidise I. Implantable artificial cell: theory and practice. In Shafrir E, Renold AE, eds. Lessons from animal diabetes. London: Libbey, 1984, p 648–654.

98. Bessman SP, Schultz RD. Progress toward a glucose sensor for the artificial pancreas. In Ion selective microelectrodes. New York: Plenum Press, 1974, p 184–197.

99. Layne EC, Schultz RD, Thomas LJ, Salma G, Sayler DF, Bessman SP. Continuous extracorporeal monitoring of animal blood using the glucose electrode. Diabetes 1976; 25:81–89.

100. Dicke JM, Henderson GI. Placental amino acid uptake in normal and complicated pregnancies. Am J Med Sci 1988; 295:223–227.

4

Fuel Metabolism in Pregnancy—Clinical Aspects

Lois Jovanovic-Peterson and Charles M. Peterson

Fuel metabolism in pregnancy changes in response to the needs of the fetus and the mother. The flow of fuels to the fetus is influenced by the sequential rise of diabetogenic hormones. In other words, the cascade of hormonal events in pregnancy is orchestrated to promote either maternal glucose production or decreased peripheral utilization and, thus, provides more fuel for the fetus.

Exercise has known effects on both aspects of fuel metabolism. Exercise not only decreases postprandial glucose levels, but it also facilitates glucose utilization. When the diabetogenic hormones of pregnancy result in maternal diabetes in the process of mediating fuel to the fetus, exercise may be used to advantage. Gestational diabetes is the result of a maternal defect in insulin secretion and in glucose utilization that occurs when the diabetogenic hormones rise to their peak levels.

This chapter will outline the relationship between the hormones of pregnancy and maternal glucose homeostasis; it will also explain the pathology of the mother and the fetus, which occurs when maternal glucose levels rise excessively in response to rising diabetogenic hormones. The last section will be a discussion of the utility of exercise as a treatment modality when maternal hyperglycemia occurs as in the case of gestational diabetes.

FIRST TRIMESTER CHANGES (Table 4.1)

Normal Response to Pregnancy

With (and perhaps antecedent to) implantation of the trophoblast, the production of pregnancy-related hormones begins. These hormones immediately alter the metabolism of nutrients to shift the priority of metabolic products toward the growing fetus. A buffering mechanism must be initiated early in

Table 4.1. First Trimester Changes

Maternal	Fetal
Normal Pregnancy	
Increased insulin demand	Insulin secretion
Increased diabetogenic hormones	Glucagon secretion
Prolactin	Glucose sensitivity
hCS	
Estrogens	
Progesterones	
Cortisol	
Potential Pathology	
Type I diabetes mellitus	Macrosomia
Type II diabetes mellitus	Intrauterine growth retardation
	Spontaneous abortion
	Congenital malformations

pregnancy to prevent the mother from suffering deleterious hypoglycemia between feedings as her reserves continue to flow to her unborn child. Maternal glucose homeostasis is sustained by a delicate interplay of maternal hormones designed to increase fat storage, decrease energy expenditure, and delay glucose clearance. In addition, fetal needs are met through the fetal control of nutrients mediated via a variety of messages, chiefly by fetal hormones. Hormonal messages from the conceptus can affect metabolic processes, uteroplacental blood flow, and cellular differentiation.

Maternal Changes

Immediately after ovulation, the corpus luteum is converted into a factory that makes 17 OH- progesterone. Luteinizing hormone (LH) from the pituitary is necessary to keep the corpus luteum functioning. Once conception and subsequent implantation occur, human chorionic gonadotropin (hCG) stimulates the corpus luteum's production of 17 OH- progesterone until the placental production of steroids is adequate. Thus, hCG is only needed for the first 12 weeks of gestation as the corpus luteum is needed only during these early phases of placental growth (1). hCG does not seem to have any effect on glucose homeostasis. Other hormones that do promote production of glucose are, therefore, urgently needed early in pregnancy.

The adult ovary is capable of making steroids directly from acetate, but this capability is not true of the placenta. Estrogen formation by the placenta is dependent on precursors that reach it from both the fetal and maternal compartments. To form estrogens, the placenta aromatizes the androgens coming primarily from the fetus. The fetal adrenal gland provides dihydroepiandrosterone (DHEA) that proceeds through a series of hydroxylations and then double bond formation or aromatization into estrone and 17-β estradiol. In addition, some of the fetal DHEA undergoes 16-α hydroxylation in the fetal liver and/or fetal adrenal gland to become 16-α hydroxydihydroepiandrosterone (HDHEA) sulfate, which is cleaved in the placenta to 16-α OH HDHEA and aromatized to estriol (2). The time course of the appearance of estrogens during pregnancy are listed in Table 4.2. As can be seen, estrogens rise within 32 days of conception.

Estrogens have weak anti-insulin properties. Table 4.2 ascribes relative diabetogenic

properties to the hormones. In this table, estrogen has a relative potency of 1 on a scale of 1–5. Estrogen's major gluconeogenic property is derived from its stimulating effect on liver production of cortisol-binding globulin (CBG). As CBG is increased, the maternal adrenal gland secretes more cortisol to saturate the elevated CBG and produces, in addition, enough cortisol to increase the level of free cortisol. Hypercortisolemia causes insulin resistance, delayed glucose clearance, and thus more available glucose for fetal use. In Table 4.2, the appearance of cortisol is timed to contribute to the rising demand for glucose at 50 days. Cortisol has the strongest diabetogenic property of the hormones listed.

In contrast to estrogen, progesterone production by the placenta is independent of the quantity of precursor available, uteroplacental perfusion, fetal well-being, or even the presence of a live fetus. Thus, progesterone is not useful as a marker of impending abortion (3). The majority of placental progesterone is derived from cholesterol that is readily available. The placenta does not make 17 OH-progesterone until the 32nd week. Once the corpus luteum deteriorates, progesterone arising from the placenta is the major form of the hormone. Progesterone has a direct effect on glucose metabolism (4). When progesterone is administered to normal fasting women, the serum insulin concentration rises while glucose remains unchanged. In monkeys, progesterone increases both the early and total insulin secretory responses to glucose (5). Progesterone does not peak until the 32nd week of gestation. Those women who screen negative on a glucose screening test for gestational diabetes at 26 weeks may not pass the test at 32 weeks due to the diabetogenic properties of progesterone (a 4 on the scale of 1–5) (Table 4.2).

Two other pregnancy-related hormones warrant discussion. They are peptide hormones. The first hormone is prolactin (hPRL) and the second hormone is human chorionic somatomammatropin (hCS).

Barberia and associates (6) showed that the initial rise in hPRL in pregnancy occurs within a few days after the estradiol levels start to increase above nonpregnant levels (30–33 days

Table 4.2. Sequential Rise and Potency of the Diabetogenic Hormones of Pregnancy

Hormone	Onset of Elevation (Days)	Peak Elevation (Weeks)	Relative Diabetogenic Potency on a Scale of 1 (Weak)- 5 (Strong)
Estradiol	32	26[a]	1
Prolactin	36	10	2
Human chorionic somatomammo- tropin	45	26[a]	3
Cortisol	50	26[a]	5
Progesterone	65	32[b]	4

[a]Optimal time to screen for GDM.
[b]Optimal time to rescreen for GDM in those women who screen negative at 26 weeks.

after the LH peak), whereas the rise in hPRL levels above the nonpregnancy luteal phase levels occurs 32–36 days after the LH peak (Table 4.2). The estrogen level seems to initiate the "turning on" of prolactin. Without a rise in estrogen with a resultant rise in prolactin levels, spontaneous abortion seems imminent (3). What is the function of prolactin so early in pregnancy? Prolactin is so named because it is necessary for lactation, a third trimester event. What is a lactation-promoting hormone doing in the first few days of pregnancy? Some researchers believe that prolactin is "luteotropic" and works in concert with hCG to nourish the corpus luteum (7). Others (8) have suggested that prolactin enhances cell-to-cell communication among the β-cells in pancreatic islets. These investigators have shown a 10-fold increase in β-cell coupling, independent of glucose stimulation. Thus, prolactin may be necessary early in pregnancy to stimulate both maternal and fetal β-cell hypertrophy. In Table 4.2, prolactin has a diabetogenic potency of 2 on the scale of 1–5.

hCS is a protein hormone with immunological epitopes and biological properties similar to pituitary growth hormone (hGH). The original name, human placental lactogen, was so named because of its lactogenic properties in animals; however, such properties in women have not been confirmed. Josimovich (9) found that hCS has luteotropic properties that would explain the rise of this hormone so early in pregnancy. Similar to prolactin, hCS has an effect on glucose metabolism. hCS rates a potency of 3 in the diabetogenic property scale (Table 4.2).

hCS does have hGH-like effects on tibial epiphysial growth, body weight gain, and sulfate uptake by costal cartilage in the hypophysectomized rat, although the effective dose required is 100–200 times that of hGH (10, 11).

The effects of hCS on fat and carbohydrate metabolism are similar to those after treatment with hGH. There is inhibition of peripheral glucose uptake and stimulation of insulin release (12). A comparable maximal increase in plasma free fatty acids occurs after administration of hCS or hGH in hypopituitorism. In addition, infusion of hCS into an hypophysectomized, diabetic man caused the blood glucose to rise 4-fold above baseline (13).

In summary, the hormonal changes early in pregnancy can be viewed as a serial rise in hormones intended to maintain a constant glucose supply to the fetus. As the fetal metabolic requirements increase, the gluconeogenic properties and concentration of hormones rise. The order of hormonal presentation in pregnancy is inverse to its relative gluconeogenic property. The first hormone, hCG, has no gluconeogenic effect and cortisol, a relatively late-appearing hormone, has the most potent gluconeogenic effect. Table 4.2 lists the order of rise of each of these hormones in early pregnancy, and shows the relative potency of each to supply glucose to the fetus. The sole purpose of the sequential rise could be so ordered as to provide glucose substrate to the fetus, rather than for any other purpose.

PATHOLOGICAL RESPONSE TO PREGNANCY-RELATED GLUCONEOGENIC HORMONES

Maternal Pathology

During the course of pregnancy, the insulin requirement rises progressively (14). Carbohydrate tolerance is minimally affected in normal pregnant women because the normal pancreas can increase insulin production to compensate for the diabetogenic stresses of pregnancy. Kuhl and Hornnes (15) investigated the cause of hyperglycemia in the 1% of their population who failed to be able to maintain normoglycemia during pregnancy. They found that the insulin response of their hyperglycemic pregnant women differed from their normoglycemic pregnant women in two pertinent ways. They observed first, a delayed insulin response to a carbohydrate load, and second, that the insulin response per unit of glycemic stimulus was significantly lower than that seen in normoglycemic women. They also found that insulin degradation was unaffected by pregnancy and the proinsulin share of the total plasma insulin immunoreactivity did not increase during pregnancy. They concluded that the main cause of gestational diabetes, or that diabetes which is uncovered in pregnancy, is insulin resistance. Gestational diabetes occurs when a pregnant woman has a limited insulin secretory capacity and thus cannot produce enough insulin to compensate for the diabetogenic hormones: estogen, hPRL, hCS, cortisol, and progesterone.

Those women who have diabetes before pregnancy need to increase their exogenous insulin doses to compensate for the rising diabetogenic hormones of pregnancy. In the case of type I, or insulin-dependent diabetes, the prepregnant insulin requirement of 0.6 units/24 hours rises to 0.7 units/kg/24 hours in the first few weeks of pregnancy. By the second trimester, the insulin requirement rises to 0.8 units/kg/24 hours. By term, the insulin requirement is 0.9–1.0 units/kg/24 hours. If the doses of insulin are not increased appropriately, maternal hyperglycemia occurs. Because hyperglycemia is harmful to the process of organogenesis, which occurs in the first 8 weeks of pregnancy (16), type I women should normalize their blood glucose levels before conception (17).

Diabetic women who have glucose levels twice the normal range at the time of conception have been shown to have subnormal levels of hCG, estradiol, and hPRL (18). The three hormone levels were shown to return to normal range within 2–6 weeks after normoglycemia was achieved. These observations lend support to the claim that normoglycemia in diabetic women results in a normal pregnancy (19).

There is evidence that maternal hormone levels in the first trimester reflect the integrity of the trophoblastic implantation and the subsequent vascular status of the placental-maternal interchange (20). The reason for subnormal hormonal levels in women whose diabetes is out of control is not known; however, possibilities include poor implantation, poor vascular status, small placenta, or glycosylation of these hormones resulting in inaccurate assay by antibody or receptor techniques. Whatever the reason for a subnormal hormonal profile, there is reason to suspect that the consequence would be a poor prognosis for the fetus. Recent studies indicate that hyperglycemia during the first trimester is associated with a higher risk of congenital malformations (17, 21, 22). Whether these malformations are the result of hyperglycemia, hormonal imbalance, or other unknown aspects of poor control remains to be elucidated.

The situation appears to be different for testosterone and androstenedione. Despite normoglycemia, diabetic women have significantly higher testosterone levels shortly after conception and generally higher androgen levels throughout the 12-week period studied. hCG levels are not higher in diabetic than in control subjects and, unlike the situation in nonhuman primates (23), rising hCG levels do not stimulate an increase in androgen production. Because sex hormone-binding globulin is known to be elevated in diabetic pregnancies (24), the increased testosterone may be the result of sequestration by the binding protein with consequent decreased metabolic degradation.

Alternatively, the increased androgen levels may not be related to pregnancy. Increased androgen levels have been reported in nonpregnant diabetic women (25, 26) and in female streptozocin-diabetic rats (27). In vitro studies suggest that insulin may stimulate ovarian androgen production (28); it is possible that the peripheral hyperinsulinemia produced by exogenous insulin administration could lead to elevated androgen levels.

Because hCG and prolactin levels may reflect the integrity of trophoblastic implantation (3), the finding that these hormones can be normalized by better diabetes control before conception may be of considerable clinical importance. Diabetic women who achieve normoglycemia before conception may be able to reduce their risk for a fetal loss. The NIH-DIEP study showed that the spontaneous abortion rate in normoglycemic women is 9.5%; in slightly hyperglycemic women, it is 14.5%; and in severely hyperglycemic women, the rate is greater than 21%. Their normal control population had a spontaneous abortion rate of 16% (29).

In the case of type II diabetes mellitus, the patient may be managed with diet and exercise alone or an oral agent may be prescribed. Once pregnancy occurs, hyperglycemia will result, unless insulin is added. Oral agents during pregnancy are contraindicated in the United States because they cross the placenta and may impact on fetal pancreatic function in the third trimester. Studies of fetal pancreatic response to glipizide in the first and second trimesters have shown no effect (30).

Gestational diabetes (GDM) does not occur until the diabetogenic forces overwhelm the deficient maternal pancreas. GDM usually presents in the second trimester, but it is possible that all GDM may be undiagnosed type II diabetes (31). First trimester hyperglycemia is so deleterious to the growing fetus that all women in their childbearing years should perhaps be tested for diabetes before beginning a pregnancy.

NORMAL FETAL GROWTH AND DEVELOPMENT

Glucose crosses the placenta by carrier-mediated facilitated diffusion. Battaglia and Meschia and their associates (32, 33) reported that the fetal lamb receives only one-third of the glucose that the uterus takes up from the maternal circulation. Their data indicate that the uterus and placenta are important sites of glucose utilization.

In contrast, amino acids are actively transported to the fetus (34). Phelps and associates (35) have measured around-the-clock amino acids profiles in normal pregnant and nonpregnant women and report that alanine and leucine are significantly lower in pregnant women at all periods of the 24-hour day.

Free fatty acids cross the placenta in small amounts by gradient-dependent diffusion and are esterified to triglyceride by fetal adipocytes. In perfusion studies of human placenta, Hull and Elphick (36) reported that there was little evidence for selective transfer of different fatty acids and that the net transfer from mother to fetus was sensitive to free fatty acid concentration on the maternal side.

Insulin, a large polypeptide, binds to microvillous membranes of the placenta, in which it is degraded but not transported to the fetus (37). The role of maternal insulin in placental regulation of metabolic fuels has not been established. Steel and associates (37) suggested that the abundance of placental insulin receptors might suggest a role for insulin in regulation of glucose uptake, glycogen metabolism, or lipolysis, because these are physiological effects of the hormone in other tissues.

When the fetus receives too much glucose from the mother, development can be halted and a spontaneous abortion may occur; or development can be aberrant and produce structural and/or functional abnormalities.

PATHOLOGICAL FETAL DEVELOPMENT

Structural Anomalies

In the NIH-DIEP study, the malformation rate in those diabetic women who registered before organogenesis was completed was 4.9%. In those diabetic women who registered after organogenesis, the malformation rate was 9.0%. The normal population had a malformation rate of 2.1% (22).

It is difficult to determine causes of these high malformation rates among offspring of diabetic women. Glucose imbalance, hyperketonemia, abnormal insulin levels, and other factors have been implicated as teratogens (38, 39). Due to the interrelationship of these factors, however, animal models have provided controversial results at best. For example, induction of diabetes in laboratory animals results in an alteration of several metabolic parameters including circulating glucose and insulin levels. Likewise, infusion of glucose or insulin alters more than one metabolic parameter making it virtually impossible to monitor each altered factor independently (40).

In order to circumvent these difficulties, the technique of whole embryo culture has been employed. In this system, rat and mouse embryos develop normally and at rates similar to in vivo growth during the organogenic (teratogenic) period (41, 42). Fortuitously, the morphogenetic events that occur in cultured embryos correspond to those observed in human embryos during the 4th–6th week of gestation, i.e., the sensitive period in diabetic women. Cultured embryos develop in an environment where manipulations of blood glucose, ketone bodies, insulin, and other factors can be made independently. Studies using this approach have clearly shown that hyperglycemia is teratogenic to rat (39) and mouse embryos (43) during this early morphogenetic period, although the glucose levels required to induce malformations are very high. Other serum factors such as ketone bodies, which have been shown to be teratogenic at levels achieved during severe diabetic crisis in humans (44, 45), and somatomedin-inhibiting factor (46) may play a role as teratogens. Furthermore, serum collected from diabetic rats receiving no insulin therapy produces abnormal morphogenesis in mouse embryos at a rate directly related to the severity of the disease (46). Insulin itself is not teratogenic even at the dose of 10,000 μU/ml. These studies support the contention that insulin therapy and strict control of the diabetic state minimize the occurrence of congenital anomalies in the offspring of the diabetic woman.

Fetal Metabolic Anomalies

No matter how abundant and well balanced the nutrients, to use them, the embryo must develop suitable enzymes, a process regulated by (a) the quality and quantity of the nutrients themselves, (b) the manner in which the nutrients are obtained, and (c) the rising concentration of gluconeogenic hormones. In the first stages of fetal development, the metabolic requirements are fulfilled by nutrients continuously supplied by the placenta. This function of the placenta as a source for nutrients was called a "transitional liver" by Claude Bernard. In these early embryonic stages, there is no storage of energy and no evidence of pancreatic endocrine function or of enzymes necessary for lipogenesis and glycogen synthesis. The first histochemically differentiated α- and β-cells appear between the 7th and 10th weeks of gestation (47). Maternal hyperglycemia has been reported to increase fetal insulin secretion this early, compared to fetal insulin secreted from normoglycemic mothers. The fetal stimulatory/secretion coupling for glucose and insulin is different from the adult. Normally, fetal β-cells do not respond with an immediate bolus of insulin to a pure glucose

load. Usually, the fetal β-cells secrete insulin in response to a mixture of glucose plus amino acids (48–51). Fetal insulin is a growth factor but may not be needed until later in the pregnancy (51). Fetal pituitary hGH or insulin-like growth factors produced by the placenta may be the primary growth factors in the first trimester, and, in fact, influence insulin secretion. When the fetus experiences hyperglycemia, the fetal pancreas matures prematurely and can secrete large amounts of insulin.

Fetal hyperinsulinemia as early as the first trimester may predispose the fetus to macrosomia. In the NIH-DIEP study, first trimester postprandial hyperglycemia correlated very strongly with subsequent infant birth weight (52). The fetal pancreas, in diabetic pregnancy, often shows islet hypertrophy and hyperplasia. Other causes of fetal hyperinsulinism may be stimulation of the fetal β-cells by maternal insulin antibodies (53) and the transfer of maternal insulin to the fetus. This possibility cannot be excluded because although the normal placenta is impermeable to free insulin, bound insulin may indeed cross (54). Another factor contributing to fetal macrosomia may be excessive production of somatomedin and other growth factors that may be produced in excess by a large placenta (55).

The in vitro studies of the human fetal pancreas during the first trimester have shown that the insulin secretory response to glucose is a function of gestational age, with relative insulin secretory capacity decreasing to a nadir at 20–23 weeks and gradually increasing again thereafter. These latter findings may have implications for the development of macrosomia, because maternal hyperglycemia before 18 weeks may initiate excess fetal insulin secretion despite normal maternal glucose levels in the second and third trimesters (56).

SECOND TRIMESTER: TABLE 4.3

Maternal Response

The hormonal profile in the second trimester is at its peak for all five diabetogenic hormones, specifically estrogen, hPRL, hCS,

Table 4.3.   Second Trimester

Maternal	Fetal
Normal Pregnancy	
Peak of diabetogenic hormones	Pancreatic insulin secretion
	Growth hormone secretion
Potential Pathology	
Gestational diabetes	Macrosomia
	Hyperinsulinemia
	Fetal wastage

cortisol, and progesterone (Table 4.2). It is not surprising, therefore, that the highest prevalence of gestational diabetes occurs at weeks 24–28 of gestation (57). The literature still reflects the controversy as to the true defect in gestational diabetes. Some reports indicate that women are normoinsulinemic, and some that GDM women are insulinopenic. The controversy may arise from the fact that GDM women constitute a heterogeneous group with varying patterns of insulin secretion.

During pregnancy, three major groups of patients with carbohydrate intolerance are recognized. Type I insulin-dependent women are insulin deficient. The exogenous insulin taken by these patients must be titrated upward to compensate for the nutrient demands, the increased weight, and the anti-insulin hormones.

In contrast, the generally older and heavier women with type II diabetes (noninsulin-dependent diabetes mellitus) who have normal, decreased, or even higher than normal amounts of endogenous insulin are usually asymptomatic during the first trimester. They are noninsulin dependent when not pregnant, but require exogenous insulin during gestation to maintain euglycemia. Their increment in insulin requirement during pregnancy is large (98%) and not accompanied by a proportional reduction in 24-hour integrated glucose values (58). Thus, they demonstrate a more marked resistance to insulin during pregnancy than do women with type I diabetes. These patients are not prone to ketosis during gestation and do not have ketonuria even when dietary intakes are as

low as 1600–1800 kcal/day (59). Increasingly, it is recognized that type II diabetes may occur at all ages.

Pregnancy represents a severe stress test of carbohydrate tolerance, the most severe test for diabetes that a woman will experience in her entire lifetime. Of all pregnant women, 1–12% may fail this test and develop gestational diabetes (59). These patients may be obese or of normal weight. Metzer et al. (60) reported that even these mildly diabetic women have distinctly abnormal alterations in every type of metabolic fuel. These include elevated levels of plasma glucose, fasting plasma triglycerides, and fasting free fatty acids. They also noted that plasma values for the gluconeogenic amino acid, serine, tended to stabilize at slightly higher levels during overnight fasting, whereas postprandial increments in the plasma values for the branched chain amino acid, isoleucine, seemed to persist longer after every meal.

A normal woman has a progressive rise of insulin levels into the third trimester. The average total insulin level in normal pregnant women at 12 weeks' gestation is four times greater than nonpregnant women. The peak level reached by 32 weeks is correlated with percentage of body fat, although, Nordlander et al. (61) found that urinary C-peptide was not related to maternal weight, weight gain, or skinfold thickness. They did note that C-peptide correlated with the maternal postpartum weight, however. Rat studies clearly show that the rise in serum insulin is correlated to pancreatic islet hypertrophy (62). Type I diabetic women have no endogenous insulin and, therefore, must mimic this rise with increasing exogenous doses of insulin. Type II diabetic pregnant women tend to have higher baseline insulin levels than normals, a delayed response to meal stimulation, and a lower total insulin concentration over 24 hours than normal women. Women with gestational diabetes have a varied pattern of insulin secretion. The most consistent pattern is normal to elevated fasting insulin levels, but a decreased insulin response to meals (58).

Hollingsworth and Grundy (63) have reported an interesting finding. In their study of type II diabetic women, they found a significantly higher total fasting triglyceride in the second trimester than normal pregnant woman (63). They reported that gestational diabetic women have a cortisol and triglyceride pattern similar to type II patients.

The accentuated hypertriglyceridemia of pregnant type II patients is probably the result of combined overproduction induced by the combination of pregnancy and diabetes. These patients have an enhanced synthesis of very low-density lipoprotein that may be due to increased free fatty acids, hypertriglyceridemia, and increased caloric intake. These same factors may contribute to an overproduction induced by pregnancy. Knopp and Worth (64) have also observed pregnancy-associated hypertriglyceridemia in non-insulin-dependent diabetes mellitus. Thus, women with type I and women with type II diabetes differ from each other in respect to lipid metabolism; and during pregnancy, women with type II or gestational diabetes exhibit a marked pregnancy-associated hypertriglyceridemia that is significantly greater than that of normal or type I diabetic women. These differences may result in alterations in metabolic fuels available to the fetus.

Fetal Response

In vivo and in vitro experiments in rodents clearly show that mild maternal diabetes in the second trimester produces marked fetal pancreatic islet hypertrophy (65, 66). Fetal islet cell hypertrophy may be initiated by hyperglycemia, but hGH is a necessary factor. hGH is necessary for increasing cell multiplication. Freak accidents of nature have suggested this role of hGH: anencephalic fetuses are not macrosomic despite documented maternal hyperglycemia (67).

Hyperglycemia not only stimulates hyperinsulinemia, but also initiates the first phase of insulin secretion. Second trimester fetal islets do not normally have an initial phase of insulin secretion in response to glucose. In vitro studies show that fetal islets cultured in 2.8 mM glucose demonstrated no first phase of insulin secretion to an acute glucose load, whereas islets cultured in 11.1 mM glucose demonstrated a biphasic response (68).

Extremes of hyperglycemia may, in fact,

result in growth-retarded fetus. The clinical literature reports that infants of diabetic mothers with the most severe forms of diabetes were actually small for gestational age. As treatment programs improved maternal glycemic levels, intrauterine growth retardation no longer seemed to be a complication of vascularly compromised diabetic women (69). In vitro studies confirm this clinical observation. Swenne and Ericksson (70) showed that fetuses from severely diabetic rats had cell division rates of the endocrine pancreas markedly below normal. In addition, these two investigators showed that the fetuses from the severely diabetic women had a lower β-cell mass than the controls. Of note, insulin treatment of the diabetic mothers normalized the fetal pancreatic findings (71).

One confusing aspect of the regulation of fetal pancreatic insulin secretion is the observation by Philipps et al. (72) that hyperglycemia produced by infusion of glucose into fetal lambs is significantly related to an increase in fetal O_2 consumption and to a decrease in fetal arterial blood O_2 content, but is not significantly related to an increase in insulin concentration (72). They hypothesized that the hypoxemia may have blunted the insulin secretion response. The mechanism for this effect is obscure but studies in adults of a variety of species have demonstrated that β-cell function is, in part, regulated by the functional activity of the sympathetic nervous system and by circulating catecholamines (73). Furthermore, epinephrine infusions can reduce basal rates of insulin secretion and block the release of insulin that occurs in response to hyperglycemia. Because epinephrine secretion increases during fetal hypoxemia, it seems reasonable that fetal insulin secretion can be regulated by a variety of conditions that occur as a result of maternal and fetal hyperglycemia, including hyperglycemia itself, hypoxemia, increased sympathetic nervous activity, and changes in amino acid concentration.

THIRD TRIMESTER (TABLE 4.4)

Maternal Response

During late pregnancy, fasting in normal women results in increased concentrations of

Table 4.4. Third Trimester Normal Pregnancy

Maternal	Fetal
Normal pregnancy	
Increased metabolic demand	Increased fetal mass
Increased maternal mass	Increased glucose sensitivity
Increased insulin output	
Increased peripheral glucose utilization	
Decreased hepatic glucose output	
Potential Pathology	
Gestational diabetes	Macrosomia
	Hyperinsulinemia
	Hypokalemia

fatty acids and ketoacids to levels greater than observed in nonpregnant women (74). In the pregnant diabetic woman, these fasting-induced substrate concentration changes are augmented when insulin is insufficient and diabetic control is poor (75). In addition, glucagon levels are reported to peak in the third trimester (76). The extent to which such increases in fatty acid and ketoacid concentrations affect fetal metabolism depends largely on the permeability of the placenta and the maternal and fetal arterial concentrations of these substrates. Rapid placental transport of free fatty acids from mother to fetus has been demonstrated in human and in other species, such as the guinea pig and the rabbit (77). However, there remains no evidence that free fatty acids are transferred to the fetus in these species in amounts that exceed accretion in the tissues as structural lipids and in the adipose tissue stores. This is particularly true for the human in whom, during the last third of gestation, body fat content increases to 16–18% of fetal body weight (78). This observation suggests that free fatty acids are not used extensively by the fetus as fuels, but contribute primarily to fat deposition (79). Nevertheless, negligible to small rates of fatty acid oxidation have been observed in several species. Fetal rhesus monkey tissues can oxidize fatty acids to a limited extent (80), as can human fetal brain, liver, placenta, and lung tissue slices in vitro (81). It is less clear to what extent fatty acid oxidation would

occur in the fetus of the pregnant diabetic woman because, as previously discussed, the combination of hyperglycemia and hyperinsulinemia may direct glucose to oxidative metabolism as a substitute for fatty acid oxidation, and may direct both glucose and fatty acids into lipid synthesis. Similar considerations apply to ketone bodies to which the human placenta is highly permeable (82).

Limited fatty acid oxidation in fetal tissues has also been suggested to result from deficiency in the transport of fatty acids into mitochondria (83). This process requires sufficient amounts of carnitine and the enzyme carnitine palmitoyl transferase a and b in order to form palymitoyl carnitine (84). Cytosolic concentrations of carnitine increase throughout the latter part of gestation consistent with a decreased ability of premature newborn humans to clear fat from the plasma (83). Addition of carnitine to in vitro cell cultures results in an increase of fatty acid oxidation (85). A similar augmentation of fatty acid oxidation in premature newborns supplemented with carnitine has also been observed (86).

Thus, for a variety of reasons, it appears that fatty acid transport to the fetus results primarily in increasing rates of fat deposition. It remains to be determined to what extent these processes are regulated by fatty acid concentrations relative to glucose concentrations, and how insulin may modulate these processes.

Hay and co-workers (87) have shown that during late pregnancy in the sheep, glucose utilization is reduced. In addition, insulin resistance is present in nonuterine tissues, but uterine glucose uptake and uterine glucose utilization were not different from normal nonpregnant sheep and were not altered by changes in maternal insulin concentration. This study is interesting in light of the clinical observation that, during the increased uterine work of labor, the insulin requirement drops (88).

A late third trimester change in insulin requirement has been noted by us in a group of more than 300 insulin-dependent diabetic women. The insulin requirement continues to increase into the third trimester to 1.0 ± 0.2 units/kg/24 hours (14). Then, about 10–

14 days before the onset of labor, the overnight insulin requirement begins to drop; however, the daytime insulin requirement continues to increase, which results in no overall change in the 24-hour requirement. This overnight drop in insulin requirement may be due to large quantities of glucose siphoning to the rapidly growing fetus. During the times a woman is not eating, she may experience hypoglycemia if she does not lower her insulin doses. An alternative hypothesis may be that some unknown hormone that initiates labor potentiates glucose utilization. Perhaps increased uterine activity could also be responsible for the increased glucose utilization. During active labor, the insulin requirement drops to zero. The glucose utilization rate rises 8-fold above baseline to a level of 2.55 mg/kg/min (88). The increased need for glucose, coupled with a fall in insulin requirement, parallels the work of labor.

Fetal Response

Even short-term hyperglycemia can affect fetal β-cell function. The effects of gestational hyperglycemia on β-cell function were studied in near-term fetuses from unrestrained pregnant rats made slightly or highly hyperglycemic using continuous glucose infusion during the last week of pregnancy (89). Compared with controls, slightly hyperglycemic fetuses showed increased pancreatic and plasma insulin concentrations and similar insulin release in response to glucose in vitro. In highly hyperglycemic fetuses, pancreatic and plasma insulin concentrations were unchanged compared with controls, and insulin release in vitro was insensitive to glucose and to the mixture of glucose plus theophylline. These results confirm that glucose is able to stimulate insulin secretion in normal or slightly hyperglycemic fetuses and suggest that severe hyperglycemia per se, without the association of other metabolic disorders or toxic injuries, profoundly alters the stimulus-secretion coupling of the fetal rat β-cell. The nadir of the blood glucose level of the neonate is inversely proportional to the peak maternal glucose level during delivery. Thus, maternal glucose balance during labor and delivery is important in the prevention of neonatal hypoglycemia (90).

POSTPARTUM

Maternal

The normal postpartum change in glucose tolerance was studied by Hubinont and co-workers (91). They observed a marked decrease in basal plasma insulin and C-peptide concentrations, as well as in the β-cell secretory response to hyperglycemia at the 5th day postpartum, compared to the high values recorded in late pregnancy. Except for a higher basal C-peptide level and a lower plasma prolactin concentration, there was no major difference between early lactation and postlactation. At the 5th day after delivery, the insulin response to hyperglycemia was lower in lactating than in nonlactating women (14 subjects in each group). They concluded that, in normal women, pancreatic β-cell function undergoes a rapid normalization during the postpartum period.

Botto and co-workers (92), studied β-cell secretion and peripheral insulin resistance during pregnancy and after delivery in GDM women with obesity. During the oral glucose tolerance test (OGTT), C-peptide and insulin values in the late phase of the OGTT were lower than in controls, both during pregnancy and postpartum. Moreover, in the GDM women there was an inverse correlation between these late-phase insulin levels on the OGTT and ponderal index after delivery. This study shows that both a decreased insulin response to glucose and the degree of adiposity play a role in abnormal β-cell response in GDM.

Ward and co-workers (93) found that abnormalities of islet cell function in women with histories of gestational diabetes related not only to the degree of adiposity, but also to their fat distribution. They found that insulin sensitivity in lean former GDM women was similar to controls. In contrast, insulin sensitivity in obese former GDM women was significantly less than the controls.

To assess whether differences in fat distribution and fat cell size were associated with these differences in insulin sensitivity, the waist to thigh circumference ratio, the waist to hip ratio, and abdominal fat cell diameter were measured. All three were significantly greater in the obese former GDM women than in controls. Thus, an abnormal central distribution of adiposity appears to be associated with the insulin action defect in obese former GDM women. This study supports the clinical observation that obese former GDM women have a 50–60% prevalence of type II diabetes as they age (94), whereas lean former GDM women have less than a 25% prevalence rate of type II diabetes as they age (95).

LACTATION AND PANCREATIC FUNCTION

Marynissen and co-workers (96) investigated the influence of lactation on morphometric and secretory variables in pancreatic β-cells of mildly diabetic rats. In nondiabetic rats, lactation accelerates the restoration of pancreatic β-cell function after the period of increased secretory activity associated with pregnancy. In the mildly diabetic animals, the changes in endocrine pancreatic function normally associated with pregnancy and lactation were greatly attenuated, albeit not completely eliminated. The increased biosynthetic and secretory activity imposed on surviving β-cells after streptozocin administration tends to mask the adaptive changes in β-cell function otherwise seen during the postpartum and lactation period. They further noted (97, 98) that a lower plasma insulin level, a lower percentage of endocrine tissue, and a lower volume density of β-cells are found in lactating, compared to nonlactating normal rats. In addition, they have reported that islets isolated from lactating rats as compared to islets from nonlactating rats release less insulin when incubated in the absence of exogenous nutrient or the presence of glucose and aminoacids. It is speculated (99) that the decreased secretory activity in islets removed from lactating rats may be accounted for by a decreased calcium content of the islets.

Clinically, we find that the overnight insulin requirement is reduced in lactating type I insulin-dependent women (100). In addition, maternal milk glucose and insulin concentration is positively correlated with maternal serum insulin and glucose levels. The nutritional meaning to the infant of these variations in glucose and insulin levels in milk remains to be determined (101).

UTILITY OF EXERCISE AS A TREATMENT FOR GESTATIONAL DIABETES

GDM is the most common medical complication of pregnancy. Current management consists of diet and careful monitoring of fasting and postprandial glucose levels. The goal of therapy is maintenance of euglycemia. When euglycemia is not achieved by diet alone, insulin therapy is recommended (102). GDM is considered to be, in part, a disease of glucose clearance, although it has been shown that this disorder is a heterogeneous entity (60). Initiation of insulin therapy per se is palliative, but does not speak to the primary defect(s) that may include hyperinsulinemia. Rather, treatment modalities that overcome a peripheral resistance to insulin such as sulfonylurea treatment or exercise might be preferable. Although the sulfonylurea agents are reported to increase insulin sensitivity (103), these agents are contraindicated for use in GDM in the United States (104).

Cardiovascular conditioning exercise facilitates glucose utilization inter alia by increasing insulin binding to and affinity for its receptor (105). Although exercise during pregnancy has been gaining acceptance (106), it remains controversial (107–115). Specifically, maternal exercise on a bicycle ergometer has been associated with fetal bradycardia (107, 111). We, therefore, designed a study, utilizing arm ergometry (AE), which has not been associated with either uterine activity or fetal bradycardia (116), to evaluate the impact of a training program on glucose tolerance in GDM (117).

GDM women (N = 19) were randomized into either group 1, a 6-week diet alone group (24–30 kcal/kg/24 hours; 20% protein, 40% CHO, 40% fat), or group 2, the same diet plus exercise (20 minutes 3×/week for 6 weeks) utilizing an AE to maintain heart rate in the training range. Glycemic response was monitored by glycosylated hemoglobin (HbA_{lc}), a 50-g oral glucose challenge (GCT) with a fasting (FPG) and 1-hour (1hpc) plasma glucose; and self blood glucose monitoring (SBGM) fasting and 1hpc. Week 1 glycemic parameters were equal between groups. Week 6 data (mean ± SD) were: group 1 HbA$_{1c}$ 4.7 ± 0.2% vs. group 2 4.2 ± 0.2%, p<0.001; group 1 GCT FPG 87.6 ± 6.2 mg/dl vs. group 2 70.1 ± 6.6 mg/dl, p<0.001; group 1 GCT 1hpc 187.5 ± 12.9 mg/dl vs. group 2 105.9 ± 18.9 mg/dl, p<0.001 (Fig. 4.1). The glycemic levels diverged between the groups at week 4.

This study documented that women with GDM can train using AE and that such a program of cardiovascular conditioning exercise results in lower levels of glycemia than a program of diet alone. The effects of exercise on glucose metabolism became apparent after 4 weeks of training and appeared to impact both hepatic glucose output (as reflected by fasting glucose levels) as well as glucose clearance (as reflected by glucose values after a 50-g oral GCT).

Our observations appear contrary to the literature asserting that the natural progression of glucose intolerance during gestation is deterioration with increasing gestational week (118) and that walking exercise in type I insulin-dependent diabetic pregnant women is associated with no improvement (119). However, neither of the previous studies addressed the issue of GDM with its unique problems of glucose homeostasis.

The implications of our study for the health care of women with GDM remain to be determined. Compliance with the protocol was 100% and there was no maternal or infant morbidity associated with the training program in this small series. The present results also imply that a cardiovascular conditioning program might obviate insulin treatment in many women with GDM. The economic and health care implications of these observations, therefore, warrant further testing.

SUMMARY

The changes in the endocrine pancreas of the mother and the fetus are truly a remarkable adaptation to the mutual increase in nutrient demands. Although the fetus seems to get priority for fuels, the mother's glucose homeostasis adapts to provide a constant source of nutrients even in times of food deprivation. The changes in the endocrine pancreas of the mother and fetus are exquisitely designed to compensate for the sequential rise of the diabetogenic hormones of pregnancy: hPRL, hCS, cortisol, and progesterone. When maternal glucose homeostasis goes awry, there are maternal and fetal consequences in each trimester. Exercise as a treatment modality was presented as an option to treat the hyperglycemia of GDM. This chapter reviewed the metabolic and hormonal changes required in each trimester and the fetal pathology that may result. The conclusion from this review is that even minor perturbations of maternal glucose outside the normal range can produce major fetal pathology. The logical clinical conclusion is that all pregnant women need to keep their blood glucose in the normal range before, during,

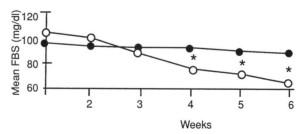

Figure 4.1. Weekly mean fasting blood glucose (*FBS*, mg/dl) of the self blood glucose monitored results from weeks 1–6 of the protocol. The *closed circles* represent mean values for group 1 (diet alone) and the *open circles* represent group 2 (diet and exercise). The symbol (*) indicates a significance of p<0.001. (Adapted from Jovanovic-Peterson L, Durak E, Peterson CM. Randomized trial of diet versus diet plus cardiovascular conditioning on glucose levels in gestational diabetes. Am J Obstet Gynecol 1990;754–756.)

and in between their pregnancies. In addition, all pregnant women need to be tested for GDM to discover and treat hyperglycemia, perhaps with an exercise program, as soon as possible.

REFERENCES

1. Csapo AL, Pulkkinen MO, Wiest WG. Effects of luteectomy and progesterone replacement in early pregnant patients. Am J Obstet Gynecol 1973; 115:759.
2. Jaffe RB. The endocrinology of pregnancy. In: Yen SSC, Jaffee RB, eds. Reproductive endocrinology: physiology, pathophysiology, and clinical management. Philadelphia: WB Saunders, 1978; 521–536.
3. Jovanovic L, Dawood MY, Landesman R, Saxena BB. Hormonal profile as a prognostic index of early threatened abortion. Am J Obstet Gynecol 1978; 130:274–276.
4. Hiriis-Nielsen J, Nielsen V, Molsted-Pedersen L, Deckert T. Effects of pregnancy hormones on pancreatic islets in organ culture. Acta Endocrinol (Copenh) 1986; 111:336–341.
5. Kalkhoff RK, Jacobson M, Lemper D. Progesterone, pregnancy and the augmented plasma insulin response. J Clin Endocrinol Metab 1970; 31:24.
6. Barbieri RL. Whu-Fadil S, Kletzky OA, Nakamura RM, Mishell DR. Serum prolactin patterns in early human gestation. Am J Obstet Gynecol 1975; 121:1107.
7. Ho Yuen B, Cannon W, Lewis J, Sy L, Woolley S. A possible role for prolactin in the control of human chorionic gonadotropin and estrogen secretion by the fetoplacental unit. Am J Obstet Gynecol 1980; 136:286.
8. Michaels RL, Sorenson RL, Parsons JA, Sheridan JD. Prolactin enhances cell-to-cell communication among beta-cells in pancreatic islets. Diabetes 1987; 36:1098–1103.
9. Josimovich JB. Placental lactogenic hormone. In: Endocrinology of pregnancy, New York: Harper & Row, 1971; p 184–196.
10. Josimovich JB, MacLaren JA. Presence in the human placenta and term serum of a highly lactogenic substance immunologically related to pituitary growth hormone. Endocrinology 1962; 71:209.
11. Spellacy WN, Buhi WC, Schram JC, Birk SA, McCreary SA. Control of human chorionic somato-mammotropin levels during pregnancy. Obstet Gynecol 1971; 37:567.
12. Kim YJ, Felig P. Plasma chorionic somatomammotropin levels during starvation in mid-pregnancy. J Clin Endocrinol Metab 1971; 32:864.
13. Gaspard VJ, Sandront HM, Luyckx AS, Lefebvre PJ. The control of human placental lactogen (HPL) secretion and its interrelation with glucose and lipid metabolism in late pregnancy. In: Camerini-Davalos RH, Coles HS, eds. Early diabetes in early life. New York: Academic Press, 1975; p 273–278.
14. Jovanovic L, Druzin M, Peterson CM. Effect of euglycemia on the outcome of pregnancy in insulin-dependent diabetic women as compared with normal control subjects. Am J Med 1981; 71:921–927.
15. Kuhl C, Hornnes PJ. Endocrine pancreatic function in women with gestational diabetes. Acta Endocrinol (Suppl) (Copenh) 1986; 277:19–23.
16. Mills JL, Baker L, Goldman A. Malformations in infants of diabetic mothers occur before the seventh gestational week. Implications for treatment. Diabetes 1979; 23:292–293.
17. Fuhrmann K, Ruher H, Semmler K, Fischer F, Fisher M, Glockner E. Prevention of congenital malformations in infants of insulin dependent diabetic mothers. Diabetes Care 1983; 6:219–223.
18. Jovanovic L, Peterson CM, Saxena BB, Dawood Y, Saudek CD. Feasibility of maintaining normal glucose profiles in insulin-dependent pregnant women. Am J Med 1980; 68:105–112.
19. Jovanovic L, Peterson CM. Preface. In: Jovanovic L, Peterson CM, eds. Diabetes and pregnancy: teratology, toxicology and treatment. Philadelphia: Praeger, 1985.
20. Sadler TW, Horton WE. Effects of maternal diabetes on early embryogenesis: the role of insulin and insulin therapy. Diabetes 1983; 32:1070–1074.
21. Miller E, Hare JW, Clogerty JP, Dunn PJ, Gleason RE, Soeldner J, Kitzmiller JL. Elevated maternal hemoglobin A_{lc} in early pregnancy and major congenital anomalies in infants of diabetic mothers. N Engl J Med 1981; 304:1331–1334.
22. Mills JL, Knopp RH, Simpson JL, et al. Lack of relationship of malformation rates in infants of diabetic mothers to glycemic control during organogenesis. N Engl J Med 1988; 318:671–676.
23. Castracane VD, Jovanovic L, Mills JL. Effect of normoglycemia before conception on early pregnancy hormone profiles. Diabetes Care 1985; 8:473–476.
24. DeHertogh R, Thomas K, Vanderheyden I. Quantitative determination of sex hormone-binding globulin capacity in the plasma of normal and diabetic pregnancies. J Clin Endocrinol Metab 1976; 42:773–777.
25. Gibson M, Schiff I, Tulchinsky D, Ryan KJ. Characterization of hyperandrogenism with insulin-resistant diabetes type A. Fertil Steril 1980; 33:501–505.
26. Szpunar WE, Blair AJ, McCann DS. Plasma androgen concentrations in diabetic women. Diabetes 1977; 26:1125–1129.
27. Leaming AB, Mathur RS, Levine JH. Increased plasma testosterone in streptozotocin-diabetic female rats. Endocrinology 1982; 111:1329–1333.
28. Barbieri RL, Makris A, Ryan KJ. Effects of insulin on steroidogenesis in cultured porcine ovarian theca. Fertil Steril 1983; 40:237–241.
29. Mills JL, Simpson JL, Driscoll SG, Jovanovic-Peterson L, et al. Incidence of spontaneous abortion among normal women and insulin dependent diabetic women whose pregnancies were identified within 21 days of conception. N Engl J Med 1989; 319:1617–1623.
30. Peterson CM, Miller N, Walker L, Formby B. Effect of glipizide on insulin secretion from cultured human fetal pancreatic islets. Diabetes Care 1986; 5:556–557.
31. Weiss PAM. Gestational diabetes—a survey. In: Weiss PAM, Coustan DR, eds. Gestational diabetes. Vienna: Springer-Verlag, 1988; p 1–58.
32. Battaglia FC, Meschia G. Principal substrates of fetal metabolism. Physiol Rev 1978; 58:499.
33. Meschia G, Battaglia FC, Hay WW, Sparks JW. Utilization of substrates by the ovine placenta in vivo. Fed Proc 1980; 39:245.
34. Battaglia FC. Principal substrates of fetal metabolism: fuel and growth requirements of the ovine fetus. In: Pregnancy, metabolism, diabetes and the

fetus. Amsterdam: CIBA Foundation Symposium 63 (new series), 1979; p 57–74.

35. Phelps RL, Metzger BE, Freinkel N. Carbohydrate metabolism in pregnancy. XVIII. Diurnal profiles of plasma glucose, insulin, free fatty acids, triglycerides, cholesterol and individual amino acids in late normal pregnancy. Am J Obstet Gynecol 1981; 140:730.

36. Hull D, Elphick MG. Evidence for fatty acid transfer across the human placenta. In: Pregnancy, metabolism, diabetes and the fetus. Amsterdam: CIBA Foundation Symposium 63 (new series), Excerpta Medica, 1979; p 75–91.

37. Steel RB, Mosley JD, Smith CH. Insulin and placenta: degradation and stabilization, binding to microvillous membrane receptors, and amino acid uptake. Am J Obstet Gynecol 1979; 135:522.

38. Zwilling E. Micromelia as a direct effect of insulin-evidence from in vitro and in vivo experiments. J Morphol 1959; 194:159–179.

39. Cockroft DL, Coppola PT. Teratogenic effects of excess glucose on head-fold rat embryos in culture. Teratology 1977; 16:141–146.

40. Van Lancker JL. Molecular and cellular mechanisms in disease. New York: Springer-Verlag, 1976; p 423–457.

41. New DAT. Whole embryo culture and the study of mammalian embryos during organogenesis. Biol Rev 1978; 53:81–122.

42. Sadler TW. Culture of early somite mouse embryos during organogenesis. J Embryol Exp Morphol 1979; 49:17–25.

43. Sadler TW. Effects of maternal diabetes on early embryogenesis II Hyperglycemia-induced exencephaly. Teratology 1980; 21:349–356.

44. Horton WE, Sadler TW. Effects of maternal diabetes on early embryogenesis alterations in morphogenesis produced by the ketone body B-hyroxybutyrate. Diabetes 1983; 32:610–616.

45. Sadler TW, Horton WE, Warner CW. Whole embryo culture: a screening technique for teratogens? Terat carcin Mutagen 1982; 2:243–253.

46. Cockroft DL, Freinkel N, Philbos LS, Shambaugh GE. Metabolic factors affecting organogenesis in diabetic pregnancy. Clin Res 1981; 29:577A.

47. Gasparo M de, Van Assche FA, Gepts W, Hoet JJ. The histology of the endocrine pancreas and the insulin content in the microdissected islets of fetal pancreas. Rev Fr Etude Clin Biol 1969; 9:904–906.

48. Van Assche FA, Hoet JJ, Jack PMB. Endocrine pancreas of the pregnant mother, fetus, and newborn. In: Beard RW, Nanthanielsz PW, eds. Fetal physiology and medicine, 2nd ed. New York: Dekker, 1984; p 127–152.

49. Fowden AL. Effects of arginine and glucose on the release of insulin in the sheep fetus. J Endocrinol 1980; 85:121–129.

50. Fowden AL. Effects of adrenaline and amino acids on the release of insulin in the sheep fetus. J Endocrinol 1980; 87:113–121.

51. Young M, Horn J, Noakes DL. Protein turnover rate in fetal organs. The influence of insulin. In: Visser HKA, ed. Nutrition and metabolism of the fetus and infant. The Hague: Mardrums Nijhoff 1979; p 19–27.

52. Jovanovic-Peterson L. The relationship between glucose levels and macrosomia: The diabetes in early pregnancy study. Abstract submitted to the Annual Meeting of the American Diabetes Association, June, 1989.

53. Tamas G, Bekefi D, Gaal O. Insulin antibodies in diabetic pregnancy. Lancet 1975; 1:521.

54. Bauman WA, Yalow RS. Transplacental passage of insulin complexed to antibody. Proc Natl Acad Sci 1981; 78:4588–4590.

55. Girard JR. Factors affecting the secretion of insulin and glucagon by the rat fetus. Diabetes 1974; 23:310–317.

56. Dudek RW, Kawabe T, Brinn JE, Poole MC, Morgan CR. Effects of growth hormone on the in vitro maturation of fetal islets. Proc Soc Exp Biol Med 1984; 177:69–76.

57. Josimovich JB. Placental lactogenic hormone. In: Endocrinology of pregnancy. New York, Harper & Row, 1971: p 184–196.

58. Hollingsworth DR: Alterations of maternal metabolism in normal and diabetic pregnancies: Differences in insulin-dependent, non-insulin-dependent, and gestational diabetes. Am J Obstet Gynecol 1983; 146:417–427.

59. Hadden DR. Geographic, ethnic, & racial variations in the incidence of gestational diabetes. Diabetes 1985; 34 (suppl 2):8–12.

60. Metzger BE, Bybec DE, Frienkel NO, Phelps RL, Radvany RM, Vaisrub N. Gestational diabetes mellitus: correlations between phenotypic and genotypic characteristics of the mother and abnormal glucose tolerance during the first year post partum. Diabetes 1985; 34(suppl 2):111–115.

61. Nordlander E, Hanson U, Persson B, Stangenberg M. Pancreatic B-cell function during normal pregnancy. Diabetes Res 1987; 6:133–136.

62. Swenne I. Glucose-stimulated DNA replication of the pancreatic islets during the development of the rat fetus: effects of nutrients, growth hormone, and triiodothyronine. Diabetes 1985; 34:803–807.

63. Hollingsworth DR, Grundy SM. Pregnancy associated hypertriglyceridemia in normal and diabetic women: Differences in type I, type II and gestational diabetes. Diabetes 1982; 31:1092.

64. Knopp RH, Warth M. Lipoprotein changes in pregnancy. A distinct endogenous hypertriglyceridemia. J Clin Invest 1973; 42:48a.

65. Ziegler B, Lucke S, Besch W, Hahn HJ. Pregnancy-associated changes in the endocrine pancreas of normoglycaemic streptozotocin-treated Wistar rats. Diabetologia 1985; 28:172–175.

66. Reusens-Billen B, Remacle C, Daniline J, Hoet JJ. Cell proliferation in pancreatic islets of rat fetuses and neonates from normal and diabetic mothers. An in vitro and in vivo study. Hormone Metab Res 1984; 11:565–571.

67. Hoet JJ. The etiology of congenital malformations in infants of diabetic mothers: Environmental and genetic interaction. In: Jovanovic L, Peterson CM, Fuhrmann K, eds. Diabetes and pregnancy: teratology, toxicology, and treatment. New York: Praeger, 1986; p 72–82.

68. Dudek RW, Kawabe T, Brinn JE, O'Brien K, Poole MC, Morgan CR. Glucose affects in vitro maturation of fetal rat islets. Endocrinology 1984; 114:582–587.

69. Jovanovic L, Peterson CM. Is pregnancy contraindicated in women with diabetes mellitus? Diabetic Nephropathy 1984; 3:36–38.

70. Swenne I, Eriksson U. Diabetes in pregnancy: Islet

cell proliferation in the fetal rat pancreas. Diabetologia 1982; 23:525–528.

71. Eriksson U, Swenne I. Diabetes in pregnancy: Growth of the fetal pancreatic β cells in the rat. Biol Neonate 1982; 42:239–248.

72. Philipps AF, Dubin JW, Raye JR. Fetal metabolic response to endogenous insulin release. Am J Obstet Gynecol 1981; 139:441–445.

73. Woods SC, Porte D. Neural control of the endocrine pancreas. Physiol Rev 1974; 54:596–619.

74. Freinkel N, Metzger BE, Nitzan M, et al. "Accelerated starvation" and mechanism for the conservation of maternal nitrogen during pregnancy. Isr J Med Sci 1972; 8:426–439.

75. Hollingsworth DR. Endocrine and metabolic homeostasis in diabetic pregnancy. Clin Perinatol 1983; 10:593–614.

76. Fiore R, Maldonato A, Zicari D, et al. Endocrine pancreatic function in insulin-dependent diabetic pregnant women. Acta Endocrinologica (Suppl) 1986; 277:31–36.

77. Hull D, Elphick MC. Evidence for fatty acid transfer across the human placenta. In: Pregnancy metabolism, diabetes and the fetus. Amsterdam: Ciba Found Symp: Exerpta Medica, 1979; p 75–91.

78. Widdowson EM. Chemical composition of newly born mammals. Nature 1950; 166:626–627.

79. Sparks JW, Girard JR, Battaglia FC. An estimate of the caloric requirements of the human fetus. Biol Neonate 1980; 38:113–119.

80. Roux JF, Myers RE. In vitro metabolism of palmitic acid and glucose in the developing tissue of the rhesus monkey. Am J Obstet Gynecol 1974; 118:385–392.

81. Yoshioka T, Roux JF. In vitro metabolism of palmitic acid in human fetal tissues. Pediatr Res 1972; 6:675–681.

82. Robinson AM, Williamson DH. Physiological roles of ketone bodies as substrates and signals in mammalian tissues. Physiol Rev 1980; 60:143–189.

83. Warshaw JB, Terry ML. Cellular energy metabolism during fetal development. II. Fatty acid oxidation by the developing heart. J Cell Biol 1970; 44:354–360.

84. Bailey E, Lockwood E. Some aspects of fatty acid oxidation and ketone body formation and utilization during development of the rat. Enzyme 1973; 15:239–253.

85. McGary JD, Robles-Valdes C, Foster DW. Role of carnitine in hepatic ketogenesis. Proc Natl Acad Sci 1975; 72:4385–4388.

86. Schmidt-Sommerfeld E, Penn D, Wolf H. Carnitine deficiency in premature infants receiving total parenteral nutrition. Effect of L-carnitine supplementation. J Pediatr 1983; 102:931–935.

87. Hay WW, Lin CC, Meznarich HK. Effect of high levels of insulin on glucose utilization and glucose production in pregnant and nonpregnant sheep. Proc Soc Exp Biol Med 1988; 189:275–284.

88. Jovanovic L, Peterson CM. Insulin and glucose requirements during the first stage of labor in insulin-dependent diabetic women. Am J Med 1983; 75:607–612.

89. Bihoreau MT, Ktorza A, Kervran A, Picon L. Effect of gestational hyperglycemia on insulin secretion in vivo and in vitro by fetal rat pancreas. Am J Phys 1986; 251:E86–91.

90. Cornblath M, Tildon JT, Wapnir RA. Metabolic adaptation in the neonate. Isr J Med Sci 1972; 8:453.

91. Hubinont CJ, Balasse H, Dufrane SP, Leclercq-Meyer V, Sugar J, Schwers J, Malaisse WJ. Changes in pancreatic β cell function during late pregnancy, early lactation and postlactation. Gynecol Obstet Invest 1988; 25:89–95.

92. Botto RM, Sinagra D, Donatelli M, Amato MP, Angelico MC, Cangemi C, Bompiani G. Evaluation of β-cell secretion and peripheral insulin resistance during pregnancy and after delivery in gestational diabetes mellitus with obesity. Acta Diabetol Lat 1988; 25:81–88.

93. Ward WK, Johnston CL, Beard JC, Benedetti TJ, Porte D Jr. Abnormalities of islet β-cell function, insulin action, and fat distribution in women with histories of gestational diabetes: relation to obesity. J Clin Endocrinol Metab 1985; 61:1039–1045.

94. Mestman JH, Anderson CV, Guadalupe V. Followup of 360 subjects with abnormal carbohydrate metabolism during pregnancy. Obstet Gynecol 1972; 39:421–425.

95. O'Sullivan JB. Body weight and subsequent diabetes mellitus. JAMA 1982; 248:949.

96. Marynissen G, Malaisse WJ, Van-Assche FA. Influence of lactation on morphometric and secretory variables in pancreatic beta-cell of mildly diabetic rats. Diabetes 1987; 36:883–891.

97. Marynissen G, Aerts L, Van Assche FA. The endocrine pancreas during pregnancy and lactation in the rat. J Dev Physiol 1983; 5:373–381.

98. Marynissen G, Malaisse WJ, Van Assche FA. Ultrastructural changes of the pancreatic beta-cell and the insulin secretion by islets from lactating and non-lactating rats. J Dev Physiol 1985; 7:17–23.

99. Hubinont CJ, Dufrane SP, Garcia MP, Valverde I, Sener A, Malaisse WJ. Influence of lactation upon pancreatic islet function. Endocrinology 1986; 118:687–694.

100. Jovanovic-Peterson L, Peterson CM. Insulin requirements for nursing mothers. Diabetes Professional 1988; Summer:7.

101. Jovanovic-Peterson L, Peterson CM. Maternal milk and plasma glucose and insulin levels: studies in normal and diabetic subjects. J Am College Nut 1989; 8:125–131.

102. Summary and Recommendations of the Second International Workshop-Conference on Gestational Diabetes Mellitus. Diabetes 1985; 34(suppl 2): 123.

103. Peterson CM, Sims RV, Jones RL, Rieders F. Bioavailability of glipizide and its effect on blood glucose and insulin levels in patients with non-insulin dependent diabetes. Diabetes Care 1982; 5:497–500.

104. Jovanovic L. Preface. In: Jovanovic L, ed. Controversies in diabetes and pregnancy. New York: Springer-Verlag, 1988: p vii.

105. Pedersen O, Beck-Nielsen M, Heding L. Increased insulin receptors after exercise in patients with insulin-dependent diabetes mellitus. N Engl J Med 1980; 302:886–892.

106. American College of Obstetrics and Gynecology: Home exercise programs. Published by the American College of Obstetrics and Gynecology. May, 1986.

107. Artal R, Romem Y, Wiswell R. Fetal bradycardia induced by maternal exercise. Lancet 1984; 2:258–260.

108. Hon EH, Wohlgemuth R. The electronic evaluation of fetal heart rate. IV. The effect of maternal exercise. Am J Obstet Gynecol 1961; 81:361–371.

109. Pomerance JJ, Gluck L, Lynch VA. Maternal exercise as a screening test of uteroplacental insufficiency. Obstet Gynecol 1974; 44:383–387.

110. Dale E, Mullinax K, Bryan D. Exercise during pregnancy: Effect on the fetus. Can J Ap Sports Sci 1982; 7:98–103.

111. Jovanovic L, Kessler A, Peterson CM. Human maternal and fetal response to graded exercise. J Appl Physiol 1985; 58:1719–1722.

112. Collings C, Curet LB. Fetal heart rate response to maternal exercise. Am J Obstet Gynecol 1985; 151:498–501.

113. Hauth JC, Gilstrap LC, Widmer CK. Fetal heart rate reactivity before and after maternal jogging during the third trimester. Am J Obstet Gynecol 1982; 142:545–547.

114. Edwards M, Metcalfe J, Dunham M, Paul M. Accelerated respiratory response to moderate exercise in late pregnancy. Respir Physiol 1981; 45:229–241.

115. Dressendorfer E, Goodlin R. Fetal heart rate response to maternal exercise testing. Phys Sportsmed 1980; 8:91–94.

116. Jovanovic L, Peterson CM, Board PJ, Dyer CR. Arm ergometry is a safe form of training for pregnant women. Clin Res 1987; 35:289A.

117. Jovanovic-Peterson L, Durak E, Peterson CM. Randomized trial of diet versus diet plus cardiovascular conditioning on glucose levels in gestational diabetes. Am J Obstet Gynecol 1990; 162:754–756.

118. Jovanovic L, Peterson CM. Screening for gestational diabetes: optimal timing and criteria for retesting. Diabetes 1985; 34 (suppl 2):21–23.

119. Hollingsworth DR, Moore TR. Postprandial walking exercise in pregnant insulin-dependent (type I) diabetic pregnant women: reduction of plasma lipid levels but absence of a significant effect on glycemic control. Am J Obstet Gynecol 1987; 157:1359–1363.

5

Maternal Hemodynamics in Pregnancy

Mark J. Morton

CARDIAC OUTPUT

Maternal cardiac output increases during mammalian pregnancy; however, a quantitative description of that generalization is difficult for humans. The following statements appear tenable at this time. First, cardiac output increases before and in excess of the increment in uterine blood flow. Second, the increase in cardiac output is accomplished by cardiac enlargement and increased heart rate rather than by changes in loading or contractility. Third, posture dominates the control of cardiac output late in pregnancy because of its influence on venous return. Finally, exercise capacity is reduced in pregnancy because a portion of cardiac output is committed to nonmuscular tissues and because venous return may be impaired.

Time Course, Magnitude, and Effects of Posture

The clinician who examines a young, healthy woman in the second trimester of pregnancy receives many clues to the presence of a hyperkinetic circulation. The rosy cheeks, warm skin, active precordium, ejection murmur, and bounding peripheral pulses support this impression. It is not surprising, therefore, that most values for resting cardiac output are 30–50% greater during midpregnancy (1–6) than nonpregnant values. Cardiac output is increased and probably does not increase further after the second trimester. This time course has clinical relevance when considering the interaction between pregnancy and cardiac pathophysiology; the maximal stress on the cardiovascular system probably occurs by the second trimester. The fact that cardiac output reaches maximum values by midpregnancy also suggests that mechanisms other than increased uterine blood flow are responsible.

The techniques used for the measurement of cardiac output during human pregnancy are shown in Table 5.1. The strengths and weaknesses of each technique are worth considering when attempting to rationalize the different results and conclusions that various investigators have reported in the past 45 years. Unlike patients with severe cardiac disease, young healthy people have very labile cardiac outputs that are importantly affected by emotional state in addition to the

Table 5.1. Cardiac Output Measurement Techniques Used in Human Pregnancy

Technique	Requirements	Accuracy
Direct Fick	Oxygen consumption, mixed venous and arterial blood O_2 contents	++++
Indirect Fick		
Dye dilution	Indicator injection proximal to a mixing chamber (ventricle) with concentration sampling distally	++++
Thermal dilution	Indicator injection proximal to a mixing chamber (ventricle) with concentration sampling distally	++++
Rebreathing	Accurate measurement of respiratory gases and soluble indicator, subject cooperation with rapid rebreathing, no lung disease	+++
Doppler	Integrated velocity, orifice area, heart rate	+++
2-D echo	High quality orthoganol, apical views for area-length or Simpson's rule assessment, heart rate	++
M-mode echo	High quality minor axis dimension measurement, heart rate	++
Impedence	dz/dt, ejection time, electrode distance, hematocrit, heart rate	+

underlying condition (pregnancy) that is being investigated. Thus, it is very important that the subject being studied be allowed as much separation from the trauma of an invasive technique as possible in order that a basal state may be reached. Occlusive nose clips and mouthpieces or hoods and the imposing equipment and chest exposure associated with echocardiographic and Doppler techniques may likewise cause anxiety. Because cardiac output literally varies from beat to beat, it is important to know over what period of time each technique measures output or stroke volume. The direct Fick technique usually measures flow over about 15–30 seconds, depending upon the amount of time necessary to draw the mixed venous and arterial blood samples. Green dye dilution measurements integrate concentration over a similar time period while thermodilution is somewhat shorter. The ease of repeat measurements with the indicator-dilution methods allows two or three samples to be averaged resulting in a cardiac output that represents a mean flow over several minutes. In contrast, Doppler, two dimensional (2-D), and M-mode echocardiographic and impedance techniques measure stroke volumes of individual beats. The result of each beat analysis is then averaged over, for example, six beats and the mean stroke volume is multiplied by the average heart rate during that period. Because the analysis of each beat is frequently laborious, cardiac output measurements encompassing a long period of time and thus smoothing out normal variability are less likely to be reported than with the indicator-dilution techniques.

The direct (7) and indirect (8, 9) Fick techniques are the gold standard for the measurement of cardiac output. The theory of these measurements is rigorous and the actual component measurements, for example, oxygen consumption, oxygen content, dye concentration, or temperature can be made with accuracy. There is little room for observer error in these measurements. Soluble gas disappearance from rapidly inhaled, known gas mixtures and volumes can also give reliable estimates of pulmonary capillary blood flow from indirect Fick principles (10).

The availability of accurate gas concentration measurements "on line" with a mass spectrometer has made "rebreathing" techniques utilizing acetylene or dimethyl ether practical. Subject cooperation is critical for these studies. The problems of recirculation and subject cooperation at high work loads limits the application of this technique during exercise. The Doppler technique is also rigorous in its theory but is subject to error (11, 12). Velocity recording must be of high quality and along the axis of flow or the angle of deviation accounted for. In addition, high quality orifice measurements must be made. The latter is the Achilles' heel of this technique. Two-dimensional and M-mode echocardiographic measurements compute stroke volume from changes in left ventricular volume during the cardiac cycle (13, 14). Empiric or geometric formulae are used to compute end-diastolic volume and end-systolic volume and their difference, stroke volume. The accuracy of echocardiographic volume measurements during pregnancy has not been independently assessed. Echocardiographic stroke volume measurements in normal subjects are quite good, using either M-mode or 2-D techniques. However, these measurements are extremely sensitive to observer error both in data acquisition and analysis. Theory regarding impedance cardiography is much less rigorous than the techniques described previously and remains an empiric technique (15). Its use in pregnancy has been questioned (16).

Early measurements of cardiac output during human pregnancy were made in supine subjects and showed a reduction of output to near postpartum levels in the third trimester (1–3). After the demonstration that the inferior vena cava is occluded in the supine position during late pregnancy (17), it was realized that posture played a crucial role in the hemodynamics of late gestation. Nevertheless, two studies (4, 18) have taken posture into account and have yielded different results, although reliable indicator-dilution techniques were used in both. Lees et al. (18) concluded from a serial study of five subjects that cardiac output did not decline in the third trimester when subjects were studied in lateral recumbency. In contrast, a serial study of 11 subjects by Ueland et al. (4) showed that cardiac output peaked in the second trimester, then fell toward postpartum levels. The fall from the second to the third trimester was greatest when women were studied supine, but also occurred in lateral recumbency and in seated subjects. In the absence of additional serial measurements of cardiac output, using invasive methods, inferential corroboration from noninvasive techniques is enlightening. A serial study of 27 women before, during, and after pregnancy by Atkins et al. (5) confirmed the findings of Ueland et al. (4): impedance cardiography, a less accepted technique, was used, but the study was well controlled. Robson and colleagues (6) have measured cardiac output serially before and during pregnancy by Doppler echocardiography in 13 subjects. Their technique has been rigorously validated and the results appear internally consistent. The results of calculated aortic flow and stroke volume, heart rate, mean arterial pressure, and systemic vascular resistance are shown for the 13 subjects as a percentage of prepregnant control values throughout

gestation in Figure 5.1. In this study, cardiac output peaked at 50% above prepregnant values at the end of the second trimester, while stroke volume peaked at the middle of the second trimester at 33% above prepregnant control values. Although stroke volume fell in the third trimester consistently by all techniques utilized in this study, the fall did not reach statistical significance. Serial M-mode echocardiographic studies have been reported from three institutions including a total of 39 subjects. Mashini et al. (19) did not demonstrate increased stroke volume, while Katz et al. (20) and Laird-Meeter et al. (21) showed progressive increases in stroke volume to term. Robson et al. (6) did not report stroke volume by the M-mode technique from their study, but it can be calculated from the dimensions supplied. Using the Teichholtz method for calculation of volumes, a reliable method for determining stroke volume (13), stroke volume was 13, 22, and 18% above prepregnant values at 12, 24, and 38 weeks, respectively. Thus, stroke volume in the third trimester is clearly dependent upon posture. However, studies performed in left lateral recumbency show stroke vol-

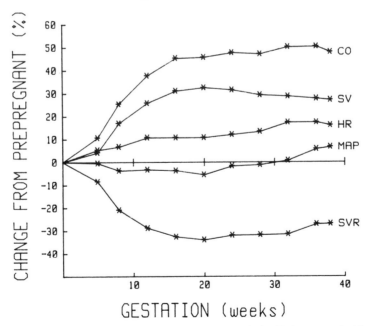

Figure 5.1. The data calculated from aortic flow from the study by Robson et al. (6) are expressed as percentage of change from prepregnant values throughout pregnancy for 13 women. CO = cardiac output, SV = stroke volume, HR = heart rate, MAP = mean arterial pressure, and SVR = systemic vascular resistance.

ume increasing, decreasing, or unchanged from second trimester values.

This persistent conflict in findings suggests that a better understanding of the maternal circulation in the third trimester is needed. As Lees (18) pointed out, "cardiac output measurements . . . are valid only for the experimental conditions under which they are made and have no universal applicability." A resurgent interest in maternal hemodynamics was evident at the 1989 meeting of the Society of Perinatal Obstetricians. Several centers reported studies of cardiac output by invasive and noninvasive techniques, in multiple positions, and during treadmill and bicycle exercise. We eagerly await the publication of these interesting studies. For now, it appears to us that the absolute value of cardiac output in the third trimester of human pregnancy is less important than the persuasive evidence that resting cardiac output is substantially increased by the second trimester and becomes highly variable in the third trimester. Assumption of a sitting or supine position causes output to fall below values measured in lateral recumbency (4). Supine recumbency may lead to symptomatic reductions of cardiac output in about 5% of pregnancies (22), the "supine hypotensive syndrome."

Determinants of Cardiac Output Changes

The reader is referred to Braunwald et al. (23) for an examination of cardiac and circulatory control.

HEART RATE

Cardiac output is the product of heart rate and stroke volume. Of the two, heart rate is more variable, ranging on average from resting values of 60/minute to almost 200/minute during maximal exercise in women of childbearing age. Because of this great range, heart rate is a powerful protector of circulatory stability. Heart rate per se may be affected by pregnancy or altered reflexly to maintain blood pressure in the face of altered vascular resistance or stroke volume.

The *intrinsic* heart rate of healthy human adults averages approximately 110 beats/min-

ute. It is normally suppressed by vagal tone and minimally supported at rest by adrenergic drive. Vagal suppression of the sinus node originates in the carotid sinus baroreceptors. Vagal release with resultant tachycardia acts to defend blood pressure; however, tachycardia alone does not increase cardiac output. For that to happen, an increase in venous return must accompany the increase in heart rate.

In human pregnancy, maternal heart rate is elevated over postpartum values in all three trimesters. Whether the mechanism is an increase in intrinsic rate, a decrease in vagal tone, or an increase in adrenergic drive (or a combination of these) is unknown. Most measurements show that heart rate increases progressively throughout pregnancy (4, 6, 19–21, 24). Using daily portable heart rate monitoring, Clapp (25) has shown that heart rate in pregnancy is increased as early as 4 weeks after the last menstrual period. Because heart rate change was not noted in the previous menstrual cycle in these women, a hormonal mechanism not normally active in the menstrual cycle is suggested.

The importance of the relative tachycardia lies in two areas. First, increased heart rate elevates myocardial oxygen requirements. This is probably not important in normal women but it may become so in the presence of important cardiovascular pathology. Second, an increased resting heart rate diminishes the increment in output that can occur with maximal exercise if maximal heart rate is unchanged; maximal work capacity falls. For example, if the maximal heart rate is 200/minute and basal heart rate increases from 60 to 80 beats/minute during pregnancy, then the maximal increment will fall from 230% to 150% of basal heart rate.

STROKE VOLUME

Stroke volume increases progressively during the first and second trimesters of human pregnancy, to a peak value approximately 30% above nonpregnant levels (4, 6). Thereafter, stroke volume becomes quite unstable and may remain the same or fall to postpartum levels, especially with changes in body position.

Left ventricular stroke volume is accomplished by the shortening and thickening of left ventricular muscle against a closed mitral valve. The determinants of muscle shortening are muscle length before shortening (preload), average muscle stress during shortening (afterload), and the intrinsic strength of the muscle (contractility). These three variables affect stroke volume on a beat-to-beat basis. Preload and contractility are regulated by the circulatory system to meet instantaneous demands. On a long-term basis, stroke volume is most affected by altering *heart size*. For example, stroke volume increases about 10-fold in the years from birth to adulthood, with unimportant changes in contractility and preload. This increment is achieved by continuous remodelling of the ventricle in order that the lumen increases progressively without a change in filling pressure. The myocytes hypertrophy producing a thickening of the wall, allowing the radius to wall thickness ratio to remain relatively constant.

PRELOAD

At the ultrastructural level, Starling's law of the heart is based upon the fact that extension of the filaments of the sarcomere during diastole increases the extent of their shortening during the subsequent systole. However, humans, when supine, are very near the "top of their Starling curve" (26); further lengthening of the sarcomere filaments evokes only minor increases in shortening. The evidence for this statement rests upon the observation that acute increases in filling pressure produce little or no change in left ventricular stroke volume of human subjects in supine recumbency. Certainly, the 30% increase in stroke volume that occurs during pregnancy could not come entirely from an increased end-diastolic pressure in the ventricle. Additionally, there is no evidence that ventricular filling pressures increase during pregnancy (1). A definitive statement regarding the importance of changes in preload as a mechanism for increasing stroke volume during pregnancy must await measurements of sarcomere length. In late gestation, however, *reduced* preload probably is important in restricting stroke volume.

AFTERLOAD

Accurate and simultaneous measurements of ventricular dimensions and pressures during systole are required to calculate muscle stress; they have not been made in pregnancy. However, we can examine several factors that affect afterload and assess the performance of the ventricle by techniques that are sensitive to changes in afterload. Extrapolation from these data suggests that reduced afterload is not responsible for the 30% increase in stroke volume during pregnancy.

Left ventricular muscle stress during systole is determined largely by the product of its radius to wall thickness ratio (r/h) and the simultaneous intraventricular pressure. In pregnancy, the r/h ratio is increased (20). Pressure during systole is determined by the volume of blood in the ventricle, its rate of ejection, and the impedance of the vascular system. The intraventricular volume and the rate of ejection are increased in pregnancy (20), but the effect of these upon afterload appears to be offset by a diminished aortic impedance. Aortic impedance, in turn, is determined by systemic vascular resistance and aortic compliance. Systemic vascular resistance falls substantially in pregnancy as evidenced by increases in cardiac output and a fall in blood pressure. Recent studies now show that the aorta enlarges and is more compliant in human pregnancy as well (27). These echocardiographic findings have been confirmed by direct measurement of aortic size in the guinea pig (28). During guinea pig pregnancy, the aorta is enlarged and more compliant and aortic impedance is reduced (28).

Five echocardiographic studies revealed mild increases in fractional shortening, ejection fraction, or normalized velocity of shortening or no change in these variables during pregnancy (6, 19–21, 29). These ejection-phase indices of ventricular function are sensitive to changes in both contractility and afterload; they are less sensitive to changes in preload. Accordingly, reduced afterload is unlikely to be important in explaining the 30% increase in stroke volume that occurs in pregnancy. Ejection fraction would need to exceed 90%

in order for either reduced afterload or increased contractility to accomplish an increase in stroke volume of this magnitude.

During pregnancy, a large, relatively thin left ventricle delivers a larger stroke volume to a compliant, low-resistance arterial circuit. Myocardial mechanics and vascular impedance are nicely matched to provide an increased cardiac output at a normal or slightly reduced arterial pressure.

CONTRACTILITY

Direct measurements of the intrinsic strength of contraction in pregnant human subjects are not available. The ejection-phase indices of function previously discussed do not show important changes in contractility. Two studies that used measurements of systolic time intervals have been reported (24, 30); both suggest that small increases in contractility occur early in pregnancy. However, the changes were small and interpretations of their significance were based on repeated applications of the t-test. If the statistical significance of these findings is in doubt, their functional importance is clear: changes in contractility that do not increase ejection fraction cannot, by themselves, increase stroke volume. Contractility changes may be more important in other species. Buttrick and colleagues (31) have shown convincingly, in the rat, that pregnancy results in increased contractility associated with increased calcium-activated myosin and actin-activated ATPase activities.

HEART SIZE

The important cardiac change during pregnancy, then, is an increase in heart size. Circumstantial evidence for this assertion comes from echocardiographic studies showing that the internal diameter of the left ventricle enlarges during pregnancy (6, 20, 21, 29). From our knowledge of filling pressure and the steep relationship between left ventricular pressure and volume, an increased filling pressure can be excluded as the mechanism causing left ventricular end-diastolic volume to increase by 30%. Investigation of pregnancy in a laboratory animal was necessary to evaluate this phenomenon further.

In guinea pigs, pregnancy is associated with a "rightward shift" of the left ventricular pressure-volume relationship; at a constant filling pressure, left ventricular volume is increased about 25% at term, compared with weight-matched controls (32); hypertrophy was not present. A subsequent study showed progressive left ventricular enlargement during guinea pig pregnancy (33). In addition, chronic estrogen administration to nonpregnant animals produced hemodynamic changes and cardiac enlargement similar to pregnancy, suggesting a hormonal mechanism for these important adaptations to pregnancy (33). A human echocardiographic study suggested that left ventricular enlargement may occur even during the transient elevations of estrogen during Pergonal administration (34). Finally, Giraud et al. (35) and Jacobson et al. (36) have recently shown conclusive evidence in chronically instrumented ewes that estrogen administration causes rapid ventricular remodelling.

In humans, it is uncertain whether there is important hypertrophy associated with cardiac enlargement in pregnancy. Katz et al. (20) showed a mild 13% increase in left ventricular mass, while Robson et al. reported a 30% (37) and 50% (6) increase in left ventricular mass at term. The latter numbers are difficult for us to accept. Wall thickness measurements by echocardiography are difficult and a different technique such as magnetic resonance imaging may be necessary to resolve this issue in humans. It is interesting that the guinea pig, which has uterine contents approaching 50% of maternal nonpregnant mass, has no change in left ventricular mass during pregnancy (32).

BLOOD VOLUME

Blood volume increases are also substantial during human pregnancy. Blood volume rises to values approximately 40–50% above control with a peak in the middle of the third trimester (38). Increases in blood volume appear to be related to the total fetal mass; thus, maternal blood volume varies with the size of the single fetus and with the number of fetuses (39). Conversely, women with a history of poor reproductive performance may have smaller blood volume increases than normal. Plasma volume increases relatively more than total hemoglobin during pregnancy, resulting in a fall in the measured hematocrit. Longo (40) proposed that the fetus and placenta regulate maternal blood volume by a feedback system that optimizes fetal development. In this scenario, estrogen production is supported by the fetal adrenal, which produces the major estrogen substrate dehydroepiandrosterone in great quantity. Estrogens, in turn, stimulate the production of renin in the liver. Increased renin production results in increased aldosterone that, in turn, increases plasma volume through renal sodium reabsorption and water retention. Other hormones, including chorionic somatomammotropin, prolactin, and progesterone, stimulate erythropoiesis and are responsible for the increase in red cell mass and total hemoglobin.

VASCULAR AND CARDIAC PRESSURES

The substantial increases in blood volume and cardiac output during pregnancy are not associated with increases in either venous or arterial pressures (1). In fact, arterial blood pressure falls during pregnancy with a decrease of approximately 10 mm Hg of mean arterial pressure by the middle of the second trimester (41). Pulse pressure is increased because diastolic pressure falls more than systolic pressure. Maternal arterial pressure normally rises to nonpregnant levels by parturition.

The lack of change in venous pressures during pregnancy is surprising. It is well known that the mean circulatory filling pressure (MCFP), the equilibrium pressure in the circulation following sudden cessation of cardiac activity, is linearly related to blood volume (42).

Because blood volume increases 40–50% during pregnancy, one would expect a proportional increase in MCFP to occur. Although two studies have concluded that MCFP is mildly elevated in pregnant anesthetized animals (43, 44), we have been unable to confirm these findings in chronically instrumented awake guinea pigs (45). In these animals, MCFP is unchanged in pregnancy although it is mildly elevated during chronic estrogen administration. The reason that MCFP is not increased despite increased blood volume is that vascular capacitance and compliance are increased during guinea pig pregnancy. Chronic estrogen administration also results in increased vascular capacitance and blood volume, suggesting a hormonal mechanism for these changes in the guinea pig. Thus, blood volume and vascular capacitance are increased in parallel and vascular filling pressures remain unchanged. It is, therefore, not possible to predict hemodynamic responses during pregnancy from acute increases in blood volume in nonpregnant animals. In human pregnancy, venous pressure below the uterus is increased (46) and undoubtedly some of the increase in vascular capacitance in human pregnancy resides in the enlarged pelvic veins and veins distal to the uterus. Nevertheless, pregnancy, estrogen, and progesterone have been reported to affect venous pressure-volume relations in the forearms of humans (47, 48). It is, therefore, possible that a sex steroid-mediated effect on vascular capacitance and compliance occurs during pregnancy.

Thus, while the initial impression of the circulation during pregnancy is one of plethora, several factors may conspire to limit venous return during human pregnancy. The first is that vascular capacitance and compliance may be increased negating the effect of increased blood volume on venous return. The second is that increased vascular capacitance and compliance on the lower extremities of humans may result in substantial reduction in venous return in the upright posture due to regional venous pooling. Lastly, the mechanical effects of the pregnant uterus may greatly add to regional venous pooling in postures other than lateral recumbency. These possibilities deserve further attention because maternal cardiovascular homeostasis and presumably fetal growth and development are dependent upon successful maintenance of maternal venous return. In addition, the ability to increase and sustain increases in venous return during upright exercise will be a crucial factor in determining maternal exercise capacity.

REGIONAL BLOOD FLOW

Burwell (49) noted earlier in this century the close resemblance between the circulation during pregnancy and in patients with arteriovenous fistula. The site of the "fistula" during pregnancy was thought to be the placenta. It is now apparent that the increases in cardiac output and uterine blood flow are out of phase in humans (50–52) and in guinea pigs (33). Cardiac output increases early in pregnancy and in excess of increases in uterine blood flow. Late in pregnancy, uterine blood flow increases rapidly while cardiac output has plateaued. Thus, early in pregnancy, blood flow to tissues other than the uterus is increased. Increased blood volume and cardiovascular remodelling produce an account that can be drawn upon as pregnancy progresses. The distribution of nonuterine blood flow in early and midpregnancy is uncertain; however, kidneys (53), skin (54), and breasts (55) are recipients of increased flow. Late in pregnancy, as uterine blood flow continues to rise, redistribution of cardiac output to the uterus from areas previously receiving excess flow occurs because cardiac output does not continue to increase. The mechanisms for the early decrease in regional vascular resistances and for the increases that result in redistribution of cardiac output to the uterus in late gestation remain to be defined.

MECHANISMS

Having acknowledged that the changes in the circulation during pregnancy are still incompletely defined, we can only speculate on the mechanisms that bring them about. One point seems clear; the cardiovascular changes of pregnancy cannot be attributed entirely to increased maternal blood flow to the uterus. Reductions in peripheral vascular resistance and increases in cardiac output and blood volume all antedate important changes in uterine blood flow. It has been demonstrated that hormonal factors are implicated in the cardiovascular adaptions to pregnancy. The hemodynamic changes that occur early in pregnancy appear to establish a circulatory reserve that can be drawn upon later in gestation to satisfy the needs of the developing fetus in the uterus.

A crucial step toward understanding cardiocirculatory physiology during pregnancy will be taken when we learn whether the generalized enlargement of the system results from plethora or is a parallel rather than a cause-and-effect phenomenon. Conventional physiological dogma would favor the former: blood volume increases in pregnancy (38); increased venous return and cardiac output follow from well-developed mechanisms (56). We are not convinced that parameters that function as powerful short-term regulators of the cardiovascular system are responsible for the major long-term adaptations of pregnancy. We support the thesis that hormonal changes early in pregnancy evoke a decrease in vascular resistance and increases in venous and arterial capacitance and heart size: simultaneously, blood volume rises and cardiac output is increased.

In the third trimester, resting cardiac output is very variable, depending upon body position. The enlarged uterus, and the distensible large veins that must drain past it, encourage venous pooling: as a result, cardiac output may fall to or below postpartum levels. The implications of this observation are clear. When cardiac output falls, the maternal organism is forced to choose between maintaining uterine blood flow at the expense of maternal tissue, or placing fetal health in jeopardy. Because women spend the majority of their time, even in the third trimester, in positions other than lateral recumbency, the maternal blood supply to the uterus probably becomes increasingly variable toward term, as venous return becomes more vulnerable.

Acknowledgments—This work was supported by NIH grants HD10034 and R01 HL40041. The advice, support, and nurturing of Dr. James Metcalfe is gratefully acknowledged. Manuscript preparation by Jean Matsumoto is greatly appreciated.

REFERENCES

1. Bader RA, Bader ME, Rose DJ, Braunwald E. Hemodynamics at rest and during exercise in normal pregnancy as studied by cardiac catheterization. J Clin Invest 1955; 35:1524–1536.
2. Roy SB, Malkani PK, Virik R, Bhatia ML. Circulatory

effects of pregnancy. Am J Obstet Gynecol 1966; 96:221–225.

3. Walters WAW, MacGregor WG, Hills M. Cardiac output at rest during pregnancy and the puerperium. Clin Sci 1966; 30:1–11.

4. Ueland K, Novy MJ, Peterson EN, Metcalfe J. Maternal cardiovascular dynamics: IV. The influence of gestational age on the maternal cardiovascular response to posture and exercise. Am J Obstet Gynecol 1969; 104:856–864.

5. Atkins AFJ, Watt JM, Milan P, Davies P, Crawford JS. A longitudinal study of cardiovascular dynamic changes throughout pregnancy. Europ J Obstet Gynecol Reprod Biol 1981; 12:215–224.

6. Robson SC, Hunter S, Boys RJ, Dunlop W. Serial study of factors influencing changes in cardiac output during human pregnancy. Am J Physiol 1989; 256:H1060-H1065.

7. Selzer A, Sudrann RB. Reliability of the determination of cardiac output in man by means of the Fick principle. Circ Res 1958; 6:485–490.

8. Hamilton WF, Riley RL, Attyah AM, Cournand A, Fowell DM, Himmelstein A, Noble RP, Remington JW, Richards DW Jr, Wheeler NC, Whitham AC. Comparison of the Fick and dye injection methods of measuring the cardiac output in man. Am J Physiol 1948; 153:309–321.

9. Ganz W, Donoso R, Marcus HS, Forrester JS, Swann HJC. A new technique for measurement of cardiac output by thermodilution in man. Am J Cardiol 1971; 27:392–396.

10. Petrini MF, Peterson BT, Hyde RW: Lung tissue volume and blood flow by rebreathing: theory. J Appl Physiol 1978; 44:795–802.

11. Stewart WJ, Jiang L, Mich R, Pandian N, Guerrero JL, Weyman AE. Variable effects of changes in flow rate through the aortic, pulmonary and mitral valves on valve area and flow velocity: impact on quantitative Doppler flow calculations. J Am Coll Cardiol 1985; 6:653–662.

12. Sahn DJ. Determination of cardiac output by echocardiographic Doppler methods: Relative accuracy of various sites for measurement. J Am Coll Cardiol 1985; 6:663–664.

13. Kronik G, Slany J, Mosslacher H. Comparative value of eight M-mode echocardiographic formulas for determining left ventricular stroke volume: A correlative study with thermodilution and left ventricular single-plane cineangiography. Circulation 1979; 60:1308–1316.

14. Starling MR, Crawford MH, Sorenson SG, Levi B, Richards KL, O'Rourke RA. Comparative accuracy of apical biplane cross-sectional echocardiography and gated equilibrium radionuclide angiography for estimating left ventricular size and performance. Circulation 1981; 63:1075–1084.

15. Kubicek WG, Kottke FJ, Ramos MU, Patterson RP, Witsoe DA, Labree JW, Remole W, Layman TE, Schoening H, Garamella JT. The Minnesota impedance cardiograph—theory and applications. Biomed Engineer 1974; 9:410–416.

16. DeSwiet M, Talbert DG. The measurement of cardiac output by electrical impedance plethysmography in pregnancy. Are the assumptions valid? Br J Obstet Gynaecol 1986; 93:721–726.

17. Kerr MG, Scott DB, Samuel E. Studies of the inferior vena cava in late pregnancy. Br Med J 1964; 1:532–533.

18. Lees MM, Taylor SH, Scott DB, Kerr MG. A study of cardiac output at rest throughout pregnancy. J Obstet Gynaecol Br Commonw 1967; 74:319–328.

19. Mashini IS, Albazzaz SJ, Fadel HE, Abdulla AM, Hadi HA, Harp R, Devoe LD. Serial noninvasive evaluation of cardiovascular hemodynamics during pregnancy. Am J Obstet Gynecol 1987; 156:1208–1213.

20. Katz R, Karliner JS, Resnick R. Effects of a natural volume overload state (pregnancy) on left ventricular performance in normal human subjects. Circulation 1978; 58:434–441.

21. Laird-Meeter K, van de Ley G, Bom TH, Wladimiroff JW, Roelandt J. Cardiocirculatory adjustments during pregnancy: an echocardiographic study. Clin Cardiol 1979; 2:328–332.

22. Kerr MG. The mechanical effects of the gravid uterus in late pregnancy. J Obstet Gynaecol Br Commonw 1965; 72:513–529.

23. Braunwald E, Ross J Jr, Sonnenblick EH, eds. Mechanisms of contraction of the normal and failing heart, 2nd ed. Boston: Little, Brown & Co, 1979.

24. Burg JR, Dodek A, Kloster FE, Metcalfe J. Alterations of systolic time intervals during pregnancy. Circulation 1974; 49:560–564.

25. Clapp JF III: Maternal heart rate in pregnancy. Am J Obstet Gynecol 1985; 152:659–660.

26. Parker JO, Case RB. Normal left ventricular function. Circulation 1979; 60:4–11.

27. Hart MV, Morton MJ, Hosenpud JD, Metcalfe J. Aortic function during normal human pregnancy. Am J Obstet Gynecol 1986; 154:887–891.

28. Hart MV, Morton MJ, Gade JN. Aortic remodelling during guinea pig pregnancy. Soc Gynecol Invest Scientif Abstr, 36th Annual Meeting, San Diego, March 15–18, 1989; p 165.

29. Rubler S, Damani PM, Pinto ER. Cardiac size and performance during pregnancy estimated with echocardiography. Am J Cardiol 1977; 40:534–540.

30. Rubler S, Schneebaum R, Hammer N. Systolic time intervals in pregnancy and the postpartum period. Am Heart J 1973; 86:182–188.

31. Buttrick PM, Schaible TF, Malhotra A, Mattioli S, Scheuer J. Effects of pregnancy on cardiac function and myosin enzymology in the rat. Am J Physiol 1987; 252:H846–H850.

32. Morton M, Tsang H, Hohimer R, Ross D, Thornburg K, Faber J, Metcalfe J. Left ventricular size, output and structure during guinea pig pregnancy. Am J Physiol 1984; 246:R40–R48.

33. Hart MV, Hosenpud JD, Hohimer AR, Morton MJ. Hemodynamics during pregnancy and sex steroid administration in guinea pigs. Am J Physiol 1985; 249:R179–R185.

34. Veille JC, Morton MJ, Burry K, Nemeth M, Speroff L. Estradiol and hemodynamics during ovulation induction. J Clin Endocrinol Metab 1986; 63:721–724.

35. Giraud GD, Morton MJ, Davis LE, Paul MS, Thornburg KL. Estrogen-induced rapid ventricular remodelling in the ewe. Submitted for publication 1989.

36. Jacobson S-L, Giraud GD, Morton MJ, Thornburg KL. The ewe, a model for the study of cardiac adaptations during estrogen administration and hypertension. Soc Gynecol Invest Scientif Abstr, 36th Annual Meeting, San Diego, March 15–18, 1989; p 176.

37. Robson SC, Hunter S, Moore M, Dunlop W. Haemodynamic changes during the puerperium: a Dop-

pler and M-mode echocardiographic study. Br J Obstet Gynaecol 1987; 94:1028–1039.

38. Hytten FE, Paintin DB. Increase in plasma volume during normal pregnancy. J Obstet Gynaecol Br Commonw 1963; 70:402–407.

39. Letsky E. The haematological system. In Hytten F, Chamberlain G, eds. Clinical Physiology in Obstetrics. Oxford: Blackwell, 1980.

40. Longo LD. Maternal blood volume and cardiac output during pregnancy: a hypothesis of endocrinologic control. Am J Physiol 1983; 245:R720–R729.

41. MacGillivray I, Rose GA, Rowe B. Blood pressure survey in pregnancy. Clin Sci 1969; 37:395–407.

42. Rothe CF. Reflex control of veins and vascular capacitance. Physiol Rev 1983; 63:1281–1342.

43. Douglas BH, Harlan JC, Langford HG, Richardson TQ. Effect of hypervolemia and elevated arterial pressure on circulatory dynamics of pregnant animals. Am J Obstet Gynecol 1967; 98:889–894.

44. Goodlin RC, Niebauer MJ, Holmberg MJ, Zucker IM. Mean circulatory filling pressure in pregnant rabbits. Am J Obstet Gynecol 1984; 148:224–225.

45. Davis LE, Hohimer AR, Giraud GD, Paul MS, Morton MJ. Vascular pressure-volume relationships in pregnant and estrogen-treated guinea pigs. Am J Physiol 1989; 257:R1205–R1211.

46. Ferris EB Jr, Wilkins RW. The clinical value of comparative measurements of the pressure in the femoral and cubital veins. Am Heart J 1937; 13:431–439.

47. Fawer R, Dettling A, Weihs D, Welti H, Schelling JL. Effect of the menstrual cycle, oral contraception and pregnancy on forearm blood flow, venous distensibility and clotting factors. Europ J Clin Pharmacol 1978; 13:251–257.

48. Goodrich SM, Wood JE: Peripheral venous distensibility and velocity of venous blood flow during pregnancy or during oral contraceptive therapy. Am J Obstet Gynecol 1964; 90:740–744.

49. Burwell CS. The placenta as a modified arteriovenous fistula, considered in relation to the circulatory adjustments to pregnancy. Am J Med Sci 1938; 195:1–7.

50. Assali NS, Rauramo L, Peltonen T. Measurement of uterine blood flow and uterine metabolism: VIII. Uterine and fetal blood flow and oxygen consumption in early human pregnancy. Am J Obstet Gynecol 1960; 79:86–98.

51. Metcalfe J, Romney SL, Ramsey LH, Reid DE, Burwell CS. Estimation of uterine blood flow in normal human pregnancy at term. J Clin Invest 1955; 34:1632–1638.

52. Lunell NO, Nylund LE, Lewander R, Sarby B. Uteroplacental blood flow in pre-eclampsia measurements with indium-113m and a computer-linked gamma camera. Clin Exp Hypertension (B) 1982; 1:105–117.

53. Lindheimer MD, Katz AI. The kidney in pregnancy. N Engl J Med 1970; 283:1095–1097.

54. Myhrman P, Jansson I, Lundgren Y. Skin blood flow in normal pregnancy measured by venous occlusion plethysmography of the hand. Acta Obstet Gynecol Scand 1980; 59:107–110.

55. Pickles VR. Blood flow estimations as indices of mammary activity. J Obstet Gynaecol Br Emp 1953; 60:301–311.

56. Guyton AC, Coleman TG, Granger HJ. Circulation: Overall regulation. Ann Rev Physiol 1972; 34:13–46.

6

Placental Oxygen Transfer with Considerations for Maternal Exercise

Brian J. Koos, Gordon G. Power, and Lawrence D. Longo

The fetus requires virtually a continuous supply of oxygen to maintain normal metabolism, growth, and development. Averaging 8 ml·min^{-1}·kg^{-1}, this oxygen requirement is derived from the maternal circulation by diffusion across the placenta. Questions arise as to what controls placental oxygen transfer under normal conditions, and how it might be affected by maternal exercise.

A number of factors contribute to oxygen transfer across the placenta and are summarized in Table 6.1. Some of these include: maternal and fetal arterial O_2 partial pressures, maternal and fetal hemoglobin affinities for O_2, maternal and fetal placental hemoglobin flow rates, the diffusing capacity of the placenta, the vascular relations of maternal to fetal vessels, and the quantity of carbon dioxide exchanged (1). This chapter will explore the role of each of these variables on oxygen transfer and identify the factors

that normally limit oxygen exchange across the placenta. The possible effects of maternal exercise on these transfer mechanisms will also be discussed.

MATERNAL BLOOD

Hemoglobin

The fetus receives oxygen by diffusion from the maternal circulation into fetal blood. Hemoglobin in maternal blood contributes considerably to the transfer of oxygen across the placenta.

Oxygen Affinity

Reduced hemoglobin binds with oxygen to form oxyhemoglobin. Because this binding is reversible, hemoglobin is able to unload oxygen as the O_2 partial pressure decreases. The ability of hemoglobin to bind oxygen depends not only upon the oxygen partial pressure but also upon the affinity of hemoglobin

Table 6.1. Major Factors Affecting Placental Oxygen Transfer

Mother	Placenta	Fetus
Arterial P_{O_2} Inspired P_{O_2} Alveolar ventilation Mixed venous P_{O_2} Pulmonary blood flow and diffusing capacity	Diffusing capacity Area O_2 diffusivity Hb reaction rates Thickness O_2 solubility	Arterial P_{O_2} Umbilical venous P_{O_2} Fetal O_2 consumption Peripheral blood flow Maternal arterial P_{O_2} Maternal placental Hg flow Placental diffusing capacity
Hb O_2 affinity pH Temperature P_{CO_2} 2,3-DPG concentration CO concentration	Spatial relation of maternal to fetal flow	Hb O_2 affinity pH temperature P_{CO_2} 2,3-DPG concentration CO concentration
Placental Hb flow rate Arterial pressure Placental vascular resistance Venous pressure Blood O_2 capacity	Amount of CO_2 exchange	Placental Hb flow rate Umbilical arterial pressure Umbilical venous pressure Placental vascular resistance Blood O_2 capacity

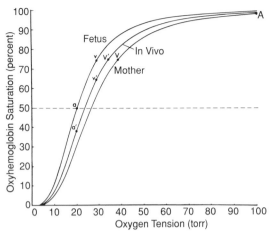

Figure 6.1. Oxyhemoglobin saturation curve under standard conditions for human maternal and fetal blood. Maternal arterial and venous values are indicated by *A* and *V*, respectively, while umbilical arterial and venous figures are represented by *a* and *v*. Maternal venous, and umbilical arterial and venous values that probably occur in vivo are indicated by *V'*, *a'*, and *v'*, respectively.

for O_2, as indicated by the sigmoid-shaped oxyhemoglobin saturation curve (2).

The P_{50} describes the partial pressure of oxygen required to half saturate hemoglobin. Under standard conditions (pH 7.4, $P_{CO_2} = 40$ torr, 37°C) the P_{50} for normal adult human blood is 26.5 torr (Fig. 6.1). However, under other conditions the position of the oxygen dissociation curve (and P_{50}) may be changed. For example, the curve shifts to the right in association with increased concentrations of CO_2, hydrogen ion (H^+), 2,3-diphosphoglycerate (2,3-DPG), adenosine triphosphate (ATP), or chloride ion. The P_{50} of maternal blood remains unchanged or is increased slightly when compared to nonpregnant values (3–8).

Oxygen Capacity

The capacity of blood for oxygen is the maximum amount of oxygen that can reversibly bind with hemoglobin. The nonpregnant woman has a hemoglobin concentration of about $14 \text{ g} \times \text{dl}^{-1}$ and an oxygen capacity of $19.1 \text{ ml} \times \text{dl}^{-1}$. During pregnancy, the red cell mass increases about 25% while plasma volume increases even more at 54% (9). As a result of this hemodilution, the hemoglobin

concentration decreases to about $12 \text{ g} \times \text{dl}^{-1}$ with an oxygen capacity of $16.4 \text{ ml} \times \text{dl}^{-1}$ (10).

FETAL BLOOD

Oxygen Affinity

In humans (11) and several other species (12–15), the fetal hemoglobin dissociation curve is shifted to the left compared to that of maternal blood under standard conditions. Figure 6.1 shows that the P_{50} for human fetal blood equals about 20 torr (5).

Under physiological conditions in vivo the fetal oxyhemoglobin curve is shifted to the right as it is slightly acidotic (pH 7.34) and hypercarbic ($P_{CO_2} = 45$ torr) as compared to standard conditions (Fig. 6.1).

Oxygen Capacity

The fetal hemoglobin concentration in humans increases from about $8.5 \text{ g} \times \text{dl.s}^{-1}$ at 10 weeks of gestation (16, 17) to a mean value of about $16.5 \text{ g} \times \text{dl}^{-1}$ at term. During this time the maternal hemoglobin concentration decreases from about 13 to $11.5 \text{ g} \times \text{dl}^{-1}$. As a result, the oxygen capacity of fetal blood exceeds that of maternal blood during the last trimester.

INTERRELATIONS OF MATERNAL AND FETAL O_2 DISSOCIATION CURVES

Oxygen Affinity

Figure 6.1 shows the oxyhemoglobin dissociation curves for human maternal and near-term fetal blood. Notice that under physiological conditions in vivo the fetal curve shifts to the right while the maternal curve shifts to the left. As a result, the maternal and fetal dissociation curves are probably nearly identical. These departures from the standard dissociation curves largely result from the slightly alkalotic and hypercarbic maternal blood and slightly acidotic and hypercarbic fetal blood. The greater temperature of the fetus (0.5°C) relative to the mother also contributes to similar oxyhemoglobin dissociation curves in vivo.

O_2 Saturation

Figure 6.2 depicts the O_2 content for human maternal and fetal blood as a function

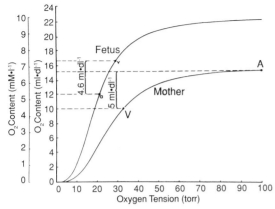

Figure 6.2. Oxygen content as a function of oxygen tension for maternal and fetal blood. The letters *A* and *V* represent values for maternal arterial and venous blood, while *a* and *v* represent those for umbilical arterial and venous blood, respectively.

of the oxygen partial pressure. This shows that normal fetal umbilical venous P_{O_2} of only about 28 torr is associated with O_2 content of $16.5 \text{ ml} \times \text{dl}^{-1}$, a value that actually exceeds the maternal content of $15.4 \text{ ml} \times \text{dl}^{-1}$. This occurs despite the fetal hemoglobin being only 75% saturated compared to 98% in the adult because of the higher O_2 capacity (greater hemoglobin concentration) of fetal blood.

The oxyhemoglobin saturation of maternal and fetal blood has important implications for placental oxygen transfer. An increase of either maternal or fetal O_2 capacity will promote placental O_2 exchange (1, 18). All other factors remaining constant, the larger the sum of maternal and fetal blood O_2 capacities, the more oxygen will be exchanged before equilibrium is reached.

Effects of Respiratory Gas Exchange

BOHR EFFECT

As fetal blood courses through the placental exchange vessels, hydrogen ions and CO_2 diffuses across the placenta resulting in a fall in P_{CO_2} and a rise in pH. This results in maternal blood becoming more acidotic and hypercarbic as it passes through the exchange areas. This increase in hydrogen ions in maternal blood shifts the oxyhemoglobin dissociation curve to the right, making more

oxygen available for transfer, while in fetal blood, the decreased hydrogen ion concentration shifts the dissociation curve to the left, promoting O_2 uptake by fetal hemoglobin. Theoretical studies by Hill and associates (19) suggest that this mechanism accounts for about 8% of the oxygen transferred to the fetus.

HALDANE EFFECT

As a result of this exchange process, the deoxyhemoglobin concentration in maternal blood increases while that in fetal blood decreases. Deoxyhemoglobin binds CO_2 to a greater extent than oxyhemoglobin; consequently, the increased concentrations of deoxyhemoglobin in maternal blood and decreased levels in fetal red cells promote CO_2 transfer from fetal to maternal blood. In fact, this "double Haldane effect" is calculated to account for 46% of placental exchange of carbon dioxide (20).

TRANSPLACENTAL DIFFUSION

Maternal and Fetal Oxygen Tensions

As shown in Table 6.1, placental oxygen exchange depends upon a number of factors. One important variable is the mean O_2 partial pressure difference between maternal and fetal exchange vessels. In fetal sheep, umbilical venous oxygen tension usually has been found to be 10–20 torr less than uterine venous values (21). But in humans the difference between umbilical and uterine venous P_{O_2} has been reported to be only about 2 torr less than that of uterine venous blood (22). These P_{O_2} measurements in humans may not reflect steady state values because the blood samples were collected at the time of cesarean section (23).

A number of factors theoretically could affect placental oxygen transfer and could account for the P_{O_2} gradient between umbilical and uterine venous blood. Such factors include the geometric relation of fetal vessels to maternal blood in the exchange areas (Fig. 6.3) and placental shunts in which arterial blood (uterine or umbilical) enters the venous circulation without passing through exchange areas. Placental blood flow in local-

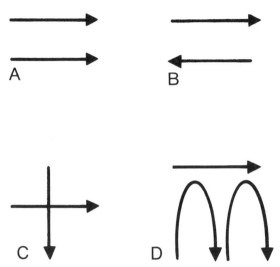

Figure 6.3.   Possible relationships of maternal and fetal blood flow within placental exchange vessels. *A,* Concurrent; *B,* countercurrent; *C,* crosscurrent, and *D,* pool flow.

ized areas of the placenta may not be the same for maternal and fetal blood. These perfusion-perfusion inequalities could also account for the greater O_2 tension in uterine venous blood than in umbilical venous blood.

Placental Diffusing Capacity

Unlike oxygen and carbon dioxide, carbon monoxide (CO) transfer across the lung and other membranes is limited by diffusion rather than blood flow. This diffusion limitation has been used to determine the CO-diffusing capacity in the lung as an index of the efficiency of pulmonary gas exchange (24), and Longo et al. (25) has applied this method to quantify gas exchange across the placenta.

Placental diffusing capacity depends upon the membrane diffusion characteristics of the placenta, such as the area, permeability, diffusivity, and thickness of the placenta. Expressed per gram of fetal weight, the placental diffusing capacity of the sheep of about $0.55 \ \text{ml} \cdot \text{min}^{-1} \cdot \text{torr}^{-1}$ (25, 26) is similar to that of the monkey (27) but significantly less than that of rodents such as the rat (B.J. Koos, R.D. Gilbert, and L.D. Longo, unpublished data), rabbit (28), and guinea pig (29, 30). The differences in cellular layers and vascular morphology probably contribute to the observed differences in the capacity for

respiratory gas transport (27). In sheep, the diffusing capacity expressed as per gram fetal weight remains remarkably constant over the last third of gestation (26).

Theoretical calculations using measured placental diffusing capacity for CO in animals has indicated that the placenta is very permeable to oxygen (25). In fact, maternal and fetal O_2 tensions are predicted to approach equilibrium during the course of a single capillary transit. Thus, under normal conditions, uteroplacental blood flow limits the total quantity of oxygen exchanged each minute across the placenta, and not the diffusion rate through the membranes.

EFFECT OF VARYING FACTORS AFFECTING OXYGEN TRANSFER

The previous discussion relates oxygen transfer to the fetus under normal conditions. However, the question arises as to what extent varying individual factors important in respiratory gas exchange affect oxygen tranfer. Such predictions can be made using mathematical equations describing placental O_2 transfer (1). An understanding of the relative importance of variables affecting placental O_2 exchange can also be determined experimentally. The observed changes in O_2 transfer would result from the experimentally altered variable as well as compensatory changes in other factors that might occur to limit the change in placental O_2 exchange.

Placental Diffusing Capacity

Under normal conditions placental diffusing capacity does not limit the rate of oxygen transfer across the placenta. However, theoretically, oxygen transfer could be affected if the diffusing capacity was reduced below a critical value. The effect on fetal blood gases of reducing the placental diffusing capacity in sheep by embolizing the uteroplacental vascular bed with microspheres was examined by Boyle et al. (31). Fetal arterial O_2 tensions did not significantly decrease until the placental diffusing capacity becomes critical at values about one-half that of normal. However, this effect may not be solely the result of reduced diffusing capacity because decreased placental blood flow and/or increased perfusion-perfusion inequalities might also have contributed. Clinically, these results suggest that decreased placental diffusing capacity in humans resulting from edematous villi associated with syphilis or erythroblastosis fetalis would have little effect on placental O_2 transfer. Moreover, they indicate that a large portion of the placenta must be affected by abruption or infarction before the normal fetus is seriously jeopardized.

Arterial Oxygen Tension

MATERNAL OXYGEN TENSION

The extent to which changes in maternal P_{O_2} affect fetal O_2 tensions depends upon the shape of the maternal and fetal oxyhemoglobin saturation curves (Fig. 6.1). For example, reducing the maternal arterial P_{O_2} from normal values (95–100 torr) to about 70 torr results in only about a 5% decrease in the oxyhemoglobin concentration of maternal blood. Such moderate reductions in maternal arterial O_2 tension may occur with high altitude or pneumonia and would be expected to have only a small effect on placental oxygen transfer and fetal arterial P_{O_2}. Further uncompensated decreases in maternal P_{O_2} are associated with much larger reductions in oxyhemoglobin concentrations and, consequently, a fall in fetal arterial oxygen tensions.

The effect of uncompensated changes in maternal arterial O_2 tensions on placental oxygen transfer has been determined experimentally by Power and Jenkins (32). Using an isolated placental cotyledon preparation, these investigators showed that the effect on oxygen exchange of increases in maternal arterial oxygen tension was minor for values greater than 70 torr, whereas a significant reduction in umbilical venous oxygen tensions occurred when maternal P_{O_2} fell below 70 torr (Fig. 6.4).

UMBILICAL ARTERIAL **PO_2**

Once fetal blood has left the placenta and supplied the fetal tissues it returns to the placenta in the umbilical arteries. Thus umbilical arterial oxygen tension is a function predominantly of placental oxygen transfer,

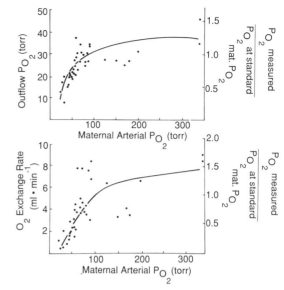

Figure 6.4.   The effect of changes in maternal arterial P_{O_2} on umbilical venous O_2 tension and exchange rate across the placenta. Samples were collected from isolated cotyledons perfused at constant umbilical flow. (From Power GG, and Jenkins F. Factors affecting O_2 transfer in sheep and rabbit placenta perfused in situ. Am J Physiol 1975;229:1147–1153.

umbilical venous O_2 tension, and fetal oxygen consumption. However, umbilical arterial P_{O_2} itself is also a major determinant of placental O_2 transfer. As umbilical arterial P_{O_2} decreases, the transplacental O_2 tension gradient increases, resulting in an increase in placental oxygen exchange rate and a fall in the end-capillary O_2 tension. Conversely, increasing umbilical arterial oxygen tension reduces the transplacental oxygen gradient and lowers the oxygen exchange rate. Theoretically, percent changes in umbilical arterial P_{O_2} affect placental oxygen transfer rate and end-capillary oxygen tension to a greater extent than similar changes in any other determinant of oxygen exchange (1). The importance of umbilical arterial oxygen tensions on transplacental oxygen transfer has also been shown experimentally by in situ perfusion of isolated cotyledons in sheep (32), as shown in Figure 6.5.

Placental Blood Flows

Oxygen transfer across the placenta depends to a great extent on the rate of placen-

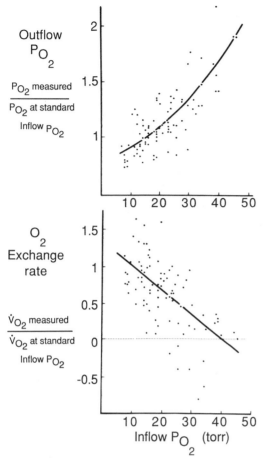

Figure 6.5. Effect of changes in umbilical arterial P_{O_2} on umbilical venous oxygen tension and O_2 exchange rate. Umbilical blood flow through the isolated cotyledon was kept constant. (From Power GG, and Jenkins F. Factors affecting O_2 transfer in sheep and rabbit placenta perfused in situ. Am J Physiol 1975;229:1147–1153.

MATERNAL FLOW

Uteroplacental blood flow increases during pregnancy from 50 ml·min^{-1} at 10 weeks (33) to about 500 ml·min^{-1} at term (34–36b). Evidence from animal studies suggests that 80–90% of this flow supplies the placenta and thus is available for transfer of oxygen and nutrients to the fetus. In the human, blood from spiral arteries enters the intervillous space

and is directed in spurts toward the chorionic plate. As the blood encounters villi it is slowed and flows laterally into venous sinuses.

Experiments in sheep (36a, 37) and monkeys (38) have shown that uterine oxygen uptake varies as a function of uterine blood flow. In sheep, fetal O_2 uptake has a curvilinear relation to changes in flow (21), as shown in Figure 6.6.

The importance of uterine blood flow on fetal oxygenation has many clinical implications. For example, placental blood flow could be reduced in women with vascular disease or pregnancy-induced hypertension. Uterine blood flow also decreases with contractions during labor, and experimental evidence in sheep indicates that the occasional mild contraction that normally occurs before labor can cause transient decreases in oxygen transfer to the fetus (39, 40).

Studies in fetal sheep have shown that reducing umbilical blood flow has little effect on the O_2 saturation of blood in the umbilical vein. However, it did reduce significantly the oxygen content of blood in the descending aorta (41) and umbilical arteries (42). In these studies, the transfer of O_2 to the fetus was found to be highly correlated with umbilical blood flow. In contrast, natural variations in umbilical blood flow (154–444 ml·min^{-1}·kg^{-1}) apparently affect arterio-

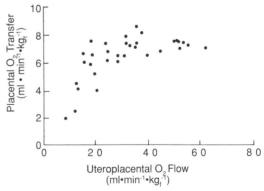

Figure 6.6 Dependence of placental O_2 transfer on uteroplacental O_2 flow. Uteroplacental O_2 delivery normally ranges between 36 and 63 ml·min^{-1}·kg^{-1}. (Redrawn from Wilkening RB, Meschia G. Fetal oxygen uptake, oxygenation, and acid-base balance as a function of uterine blood flow. Am J Physiol 1983;244:H749–H755.

tal blood flow. Both maternal and fetal blood flows contribute to this exchange, and their relative importance to placental oxygen transfer will now be considered.

venous oxygen content without changing oxygen uptake (43).

The importance of umbilical blood flow alone on placental oxygen exchange is difficult to determine in vivo because of compensating changes in other factors that affect oxygen transfer.

In an effort to minimize these problems, Power and Jenkins (32) perfused in situ an isolated cotyledon of the sheep placenta with blood of known oxygen tension and flow rate. Figure 6.7 shows the dependence of venous outflow oxygen tension and oxygen transfer on fetal cotyledonary blood flow. Outflow P_{O_2} varied inversely with cotyledonary blood flow, with higher values at lower rates of flow. In contrast, oxygen exchange rate increased with higher rates of flow.

Fetal placental blood flow normally is

thought to be proportional to the pressure difference between the umbilical arterial and umbilical venous vessels. However, because of the close association of maternal and fetal placental circulations, it is possible that changes in dimensions of one vascular bed might alter the size and thus the resistance of the other. For instance, an increase in the maternal placental blood volume might reduce the volume in fetal exchange vessels. Under these conditions, fetal placental blood flow would be proportional to the fetal inflow pressure minus that of the surrounding maternal blood. Such a "sluice" flow relation in which surrounding pressure affects vascular resistance has been described in the lung (44), and experimental evidence suggests that it also exists in the placenta (45, 46). Other evidence exists for maternal-fetal vascular interaction. For instance, fetal placental vascular compliance in sheep increased with reductions in maternal vascular pressure (47).

As a result of the sluice mechanism, elevations in uterine venous pressure might reduce umbilical blood flow. However, increasing uterine venous pressure to values up to 70 mm Hg had no significant effect on fetal limb umbilical blood flow as measured by an electromagnetic flowmeter (48). This suggests that either the sluice effect in sheep is small compared to the sensitivity of the method used to measure flow or that umbilical flow was maintained by a small rise in umbilical arterial pressure.

Whether or not there is a sluice flow pattern in the human placenta is unknown. It seems likely that fetal capillary tufts in the human placenta are surrounded by maternal blood. This arrangement should result in a greater sluice effect than observed in the sheep where stroma separates maternal and fetal capillaries. At the present time, the clinical significance of sluice flow in the placenta is not known. However, it is most likely to be of importance in postural changes of the mother that result in alterations in intervillous pressure. In the supine position, the pregnant uterus of some women compresses the inferior vena cave (49). This reduces venous return to the heart, resulting in de-

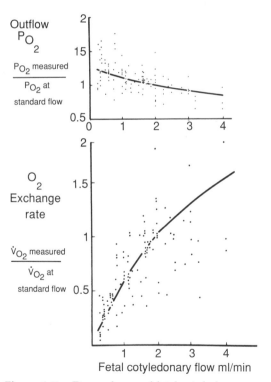

Figure 6.7. Dependence of fetal cotyledonary venous P_{O_2} and placental O_2 exchange rate on fetal cotyledonary blood flow. Umbilical arterial P_{O_2} was kept constant. (From Power GG, Jenkins F. Factors affecting O_2 transfer in sheep and rabbit placenta perfused in situ. Am J Physiol 1975;229:1147–1153.

creased cardiac output and arterial pressure. With caval compression, uterine venous outflow would be impeded, and intervillous pressure should rise. Under these conditions fetal vessels within the placenta would be compressed, resulting in increased vascular resistance and, at least initially, a reduction in fetal placental blood flow. Of course, flow might be maintained in the long-term if fetal umbilical arterial blood pressure increased sufficiently.

Hemoglobin Concentration

Alterations in the hemoglobin concentration of maternal or fetal blood could affect oxygen transfer to the fetus in several ways. For example, decreased hemoglobin concentration reduces the buffer capacity and influences oxygen transfer by the Bohr effect. A reduced hemoglobin concentration also decreases slightly the placental diffusing capacity (50) and theoretically could change the distribution of flow within placental vessels as a result of altered blood viscosity. But, these effects are minor compared to the reduced oxygen-carrying capacity of blood. Because the hemoglobin concentration determines the oxygen-carrying capacity of blood, the amount of oxygen transferred across the placenta depends to a great extent on maternal and fetal hemoglobin concentrations.

MATERNAL HEMOGLOBIN

Oxygen delivery to the placenta equals the product of placental blood flow and the O_2 content of maternal blood. A 50% reduction in maternal hemoglobin concentration would theoretically decrease by the same amount of oxygen delivery to the placenta, assuming uteroplacental blood flow remained unchanged. Therefore, reducing the hemoglobin concentration of maternal blood would be expected to have a similar effect on placental O_2 transfer as decreasing placental blood flow as far as carriage of O_2 (Fig. 6.6), but Wagner has shown that anemia and blood flow have different effects down the capillary (51). However, normal placental oxygen delivery and transfer could be maintained if a compensatory increase occurred in uteroplacental blood flow. In sheep, acute isovolemic

anemia in the ewe significantly reduces O_2 transfer to the fetus when the maternal hematocrit is lowered by at least 50% (52).

FETAL HEMOGLOBIN

Because oxygen-carrying capacity and placental blood flow determine the "oxygen flow" to the placenta, changes in fetal hemoglobin concentrations also would be expected to have similar effects on placental oxygen exchange as do changes in umbilical blood flow (Fig. 6.7). Fetal hemoglobin concentrations in sheep can be lowered more than 50% before the fetus develops a metabolic acidemia (53), and human fetuses with hemolytic anemia may develop a metabolic acidosis and hydrops with fetal hemoglobin concentrations less than 40% of normal (54, 55).

Increased fetal hemoglobin concentrations occur during hypoxia (56) or asphyxia (57). This results from a shift of water from the vascular space to the interstitial fluid compartment that accompanies vasoconstriction of certain fetal vascular beds (58). An increased number of circulating erythrocytes may also contribute. Such an increase in fetal oxygen-carrying capacity should favorably affect placental O_2 transfer under these conditions.

Variation in Hemoglobin Oxygen Affinity

As discussed earlier, hemoglobin oxygen affinity can be affected by a number of factors such as acid-base status, intraerythrocyte concentrations of 2,3-DPG, and temperature. Furthermore, the P_{50} of hemoglobin can differ from normal as the result of inherited abnormalities in hemoglobin production or as a consequence of blood transfusion.

MATERNAL BLOOD

Women with altered blood oxygen affinity due to a hemoglobinopathy apparently can give birth to normal infants. For instance, cases have been reported of women with hemoglobin Ranier ($P_{50} = 12.8$ torr) delivering infants with hemoglobin F and a normal oxygen affinity (59, 60). A normal fetus has also been reported in a mother with hemoglobin McKees Rocks, which has a P_{50} of 10 torr (61). On the other hand, a mother with hemoglobin Yakima ($P_{50} = 12$ torr) had four abortions and three stillbirths in eight pregnancies (62), but the significance of this poor reproductive history is unknown.

FETAL BLOOD

Intrauterine transfusion of the human fetus with adult red cells has developed as part of the modern management of erythroblastosis fetalis (63). In 1970, Mathers et al. (64) reported that adult hemoglobin ($P_{50} = 27.5$ torr) comprised about 75% of the total hemoglobin in newborn infants who had undergone intrauterine transfusion for hemolytic anemia within 2 weeks of delivery. Five of these six infants had a P_{50} that was within 0.5 torr of the maternal value. Novy et al. (65) also have examined the effects of intrauterine transfusion in 15 infants with severe erythroblastosis fetalis. The P_{50} of cord blood in these infants at delivery averaged 27.1 torr, a value about 6 torr greater than the mean of 20.8 in seven erythroblastotic infants who were not transfused. The transfused infants grew normally in utero and were not acidotic at birth. Thus, it is clear that decreased blood oxygen affinity is well tolerated by the human fetus.

The fetus can also survive with blood of increased oxygen affinity. For example, hemoglobin variants compatible with intrauterine development include hemoglobin Ranier ($P_{50} = 12$ torr), hemoglobin Yakima ($P_{50} = 12$ torr), and hemoglobin McKees Rocks ($P_{50} = 10$ torr). However, the fetus does not tolerate blood with very high oxygen affinity such as hemoglobin Bart's ($P_{50} = 3$ torr). This hemoglobin consists of four γ chains (66) and comprises almost all of hemoglobin in α-thalassemia major. This high oxygen affinity prevents oxygen unloading except at very low oxygen tensions and makes it of little use in oxygenating fetal tissues. Therefore, it is not surprising that fetuses with hemoglobin Bart's develop a fatal hydrops fetalis syndrome.

MATERNAL EXERCISE

As indicated previously, placental oxygen exchange is a function of maternal and fetal blood flows, placental blood hemoglobin concentrations, and arterial O_2 tensions. Several other factors affect oxygen exchange as summarized in Table 6.1. The question arises as to which of these factors are altered during maternal exercise and how such changes affect oxygen delivery to the fetus.

Lotgering et al. (67, 68) have studied the effects of exercise on pregnant ewes and their fetuses under chronic experimental conditions. During exercise (70% maximal O_2 consumption) the mean maternal arterial P_{O_2} increased by about 8%, and the maternal hemoglobin concentration rose by about 25%. However, uterine blood flow as measured by an electromagnetic flowmeter decreased by about 21% by the end of exercise period. Despite this fall in uterine blood flow, uteroplacental oxygen delivery remained unchanged as a result of the increase in maternal hemoglobin concentration.

Other changes also accompanied exercise. For example, the control values of maternal (7.45) and fetal (7.33) arterial pH increased slightly to 7.48 and 7.36, respectively. These pH changes would be expected in association with exercise hyperventilation. No significant changes occurred in fetal arterial P_{O_2} or hemoglobin concentration. The temperature of the ewe increased progressively during exercise, reaching a value of about 0.9°C greater than the control mean of 39.2°C at the end of the exercise period. After a recovery period of 20 minutes, the maternal temperature virtually returned to control values. As might be expected, the temperature of the fetus followed the maternal trend during exercise, but with some time lag.

Obviously maternal exercise affects a number of variables that determine oxygen transfer across the placenta. The net effect of these changes on oxygen exchange can be predicted using a mathematical model that describes the relative importance of these factors (1). However, the mathematical analysis requires the numerical solution of many differential equations, which consumes considerable time. In an effort to simplify such calculation, Power and Dale (unpublished data) have reduced the complex mathematical model (69) to an algebraic representation that is more easily applied to determine effects on placental oxygen transfer. As a result, placental oxygen transfer can be pre-

Table 6.2. Placental Diffusing Capacities for Carbon Monoxide[a]

Species	Diffusing Capacity (ml·min^{-1}·torr^{-1}· g fetal wt^{-1})	Reference
Rat	1.74±0.33	—[b]
Guinea pig	3.27±0.10	57
	2.28±0.13	27
Rabbit	2.33±0.21	129
Sheep	0.55±0.02	89
Monkey	0.65±0.06	26

[a]Means ± SEM for at least seven determinations.
[b]Unpublished observations of B. J. Koos, L. D. Longo and R. D. Gilbert.

dicted for changes in the following: maternal and fetal arterial P$_{O_2}$, maternal and fetal hemoglobin concentrations, maternal and fetal arterial pH, maternal and fetal blood flow, and placental diffusing capacity (Table 6.2). The fraction, p, from the standard rate of oxygen transfer may be calculated from the equation:

$$P = A \left(1 - e^{-k\Delta x}\right) \qquad (1)$$

where x is the absolute change in a single variable, and A and k are constants, the values of which depend on the variable. Table 6.3 lists the values of these variables taken as standard for the sheep and the A and k values for each variable. Ranges for each factor along with typical and maximum errors in oxygen transfer rate when compared to

the mathematical model (69) are also shown for changes in each single variable. An oxygen consumption of 24 ml·min^{-1} is taken as standard for a fetus weighting 3 kg.

When more than one factor changes, predictions can be made from the equation:

$$\dot{V}_{O_2} = 24 \pi_{i1}^n (1 + P_i) \qquad (2)$$

when n variables differ from their standard values. Placental oxygen flux ($\dot{V}_{O_2}$) can be predicted by using Equation 1 to calculate pi for i equalling 1 to n. One is added to each pi, and the results are multiplied, given the predicted fraction of the standard $\dot{V}_{O_2}$.

We have simplified the method of determining placental oxygen transfer that was used to predict the effects of exercise on placental oxygen exchange. Values for each variable were taken for control, exercise, and recovery periods for sheep exercising on a treadmill for 10 min at 70% maximum oxygen consumption (67, 68). Maternal and fetal temperature effects were included in the prediction. Placental diffusing capacity was held constant since Lotgering et al. (68) observed no change in diffusing capacity during these experiments in sheep. Fetal placental blood flow was not measured and was assumed constant at 486 ml·min^{-1}. Umbilical arterial P$_{O_2}$ also was unknown and was taken to be the standard value of 20 torr.

Figure 6.8 shows the effects of each variable on the instantaneous oxygen transfer

Table 6.3. Values Relating to Equation 1 for Sheep

Variable	Standard Value	Range	A	k	Typical Error[a]	Maximum Error[a]
Maternal arterial P$_{O_2}$ (torr)	95.0	±30.0	0.02031	0.04998	0.02	0.04
Umbilical arterial P$_{O_2}$ (torr)	20.0	±10.0	−1.839	0.04007	0.75	1.67
Maternal hemoglobin (g·100 ml^{-1})	11.0	±4.0	0.1079	0.1968	0.02	0.03
Fetal hemoglobin (g·100 ml^{-1})	12.0	±4.0	1.053	0.05997	0.02	0.04
Maternal pH	7.40	±0.30	0.1862	−2.017	0.03	0.05
Fetal pH	7.35	±0.30	0.7039	−1.627	0.30	0.53
Maternal blood flow (ml·min^{-1})	486.0	±300	0.1100	0.004555	0.08	0.18
Fetal blood flow (ml·min^{-1})	486.0	±300	0.9967	0.001518	0.11	0.20
Membrane diffusing capacily (ml·min^{-1}·torr^{-1})	2.73	±2.00	0.0005651	2.776	0.08	0.30

[a]Typical error is the standard deviation of the values calculated from Equation 1 about the actual values predicted by the model. Both typical and maximum error are in units of ml·min^{-1} oxygen flux and are valid for the ranges specified.

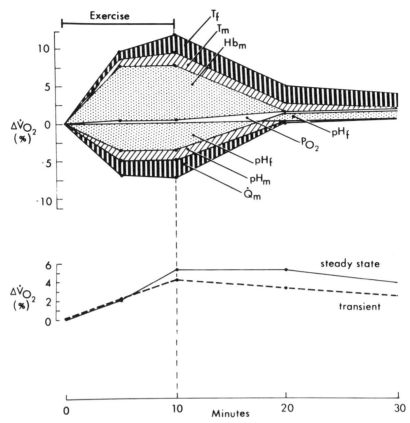

Figure 6.8. Theoretical effects of maternal exercise on placental oxygen transfer. The *top figure* shows the contribution of individual factors to the total increase or decrease in placental O_2 exchange. The *bottom figure* shows the net effect ot these changes on the transient O_2 transfer rate, as compared to changes expected under steady state conditions (T_f=fetal temperature, T_m=maternal temperature, Hb_m= maternal hemoglobin concentration, P_{O_2}=maternal arterial O_2 tension, pH_f=fetal arterial pH, pH_m=maternal arterial pH, and Q_m=uteroplacental blood flow).

rate. Notice that placental oxygen exchange is favorably affected by several factors. After 10 min of exercise, increased maternal hemoglobin concentration accounts for about 60% of this effect, while the rise in maternal and fetal temperatures is responsible for about 15% and 20%, respectively. The increase in maternal P_{O_2} also contributes, but to a lesser extent. During the recovery period, placental O_2 transfer is still favored, principally as the result of increased maternal and fetal temperatures and the slight decrease in fetal pH.

During exercise, other factors tend to reduce oxygen exchange. Decreased uterine blood flow is predicted to contribute about 31% of the total negative effect at 10 minutes. However, this was surprisingly less than the 49% contributed by the small rise in fetal arterial pH. The increase in maternal pH also tended to reduce oxygen transfer.

The net effect of exercise on transient changes in placental oxygen exchange is shown by the broken line in Figure 6.8. Under the conditions described, oxygen transfer is predicted to increase during exercise, reaching a maximum value at the end of the exercise period. During the recovery phase, transient oxygen transfer declines but is still above control values 30 minutes after starting the experiment.

In the steady state, net oxygen transfer equals fetal oxygen consumption. Assuming fetal oxygen consumption remains constant, the umbilical arterial P_{O_2} will rise, lowering placental oxygen exchange to control values. However, if the rise in fetal temperature increases fetal oxygen consumption according to van't Hoff Arrhenius' law (0.3°C rise in temperature results in a 4% increase in oxygen consumption), then net oxygen transfer under steady state conditions would be increased accordingly (Fig. 6.8).

The temperature effects on fetal metabolism theoretically would be greater during longer periods of exercise. For example, the temperature of the fetus rose 1.2°C after 40 minutes of maternal exercise at 70% maximum oxygen consumption as the maternal temperature increased 1.4°C. This temperature rise in the fetus should have increased fetal metabolism by 16%. The physiological changes accompanying exercise of this duration could account for about 6% of the increase in net oxygen transfer under steady state conditions. The remaining 10% could be provided by a 1.3-torr decrease in umbilical arterial P_{O_2}. Although it helps match placental oxygen delivery to fetal oxygen needs, such a decrease in fetal umbilical arterial P_{O_2} should result in a slightly lower umbilical venous P_{O_2}. Such a mechanism might partly explain the slight decrease in fetal arterial P_{O_2} observed at the end of 40 minutes of exercise (68). However, a caveat must be emphasized in that no experimental data exist at the present time on the effect of temperature on metabolic rate in the fetal lamb.

Summarizing, exercise induces profound physiological effects in the mother, some of which, interestingly, augment fetal oxygenation, whereas others depress it. Predominant among the favorable factors is hemoconcentration of maternal blood leading to increased oxygen-carrying capacity. Important negative factors include reduced uterine blood flow and increased pH of maternal and fetal blood. The net effect is predicted to be a balance with little change in oxygen transfer to the fetus. Whether these predictions can be confirmed in humans will require new technology and approaches.

REFERENCES

1. Longo LD, Hill EP, Power GG. Theoretical analysis of factors affecting placental O_2 transfer. Am J Physiol 1972; 222:730–739.
2. Bohr C, Hasselbalch K, Krogh A. Ueber einen in biologischer Bezeihung wichtigen Einfluss, den die Kohlensaurespannung des Blutes auf dessen Sauerstoffbindung ubt. Skand Arch Physiol 1904; 16:402–417.
3. Beer R, Bartels H, Raczkowski HA. Die Sauerstoffdissoziationskurve des fetalen Blutes und der Gasaustausch in der menschlichen Placenta. Pflugers Arch Ges Physiol 1955; 260:306–319.
4. Darling RC, Smith CA, Asmussen E, Cohen FM. Some properties of human fetal and maternal blood. J Clin Invest 1941; 20:739–747.
5. Hellegers AE, Schruefer JJP. Nomograms and empirical equations relating oxygen tension, percentage saturation, and pH in maternal and fetal blood. Am J Obstet Gynecol 1961; 81:377–384.
6. Lucius H, Gahlenbeck H, Kleine HO, Fabel H, Bartels H. Respiratory functions, buffer system, and electrolyte concentrations of blood during human pregnancy. Respir Physiol 1970; 9:311–317.
7. Prystowsky H, Hellergers A, Bruns P. Fetal blood studies; XIV. A comparative study of the oxygen dissociation curve of nonpregnant, pregnant, and fetal human blood. Am J Obstet Gynecol 1959; 78:489–493.
8. Torrance J, Jacobs P, Restrepo A, Eschback J, Lenfant C, Finch CA. Intraerythrocytic adaptation to anemia. N Engl J Med 1970; 283:165–169.
9. Longo LD, Hardesty JS. Maternal blood volume: measurement, hypothesis of control, and clinical considerations. In Scarpelli EM, Cosmi V, eds. Reviews in perinatal medicine. New York: Raven Press, 1985; p 35–59.
10. Pritchard JA, Hunt CF. A comparison of the hematologic responses following the routine prenatal administration of intramuscular and oral iron. Surg Gynecol Obstet 1958; 106:516–518.
11. Eastman NJ, Geilling EMK, Delawdner AM. Foetal blood studies; IV. The oxygen and carbon dioxide dissociation curves of foetal blood. Johns Hopkins Hosp Bull 1933; 53:246–254.
12. Barcroft J. The conditions of foetal respiration. Lancet 1933; 225:1021–1024.
13. Hall FG. A spectroscopic method for the study of haemoglobin in dilute solutions. J Physiol (Lond) 1934; 80:502–507.
14. Hall FG: Haemoglobin function in the developing chick. J Physiol (Lond) 1935; 83:222–228.
15. McCarthy EF. A comparison of foetal and maternal haemoglobins in the goat. J Physiol (Lond) 1934; 80:206–212.
16. Oski TA. Hematological problems. In Avery GB, ed. Neonatology. Pathophysiology and management of the newborn. Philadelphia: JB Lippincott, 1975; p 379–422.
17. Walker J, Turnbull EPN. Haemoglobin and red cells in the human foetus and their relation to the oxygen content of the blood in the vessel of the umbilical cord. Lancet 1953; 2:312–318.
18. Bartels H. Prenatal respiration. Amsterdam: North Holland, 1970.
19. Hill EP, Power GC, Longo LD. A mathematical model of placental O_2 transfer with consideration of hemoglobin reaction rates. Am J Physiol 1972; 222:721–729.
20. Hill EP, Power GG, Longo LD. A mathematical model of carbon dioxide transfer in the placenta and its interaction with oxygen. Am J Physiol 1973; 224:283–299.
21. Wilkening RB, Meschia G. Fetal oxygen uptake,

oxygenation, and acid-base balance as a function of uterine blood flow. Am J Physiol 1983; 244:H749–H755.

22. Wulf H. Der Gasaustausch in der reifen Plazenta des Menschen. Z Geburtshilfe Gynaekol Beilageh 1962; 158:117–134, 269–319.

23. Dawes GS. Oxygen supply and consumption in late fetal life, and the onset of breathing at birth. In Fenn WO, Rahn H, eds. Handbook of physiology; Sect. 3, Respiration; Vol. II. Washington, DC: American Physiology Society, 1965; p 1313–1328.

24. Krogh M. The diffusion of gases through the lungs of man. J Physiol (Lond) 1915; 49:271–300.

25. Longo LD, Power GG, Forster II RE. Respiratory function of the placenta as determined with carbon monoxide in sheep and dogs. J Clin Invest 1967; 46:812–828.

26. Longo LD, Ching KS. Placental diffusing capacity for carbon monoxide and oxygen in unanesthetized sheep. J Appl Physiol 1977; 43:885–893.

27. Bissonnette JM, Longo LD, Novy MJ, Murata Y, Martin Jr CB. Placental diffusing capacity and its relation to fetal growth. J Dev Physiol 1979; 1:351–359.

28. Rocco E, Bennett TR, Power GG. Placental diffusing capacity in unanesthetized rabbits. Am J Physiol 1975; 228:465–469.

29. Bissonnette JM, Wickham WK. Placental diffusing capacity for carbon monoxide in unanesthetized guinea pigs. Respir Physiol 1977; 31:161–168.

30. Gilbert RD, Cummings LA, Jachau MR, Longo LD. Placental diffusing capacity and fetal development in exercising or hypoxic guinea pigs. Am J Physiol 1979; 46:828–834.

31. Boyle JW, Lotgering FK, Longo LD. Acute embolization of the uteroplacental circulation: uterine blood flow and placental CO diffusing capacity. J Dev Physiol 1984; 6:377–386.

32. Power GG, Jenkins F. Factors affecting O_2 transfer in sheep and rabbit placenta perfused in situ. Am J Physiol 1975; 229:1147–1153.

33. Assali NS, Rauramo L, Peltonen T. Measurement of uterine blood flow and uterine metabolism; VIII. Uterine and fetal blood flow and oxygenation in early human pregnancy. Am J Obstet Gynecol 1960; 79:86–98.

34. Assali NS, Douglas Jr RA, Baird WW, Nicholson DB, Suyemoto R. Measurements of uterine blood flow and uterine metabolism; IV. Results in normal pregnancy. Am J Obstet Gynecol 1953; 66:248–253.

35. Blechner JN, Stenger VG, Prystowsky H. Uterine blood flow in women at term. Am J Obstet Gynecol 1974; 120:633–639.

36a. Caton D, Crenshaw C, Wilcox CJ, Barron DH. O_2 delivery to the pregnant uterus: its relationship to O_2 consumption. Am J Physiol 1979; 23:R52–R57.

36b. Metcalfe J, Romney SL, Ramsey LH, Burwell CS. Estimation of uterine blood flow in normal human pregnancy at term. J Clin Invest 1955; 34:1632–1638.

37. Fuller EO, Manning JW, Nutter DO, Galletti PM. A perfused uterine preparation for the study of uterine and fetal physiology. In Longo LD, Reneau DD, eds. *Fetal and newborn cardiovascular physiology; Vol. 2, Fetal and newborn circulation.* New York: Garland Press, 1978; p 421–435.

38. Parer JT, de Lannoy CW, Hoversland AS, Metcalfe J. Effect of decreased uterine blood flow on uterine

oxygen consumption in pregnant macaques. Am J Obstet Gynecol 1968; 100:813–820.

39. Harding R, Sigger JN, Wickham PJD. Fetal and maternal influences on arterial oxygen levels in the sheep fetus. J Dev Physiol 1983; 5:267–276.

40. Jansen CAM, Krane EJ, Thomas AL, Beck NFG, Lowe KC, Joyce P, Parr M, Nathanielsz PW. Continuous variability of fetal P_{O_2} in the chronically catheterized fetal lamb. Am J Obstet Gynecol 1979; 134:776–783.

41. Itskovitz J, Lagamma EF, Rudolph AM. The effect of reducing umbilical blood flow on fetal oxygenation. Am J Obstet Gynecol 1983; 145:813–838.

42. Dawes GS, Mott JC. Changes in O_2 distribution and consumption in foetal lambs with variations in umbilical blood flow. J Physiol (Lond) 1964; 170:524–540.

43. Clapp III JF. The relationship between blood flow and oxygen uptake in the uterine and umbilical circulations. Am J Obstet Gynecol 1978; 132:410–413.

44. Permutt S, Riley RL. Hemodynamics of collapsible vessels with tone: the vascular waterfall. J Appl Physiol 1963; 18:924–932.

45. Bissonnette JM, Farrell RC. Pressure-flow and pressure-volume relationships in the fetal placental circulation. J Appl Physiol 1973; 35:355–360.

46. Power GG, Longo LD. Sluice flow in placenta: maternal vascular pressure effects on fetal circulation. Am J Physiol 1973; 225:1490–1496.

47. Power GG, Gilbert RD. Umbilical vascular compliance in sheep. Am J Physiol 1977; 233:H660–H664.

48. Berman Jr W, Goodlin RC, Heymann MA, Rudolph AM. Relationships between pressure and flow in the umbilical and uterine circulations of the sheep. Circ Res 1976; 38:262–266.

49. McRoberts Jr WA. Postural shock in pregnancy. Am J Obstet Gynecol 1951; 62:627–632.

50. Longo LD, Power GG, Forster II RE. Placental diffusing capacity for carbon monoxide at varying partial pressures of oxygen. J Appl Physiol 1969; 26:360–370.

51. Wagner PD. Tissue diffusion limitation of maximal O_2 uptake: the relationship between maximal V_{O_2} and effluent muscle P_{O_2}. Fed Proc 1987; 46:811.

52. Paulone ME, Edelstone DI, Shedd A. Effects of maternal anemia on uteroplacental and fetal oxidative metabolism in sheep. Am J Obstet Gynecol 1987; 156:230–236.

53. Koos BJ, Sameshima H, Power GG. Fetal breathing, sleep state, and cardiovascular responses to graded anemia in sheep. J Appl Physiol 1987; 63:1463–1468.

54. Soothill PW, Nicolaides KH, Rodeck CH. Effect of anaemia on fetal acid-base status. Br J Obstet Gynaecol 1987; 94:880–883.

55. Soothill PW, Nicolaides KH, Rodeck CH, Clewell WH, Lindridge J. Relationship of fetal hemoglobin and oxygen content to lactate concentration in Rh isoimmunized pregnancies. Obstet Gynecol 1987; 69:268–271.

56. Born GVR, Dawes GS. Mott JC. Oxygen lack and autonomic nervous control of the foetal circulation in the lamb. J Physiol (Lond) 1956; 134:149–166.

57. Adamsons K, Beard RW, Myers RE. Comparison of the composition of arterial, venous, and capillary blood of the fetal monkey during labor. Am J Obstet Gynecol 1970; 107:435–440.

58. Dawes GS, Lewis BV, Milligan JE, Roach MR, Tay-

ner NS. Vasomotor responses in the hind limbs of foetal and new-born lambs to asphyxia and aortic chemoreceptors stimulation. J Physiol (Lond) 1968; 195:55–81.

59. Adamson JW, Parer JT, Stamatoyannopoulos G. Erythrocytosis associated with hemoglobin Ranier. Oxygen equilibria and marrow regulation. J Clin Invest 1969; 48:1376–1386.

60. Parer JT: Oxygen transport in human subjects with hemoglobin variants having altered oxygen affinity. Respir Physiol 1970; 9:43–49.

61. Winslow RM, Swenberg M-L, Gross E, Chervenick PA, Buchman RR, Anderson WF. Hemoglobin McKees Rocks ($\alpha_2\beta_2^{145tyr}x\rightarrow^{term}$) A human "nonsense" mutation leading to a shortened -chain. J Clin Invest 1976; 57:772–781.

62. Jones RT, Osgood EE, Brimhall B, Koler RD. Hemoglobin Yakima; I. Clinical and biochemical studies. J Clin Invest 1967; 46:1840–1847.

63. Liley AW. Intrauterine transfusion of foetus in haemolytic disease. Br Med J 1963; 2:1107–1109.

64. Mathers NP, James GB, Walker J. The oxygen affin-ity of the blood of infants treated by intrauterine transfusion. J Obstet Gynaecol Br Commonw 1970; 77:648–653.

65. Novy MJ, Frigoletto FD, Easterday CL, Umansky I, Nelson NM. Changes in umbilical-cord blood oxygen affinity after intrauterine transfusion for erythroblastosis. N Engl J Med 1971; 285:589–596.

66. Hunt JA, Lehman H. Haemoglobin "Bart's": a foetal haemoglobin without α-chains. Nature 1959; 184:872–873.

67. Lotgering FK, Gilbert RD, Longo LD. Exercise responses in pregnant sheep: oxygen consumption, uterine blood flow, and blood volume. J Appl Physiol 1983; 55:834–841.

68. Lotgering FK, Gilbert RD, Longo LD: Exercise responses in pregnant sheep: blood gases, temperatures, and fetal cardiovascular system. J Appl Physiol 1983; 55:842–850.

69. Hill EP, Longo LD, Power GG. Kinetics of O_2 and CO_2 exchange. In West JB, ed. Bioengineering aspects of the lung. New York: Marcel Decker, 1975; p 459–514.

7

Homeostasis of Fetal Circulation

Julian T. Parer and Denys J. Court

FETAL CIRCULATION AND ITS REGULATION

In the adult, blood travels from the left ventricle to the systemic circulation and is returned to the right side of the heart. From there it flows through the lungs for reoxygenation. This serial circulatory design is inappropriate for the fetus, because oxygenation occurs in the placenta, and a pair of parallel circulations is present. Fetal circulation is made possible by anatomic "shunts," which normally are closed rapidly at birth, when adult circulation is required (1).

The fetal circulation is illustrated in Figure 7.1 with approximate values of the percentage of saturation of blood with oxygen in various areas. Most of the physiological data presented in this section are taken from studies of chronically catheterized, unanesthetized sheep fetuses, because until recently it was rarely possible to obtain such data from the human fetus. Although species differences may occur, it is likely that the same general trends and mechanisms apply to the human fetus as apply to the sheep fetus.

Well-oxygenated blood returns from the placenta by way of the umbilical vein. This vein enters the liver, where it joins with the portal venous system. Some of the blood is shunted directly to the inferior vena cava through the ductus venosus, and some traverses the hepatic parenchyma. An average of 50% takes the latter path, but the proportion is variable (2).

The saturation of blood in the inferior vena cava is lower than that in the ductus venosus, because it has mixed with poorly oxygenated blood returning from the lower body. The inferior vena caval blood enters the right atrium, and approximately 40% is diverted immediately by way of the foramen ovale (another temporary shunt) to the left atrium. Here it mixes with a relatively small quantity

of pulmonary venous blood and enters the left ventricle and then the coronary circulation and the vessels that supply the head, neck, and upper extremities. Hence, the foramen ovale allows relatively well-oxygenated blood to supply two vital structures, the heart and the head.

Blood entering the right atrium from the superior vena cava joins with the remaining 60% of inferior vena caval blood and enters the right ventricle. From here, a small proportion enters the pulmonary circulation, but most is shunted from this bed by way of the ductus arteriosus, which joins the descending aorta. This blood supplies the gut, kidneys, and lower body and also the umbilical circulation.

Distribution of Blood Flows Within the Fetus

The distribution of blood flows in the fetus generally is described as a percentage of the cardiac output. It is a simple concept in the adult who has two essentially equal serial circulations—systemic and pulmonary. In the fetus, with two unequal parallel circulations, distribution is described as the percentage of combined ventricular output, or CVO; that is, the combined output of the left and right ventricles.

The percentage of CVO in various areas of the heart and other vessels is shown in Figure 7.2. For obvious reasons, little of this information is available from human fetuses at term; the values depicted in the figure were obtained from unanesthetized chronically catheterized term sheep fetuses.

The sheep fetus at term is the same weight as the human fetus (approximately 3 kg), but species differences occur. For example, the proportion of blood flow to the brain is considerably greater in the human than in the sheep. In the term sheep fetus, the combined

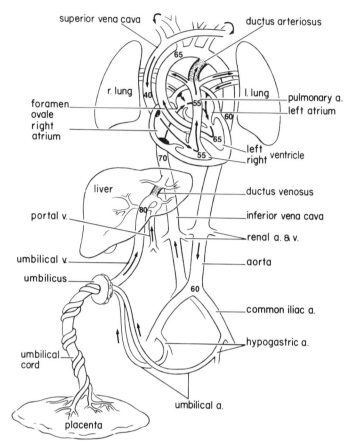

Figure 7.1.   Diagram of the fetal circulation. *Arrows* show the direction of blood flow, and *numbers* represent the approximate values of the percentage of saturation of the blood with oxygen in the fetal sheep. (From Parer JT. Handbook of fetal heart rate monitoring. Philadelphia: WB Saunders, 1983.)

ventricular output is 450 ml·min^{-1}·kg^{-1}, with twice the quantity from the right as from the left ventricle (3).

The cardiac output (CVO) in the human has been measured by noninvasive Doppler Velocimetry methods and is approximately 500 ml·min^{-1}·kg^{-1} in the third trimester, with a right to left ventricular flow ratio of approximately 1.3:1 (4, 5). This higher proportion of left ventricular flow in comparison to the fetal sheep may be explained by the greater cerebral circulation in the human.

Approximately 45% of the CVO is umbilical blood flow, i.e., approximately 200 ml·min^{-1}·kg^{-1} in the sheep fetus (3). In the human, umbilical blood flow is approximately 120 ml·min^{-1}·kg^{-1}.

Distribution of the cardiac output occurs in proportion to the vascular resistance of each

bed. These resistances are markedly changed during asphyxia, giving rise to preferential blood flow to certain vital organs, described under "Fetal Circulation during Asphyxial Stress."

Fetal Blood Pressure

The fetus is surrounded by a fluid-filled amniotic cavity, so fetal blood pressures must be related to the pressure of amniotic fluid. In the absence of uterine contractions, this pressure is generally stable.

The systemic arterial blood pressure of the fetus is considerably lower than that of the adult, averaging 55 mm Hg (systolic/diastolic, approximately 70/45 mm Hg) at term. Right ventricular pressure, 70/4 mm Hg, is slightly greater (1–2 mm Hg) than left ventricular pressure. Pulmonary arterial pressure is the

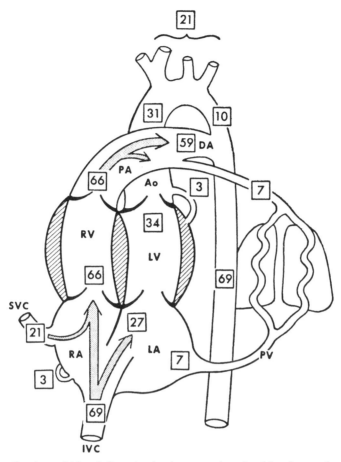

Figure 7.2.   The distribution of blood flow in the heart and major blood vessels of the fetal sheep. *Numbers* represent the percentage of combined ventricular output in various areas. (From Rudolph AM. Congenital disease of the heart. Chicago: Year Book, 1974.)

same as systemic arterial pressure. There is a slightly greater pressure in the right atrium (3 mm Hg) than in the left atrium (2 mm Hg), thus ensuring right-to-left blood flow across the foramen ovale (3).

Systemic blood pressures are somewhat lower earlier in gestation. This difference is reflected in the fact that premature newborns have a lower blood pressure than do term infants. Thus, at 30 weeks of gestation, the mean arterial blood pressure is only about 35 mm Hg (6).

Fetal Heart Rate and Its Variability

BASELINE RATE

The average heart rate in the nonmedicated term fetus before labor is 140 beats per min-

ute (bpm). Earlier in pregnancy, the heart rate is greater, although the difference is not substantial. At 20 weeks, the average fetal heart rate is 155 bpm, and at 30 weeks of pregnancy, it is 144 bpm. Variations of 20 bpm above or below these values occur in normal fetuses (7).

The fetal heart is similar to that of the adult in that it has an intrinsic pacemaker function, which results in rhythmic contractions. The sinoatrial (SA) node, which is found in one wall of the right atrium, has the fastest rate of contraction and sets the rate in the normal heart. The next fastest pacemaking rate is found in the atrium. The ventricle has a slower rate of beating than either the SA node or the atrium. In cases of complete or partial heart block in the fetus, variations in the rate below normal can be seen. Typically, a fetus with complete heart block has a rate of approximately 50–60 bpm.

Bradycardia is defined as a heart rate below 120 bpm. To distinguish it from a deceleration, the term is confined to such decreases in fetal heart rate (FHR) exceeding 2 min. A tachycardia is a baseline rate in excess of 160 bpm for at least 2 min. The mean FHR is a result of many physiological factors that modulate the intrinsic rate of the heart.

FETAL HEART RATE VARIABILITY

Fetal heart rate variability (FHRV) refers to the irregular fluctuations noted on a tracing from a cardiotachometer. The variability is due to differences in R-R intervals of the fetal electrocardiogram, and clinical FHR monitors are able to determine this to an accuracy of at least 4 msec, corresponding to a fetal heart rate difference of approximately 1 bpm at 120 bpm. Conventionally, the instantaneous FHR is displayed rather than the R-R interval. The cardiotachometer makes the calculation:

$$\text{FHR (bpm)} = \frac{60}{\text{R-R interval (sec)}}$$

and the FHR is displayed on a strip chart recorder with specific y-axis scaling (30 bpm/cm) and a paper speed of 3 cm/min. If each interval between heart beats were identical, the line would be smooth.

FHRV is clinically divided into several classes:

Short-Term Variability

Short-term variability (STV) is beat-to-beat variability, or differences between two adjacent or three serial beats. Recognition of STV requires the accurate detection of the cardiac event; only the R wave of the fetal ECG fulfills this requirement. A tracing from the Doppler ultrasound device usually contains artificial jitter; hence, this device cannot reliably be used to determine STV. Unlike the pattern presented by long-term variability the presence or absence of STV must be deliberately determined. STV is described as "present" or "absent."

Long-Term Variability

Long-term variability (LTV) consists of irregular, crude sine waves with a cycle of approximately 3–6/min. It can be detected by a direct electrode and also at times by the Doppler ultrasound method. It generally is described in terms of its approximate amplitude range in bpm.

Variability of the Oscillating Frequency

This term refers to the frequency of the sine wave-like patterns in a specific time period, generally 1 min. It is calculated by counting the number of times the heart rate tracing crosses an imaginary line drawn through the midpoint of each of the complexes.

Three basic classes of LTV are recognized: normal, decreased, and absent.

> Normal Variability—Variability in which the amplitude range of the variability is greater than 6 bpm, but less than 25 bpm.
> Decreased Variability—Variability in which the amplitude range is between 2 and 5 bpm.
> Absent Variability—Variability in which the amplitude range is less than 2 bpm, and looks "flat," or smooth.

A fourth pattern is FHRV of an amplitude greater than 25 bpm, called the saltatory pattern. This pattern consists of rapid variations in FHR, usually with a frequency of 3–6/min. It is qualitatively described as excessive variability and the excessive swings of heart rate have a strikingly bizarre appearance.

Regulation of the Fetal Circulation

This section will include a description of factors that regulate FHR, blood pressure, and distribution of blood flows. Factors causing major disturbances in the fetal circulation are described in a subsequent section.

PARASYMPATHETIC NERVOUS SYSTEM

The parasympathetic nervous system consists primarily of the vagus nerve (tenth cranial nerve), which originates in the medulla oblongata. Fibers from this nerve supply the SA node and also the atrioventricular (AV) node, the neuronal bridge between the atrium and the ventricle. Stimulation of the vagus nerve or injection of acetylcholine, the substance secreted at the nerve endings, produces a decrease in heart rate in the normal fetus as a result of vagal influence on the SA node, decreasing its rate of firing and decreasing the rate of transmission of impulses from atrium to ventricle. Similarly, blocking of this nerve in a normal fetus with a substance that competes with acetylcholine (e.g., atropine) causes an increase in the FHR of approximately 20 bpm at term (8). This effect shows that there is normally a constant vagal tone on the FHR that tends to decrease its intrinsic rate.

The vagus nerve apparently has another very important function: responsibility for transmission of impulses that cause beat-to-beat variability of the FHR. Blocking the vagus nerve with atropine results in the disappearance of this variability. Hence, it has been postulated that there are two vagal influences in the heart: a tonic influence that tends to decrease its rate and an oscillatory influence that results in fetal heart rate variability.

SYMPATHETIC NERVOUS SYSTEM

Sympathetic nerves are widely distributed in the muscle of the heart at term. Stimulation of the sympathetic nerves will release norepinephrine and will cause an increase in the FHR and an increase in the vigor of cardiac contractions. These effects result in an increase in cardiac output. The sympathetic nerves are a reserve mechanism to improve the pumping activity of the heart during intermittent stressful situations. There is normally a tonic sympathetic influence on the heart. Propranolol, a substance that blocks the action of these sympathetic nerves, causes a decrease of approximately 10–15 bpm in the FHR when it is administered to a normal sheep fetus (9). There is, however, only a small decrease in FHRV after blockade of the sympathetic nerves in primates.

It is a commonly held theory that FHRV is a result of two neuronal inputs to the fetal heart, vagal and β-adrenergic, each with a different time constant. Because atropine al-

most abolishes visually determined FHRV, and propranolol decreases it by only a little, it is very unlikely that the theory holds true for the primate or sheep (10, 11).

The responses mentioned previously refer primarily to the β-adrenergic activity. α-Adrenergic activity also is important in altering the distribution of blood flow to specific organs during stress (12). Thus, during hypoxia, there is vasoconstriction of certain vascular beds (e.g., the gut, liver, and lung), which allows preferential flow of blood with the available oxygen to vital organs (e.g., the brain, heart, and adrenals), and blood flow to the placenta is maintained.

Several factors that cause parasympathetic and sympathetic nervous systems to increase their tonic activity will be described in the following sections.

CHEMORECEPTORS

Chemoreceptors are found both in the peripheral and in the central nervous systems. They have their most dramatic effects on the regulation of respiration, but they also are important in the control of the circulation. The peripheral chemoreceptors are found in the carotid and aortic bodies, in the area of the carotid sinus and in the arch of the aorta. The central chemoreceptors are found in the medulla oblongata and respond to changes in the oxygen and carbon dioxide tensions in blood or cerebrospinal fluid perfusing this area.

In the adult, when oxygen in the arterial blood perfusing the central chemoreceptors is decreased or the carbon dioxide content is increased, there is ordinarily a reflex tachycardia. There is also a substantial increase in arterial blood pressure, which is extremely pronounced with increases in carbon dioxide concentration. Both of these effects, a tachycardia and an increase in blood pressure, are thought to be protective in attempting to circulate more blood through the affected areas, such as the brain, in order to bring about a decrease in carbon dioxide tension or an increase in oxygen. Selective hypoxia or hypercapnia of the peripheral chemoreceptors by itself in the adult produces a bradycardia, in contrast to the tachycardia and hypertension seen with central hypoxia or hypercapnia. The interactions of the central and peripheral chemoreceptors are poorly understood in the fetus and are clearly different from adult responses. The net result of hypoxia or hypercapnia in the fetus is bradycardia and hypertension (13). Recently developed techniques allow the selective study of fetal chemoreceptors, and it has been shown that the chemoreflex can be elicited in utero (14). The chemoreflex is thought to be responsible for the "reflex late deceleration" seen clinically (15).

BARORECEPTORS

Small stretch receptors in the vessel walls that are sensitive to increases in blood pressure are found in the arch of the aorta and in the carotid sinus at the junction of the internal and external carotid arteries. When pressure rises, impulses are sent from these receptors by way of the vagus or the glossopharyngeal nerve to the midbrain, resulting in further impulses by way of the vagus nerve to the heart, which tend to slow cardiac activity. This response is extremely rapid, apparent with almost the first systolic rise of blood pressure. It is a protective, stabilizing function by the body in an attempt to lower blood pressure by decreasing heart rate and cardiac output when blood pressure is increasing. This mechanism is functional in the fetus although its degree of maturity is somewhat controversial (16–18).

CENTRAL NERVOUS SYSTEM

In the adult, there are influences on heart rate from the higher centers of the brain. Heart rate is increased by certain emotional stimuli such as fear or sexual arousal. Observations on fetal lambs and monkeys have shown that the electroencephalogram or the electro-oculogram shows increased activity at times in association with variability of the heart rate and body movements. At other times, apparently when the fetus is sleeping in utero, activity slows, and the FHRV decreases, suggesting an association between these two factors and central nervous system activity (19).

The medulla oblongata contains the vasomotor centers—integrative centers at which all the inputs result in either cardioacceleration or cardiodeceleration. This center is probably also where the net result of numerous cortical and peripheral inputs is processed to form irregular oscillatory vagal impulses, giving rise to FHRV.

HORMONAL REGULATION

Adrenal Medulla

The fetal adrenal medulla produces epinephrine and norepinephrine in response to stressful situations, e.g., asphyxia. Both of these substances act on the heart and the cardiovascular system in a way similar to sympathetic stimulation. That is, they produce a faster heart rate, a greater force of contraction of the heart, and an increased arterial blood pressure. It is not clear, however, whether catecholamines exert a regulatory function in the normal, nonstressed fetus.

Adrenal Cortex

The adrenal cortex produces aldosterone in response to decreases in blood pressure in the adult. This substance causes the kidney to decrease sodium output, thus tending to increase water retention and therefore causing a blood volume increase, tending to restore blood pressure.

Vasopressin

Vasopressin, like α-adrenergic activity, has been shown to affect the distribution of blood flow in the fetal sheep (20). It appears to be particularly important during hypoxia and possibly in other stressful situations (see later).

Prostaglandins

Arachidonic acid metabolites are found in high concentrations in the fetal circulation and in many tissues. Their main role seems to be in the regulation of umbilical blood flow as well as in maintaining the patency of the ductus arteriosus during fetal life.

Renin-Angiotensin System

Angiotensin II seems to play a role in the fetal circulatory regulation at rest, but its main activity is observed during hemorrhagic stress on the fetus.

Other hormones, such as α-melanocyte-stimulating hormone, atrial natriuretic hormone, endogenous opioids, and the thyrotropin-releasing hormone (TRH), have also been described to be present in the fetus and to participate in the circulatory function regulation, but their importance is still uncertain in normal regulation.

BLOOD VOLUME CONTROL

Capillary Fluid Shift

In the adult, when the blood pressure of the body is elevated by excessive blood volume, some fluid moves out of the capillaries into the interstitial spaces, thereby decreasing the blood volume back toward normal. Conversely, if the adult loses blood through hemorrhage, some fluid shifts out of the interstitial spaces into the circulation, thereby increasing the blood volume back toward normal. There is normally a delicate balance between the pressure inside and outside the capillaries. This mechanism of regulating blood pressures is slower than the almost instantaneous regulation that occurs with the reflex mechanisms discussed previously. Its role in the fetus is not completely understood, although imbalances may be responsible for the hydrops seen in some cases of Rh isoimmunization and extreme fetal tachycardia.

Intraplacental Pressures

Fluid moves down hydrostatic pressure gradients; it also moves in response to osmotic pressure gradients. The actual values of these factors within the human placental site, where fetal and maternal blood closely approximate, is controversial. It seems likely, however, that there are some delicate balancing mechanisms within the placental site that prevent rapid fluid shifts between mother and fetus. As noted earlier, the arterial blood pressure of the mother is much higher (approximately 100 mm Hg) than that of the fetus (approximately 55 mm Hg), and osmotic pressures are not substantially different. Hence, some compensatory mechanism must be present to equalize the effective pressures at the exchange points.

Frank-Starling Mechanism

In the Frank-Starling mechanism, the amount of blood pumped by the heart is determined by the amount of blood returning to the heart. That is, the heart pumps all of the blood that flows into it without excessive damming of blood in the veins. When the cardiac muscle is stretched before contraction by an increased inflow of blood, it contracts with a greater force than before and is able to pump out more blood. This mechanism has been studied in the unanesthetized fetal lamb and it has been suggested that it is less well developed than in the adult sheep. The imperfect mechanism in the fetus is probably caused by the fact that fetal heart muscle is not as well developed as adult heart muscle. It is likely that the same is true of the human fetus, because human neonates are generally more immature than are newborn lambs. As a consequence, changes in the filling pressure or preload produce minor if any changes in CVO, suggesting that the fetal heart normally operates near the top of its function curve.

A consequence of poor development of the Frank-Starling mechanism is that in slowing of the FHR, the amount pumped per beat (stroke volume) may not increase substantially, and at values below normal, the output of the fetal heart is related to the heart rate. The same is true of modest increases in the heart rate above normal, but with greatly increased heart rates, the cardiac output is decreased because there is not sufficient time between contractions for the ventricles to fill. In other words, the cardiac output in the fetus is dependent on the heart rate, and the fetus can increase cardiac output markedly only by increasing heart rate, in contrast with the adult, who can increase cardiac output by increasing both heart rate and stroke volume.

However, studies have been done during atrial pacing, and this does not necessarily reflect the normal in vivo situation, because cardiac output depends not only on heart rate but also on preload, afterload, and contractility (21). This simple relationship does not apply to all fetal conditions (21). In particular, it appears that the fetus can, in fact, increase its stroke volume to a certain extent during hypoxic bradycardia (12), and during spontaneous changes in heart rate in the human (22).

Umbilical Blood Flow

The umbilical blood flow is approximately 300 ml/min immediately after delivery (23). This measurement, however, probably is decreased by the acute events occurring at this time and by the inevitable interference with umbilical blood flow. In comparison, the blood flow is 600 ml/min in the chronically instrumented term sheep fetus, which is approximately the same size as the human fetus at term. Recent noninvasive measurements of umbilical blood flow in term human fetuses still appear to be lower than this, i.e., about 120 $ml \cdot kg^{-1} \cdot min^{-1}$ (24). This species difference can be explained by the greater oxygen-carrying capacity of human fetal blood and the higher body temperature and, therefore, higher metabolic rate of the sheep (39° C) compared with the human (37° C).

The umbilical blood flow in sheep is approximately 45% of the combined ventricular output, and roughly 20% of this blood flow is "shunted." That is, it does not exchange with maternal blood. It either is carried through actual vascular shunts within the fetal side of the placenta or does not approach closely enough to maternal blood to exchange substances with it.

Umbilical blood flow is not affected by acute moderate hypoxia but is decreased by severe hypoxia. The umbilical cord does not have direct innervation, although umbilical blood flow decreases with the administration of catecholamines. The flow is decreased by acute cord occlusion. There are no known means of increasing umbilical flow in cases in which it is decreased chronically. Certain fetal heart rate patterns, namely, variable decelerations, however, have been ascribed to transient umbilical cord compression in the fetus during labor. Manipulation of maternal position either to the lateral or to the Trendelenburg position sometimes can abolish these patterns, the implication being that these maneuvers have

removed the fetus from the cord, thus relieving the compression.

FETAL CIRCULATION DURING ASPHYXIAL STRESS

There are relatively few comprehensive studies of the fetal circulation under conditions of moderate to severe maternal exercise, although fetal heart rate has received some attention. Such studies are described in Chapter 9.

In sheep it has been shown that uterine blood flow decreased 24% after 40 min of exercise at 70% maximal oxygen consumption (25), but uterine oxygen uptake was maintained due to increased oxygen extraction and increased oxygen capacity due to hemoconcentration. Fetal arterial oxygen pressure and content decreased moderately but heart rate and blood pressure did not change. Blood flow distribution was not altered in short-term (10 min) studies (26), nor was there stimulation of catecholamine release. It is likely that fetal oxygen uptake remained stable, and the authors concluded that maternal exercise of this degree in the sheep (presumably normally grown) did not represent a major stressful or hypoxic event to the fetus.

It is conceivable, however, that under conditions of more prolonged or intense exercise, or in the human, the reduction of uterine blood flow could result in fetal asphyxial stress. We will, therefore, review the fetal responses to hypoxia and asphyxia.

Causes of Fetal Asphyxia

Fetal asphyxia involves both hypoxia and acidosis that, if progressive and uncorrected, may lead to brain damage and fetal death. There are four basic mechanisms by which the fetus can become hypoxic: (a) insufficient blood flow to the maternal placenta (uterine blood flow), (b) insufficient blood flow to the fetal placenta (umbilical blood flow), (c) a decrease in maternal arterial oxygen tension and content (maternal hypoxia), or (d) a decrease in fetal oxygen-carrying capacity (e.g., severe fetal anemia). Rarely the hypoxia may be secondary to increased fetal oxygen requirements, as in pyrexia. The associated acidosis may initially be "respiratory," that is, secondary to reduced fetomaternal CO_2 exchange across the placenta (as in (a) or (b) above) but eventually a progressive metabolic acidosis can develop due to a change from aerobic to anaerobic metabolism in some fetal organs subsequent to inadequate tissue oxygenation.

Most experimental studies have been done using simply the imposition of hypoxia, and less information is available on the influence of deliberately imposed asphyxia. The former is achieved by giving the mother hypoxic gas mixtures to breathe, and the latter by placing adjustable occluders around the uterine artery or umbilical vessels. Hypoxia results simply in decreased O_2 tension with a metabolic acidosis that eventually develops because of the production of lactic acid as an end product of anaerobic metabolism in insufficiently perfused organs. Asphyxia (e.g., produced by reduction of uterine blood flow by 50% or more) results in a decrease in O_2 tension and an increase in CO_2 tension (giving a respiratory acidosis), and eventually a lactic acidosis. The influence of asphyxia on the fetus appears to be more detrimental than equivalent degrees of hypoxia (13).

Blood Flow Distribution

From studies such as those previously described in chronically prepared animals, a number of responses are known to occur during acute asphyxia or hypoxia in the previously normoxic fetus. There is a bradycardia caused by increased vagal activity with little change in cardiac output, and a redistribution of blood flow favoring the heart, brain, and adrenal glands (13, 27). These organs may therefore be considered the "priority organs." In addition, the placental blood flow is maintained. This initial response is presumed to be advantageous to the fetus in the same way as the diving reflex is in the adult seal, in that the blood containing the available oxygen and other nutrients is supplied preferentially to these organs. However, fetal adaptations to asphyxial stress can be sustained for a limited time only. This

time depends on the degree of asphyxia suffered. Furthermore, there may be a point beyond which the fetus is not capable of sufficient physiological adaptation and where the degree of asphyxia itself may abolish the compensatory response to hypoxia. These fetal adaptations to hypoxic and asphyxial stress will now be examined.

Distribution of the combined ventricular output occurs in proportion to the vascular resistance of each vascular bed. The "resting" vascular resistances are markedly changed during asphyxia. Thus, although cardiac output changes little with asphyxia (12, 13, 27, 28), marked vasodilation in the priority organs increases their blood flow 2 to 5-fold. The vascular resistance of the placenta is essentially unchanged by asphyxia and umbilical blood flow is maintained. The preferential redistribution of blood flow to these organs requires simultaneous vasoconstriction in vascular beds less vital for survival, namely the splanchnic organs (liver, spleen, gut, and kidney) and peripheral structures (skin and musculoskeletal tissues) (12, 13, 27, 28).

Blood flow to the priority organs in the sheep fetus during normoxia represents less than 8% of cardiac output. During hypoxia, combined flow to the priority organs may reach 20% of cardiac output, and umbilical flow remains unchanged at about 40% of cardiac output. Vasoconstriction in the nonpriority vascular beds reduces the combined blood flow to these organs from about 52% to 40%. Because cerebral blood flow is proportionately greater in human fetuses, the percentage of cardiac output to the priority organs is presumably greater during hypoxia than for the sheep fetus. This implies the need for an even greater vasoconstriction in nonpriority vascular beds of the human fetus. As these vascular beds represent the greater proportion of the total arterial tree of the fetal body, total peripheral resistance (and therefore arterial blood pressure) also rises (12).

Although this compensatory blood flow redistribution can occur for a prolonged period of time, it is not without metabolic consequences. Pyruvate and lactate accumulate from the vasoconstricted splanchnic and peripheral beds (29). The placenta may provide a pathway for clearance of excess lactate, but eventually metabolic acidosis (decreasing pH and base excess) becomes progressive unless the cause of the asphyxia is relieved.

Organ Oxygen Consumption

The oxygen consumption of an organ is proportional to its blood flow and its oxygen extraction (arteriovenous oxygen content difference). During asphyxia, arterial oxygen content is decreased. Total fetal oxygen consumption in sheep falls by up to 50–60% (30). This reduction can be maintained for up to 45 min and is completely reversible upon cessation of hypoxia. It is thought that the decrease in total oxygen consumption reflects a decrease in oxygen consumption in vascular beds that are constricted, as evidenced by the anaerobic metabolism that occurs in these organs during asphyxia. However, as an organ's oxygen consumption is proportional to its blood flow, oxygen consumption of the priority organs is largely protected by the increased flow to these organs that occurs during asphyxia.

The relationship between organ blood flow and oxygen consumption during asphyxia has been best studied in the brain and myocardium. As progressive hypoxia leads to a decreasing arteriovenous oxygen content difference across the cerebral circulation (ascending aorta minus sagittal sinus oxygen content), there is an almost exact matching of increased cerebral blood flow (31). This allows maintenance of cerebral oxygen consumption even in moderately severe hypoxia.

A similar relationship was found between blood flow and arteriovenous oxygen content difference across the myocardial circulation (ascending aortic minus coronary sinus oxygen content) in the unanesthetized fetal sheep during hypoxia (32). That is, the oxygen consumption of the myocardium remained constant because the increased blood flow exactly matched the decreased arteriovenous oxygen difference.

The above studies involved hypoxia im-posed by decreasing the ewe's inspired oxygen. As mentioned previously, a similar reduction of oxygen tension or content by an asphyxial method such as reduction of uterine blood flow may be more detrimental to the fetus. Reduction of uterine blood flow to 50% of normal for 15 min caused similar changes in blood flow redistribution to that obtained with moderately severe to severe hypoxia alone (33). However, when uterine blood flow was reduced to 25% of normal for 15 min, there was a reduction in the degree of increased cerebral and myocardial blood flow accompanied by a decrease in cardiac output. This was presumably due to a partial reversal or failure of the mechanisms regulating the compensatory blood flow responses to asphyxia in the face of overwhelming asphyxia. Cerebral oxygen consumption decreases when ascending aortic content flow falls below 1 mM·l^{-1} since both the blood flow and arteriovenous oxygen content difference are reduced (33a). Thus a "critical point" exists; when arterial oxygen delivery falls below this point, the compensatory mechanisms would no longer be able to protect the brain against reduction of oxygen consumption, and asphyxial brain damage may result.

A similar point of decompensation probably also occurs for the myocardium because with severe asphyxia, there is reduction of myocardial blood flow similar to that of the brain (33). This suggests that a critical point does occur for the myocardium and at a similar severity of asphyxia. Presumably an inability to meet myocardial oxygen consumption needs at this critical severity of asphyxia would, in time, lead to myocardial failure and further reduced cardiac output.

Metabolic Consequences of Hypoxia

The fetus depends partially on anaerobic metabolism for its energy requirements during hypoxia (29), in particular for maintaining metabolism in organs that are subjected to vasoconstriction during hypoxia/asphyxia. However, only 4 moles of ATP are generated for each mole of glucose metabolized anaerobically and 2 moles of lactate are produced, whereas 36 moles of ATP are generated per mole of glucose metabolized aerobically, without lactate accumulation. Thus, the effects of prolonged anaerobic metabolism in the vasoconstricted beds include rapid exhaustion of carbohydrate stores and progressive metabolic (lactic) acidosis. In laboratory animals, the newborn's ability to tolerate asphyxia depends upon its cardiac carbohydrate reserves (32).

Autonomic Changes during Asphyxia

Hypoxia leads to an increase in sympathetic and parasympathetic nervous system activity and an increase in the secretion of catecholamines, vasopressin, angiotensin, and other humoral agents. Many of the cardiovascular responses to hypoxia are rapidly instituted (less than 30 sec) and are probably mediated by these neural and humoral mechanisms.

Hypoxia/asphyxia leads to a marked increase in activity in all three branches of the autonomic nervous system. For example, in studies involving total or selective autonomic blockade, it is estimated from FHR responses that parasympathetic activity is augmented 3 to 5-fold and β-adrenergic activity about 2-fold (35). While the increased parasympathetic activity is all via the vagus nerve the increase in adrenergic activity arises from both sympathetic nerves (36) and adrenomedullary secretion of catecholamines (37).

The autonomically mediated cardiovascular responses to hypoxia represent a balance between vagal, α-adrenergic, and β-adrenergic influences. This counterbalancing of influences appears vital for survival. For example, simultaneous blockade of both α-adrenergic and β-adrenergic activity during hypoxia rapidly leads to fetal demise (38). This may be due to the removal of the counter-vagal influences because total blockade of all postganglianic autonomic fibers (which includes the adrenal medulla) does not result in fetal demise (39). Therefore, an important function of the increased β-adrenergic activity associated with hypoxia is limitation of the negative chronotropic effects of increased vagal activity. The aspects of the hypoxia-

induced changes that are affected by the autonomic system have been determined by the use of autonomic blocking drugs such as atropine (parasympathetic blockade), phentolamine or phenoxybenzamine (α-adrenergic blockade), or propranolol (β-adrenergic blockade).

Parasympathetic blockade during hypoxia does not cause a change in the redistribution of cardiac output that occurs during hypoxia. α-Adrenergic blockade reverses both the hypoxia-induced hypertension and the vasoconstriction of the splanchnic organs (12). β-Adrenergic blockade during hypoxia does not affect blood pressure but causes a further drop in FHR and a proportionate drop in cardiac output (28). There is an increase in placental vascular resistance and, therefore, a drop in umbilical blood flow. The hypoxia-induced increase in myocardial blood flow is halved. The increased brain and adrenal blood flow associated with hypoxia is not significantly affected by any of the above manipulations.

From these experiments, the following conclusions may be drawn: (a) The primary cardiovascular manifestation of the increased parasympathetic activity during hypoxia is a bradycardia. (b) The increased α-adrenergic activity causes systemic hypertension and vasoconstriction of the vascular beds of certain splanchnic organs (lungs, gut, liver, and spleen). This allows redistribution of blood to priority organs. (c) The umbilical circulation is spared the α-adrenergic influence because of its poor vasoconstrictive ability (40). Furthermore, the increase in β-adrenergic activity during hypoxia maintains umbilical blood flow by maintaining placental vasodilatation (28, 35). (d) Active vasodilatation of the myocardial vascular bed appears to be partially mediated by β-adrenergic activity (28) but is probably also maintained, in part, by local metabolite production. (e) Although the factors controlling adrenal and cerebral vasodilatation remain largely unknown, blood flow to the brain is inversely proportional to the arteriovenous oxygen content difference (31), and directly proportional to increases in CO_2 pressure (41). There is also evidence that arginine vasopressin dilates the cerebral vascular bed (42).

Humoral Changes during Asphyxia

Vasopressin levels are usually undetectable in normoxic sheep fetuses. However, vasopressin secretion increases with hypoxia, the levels reached correlate with the drop in arterial oxygen tension, the drop in pH, and the hypertensive response to hypoxia (42). This vasopressin response is reduced but not eliminated by sectioning vagal and sympathetic nerve trunks. Carotid body and aortic chemoreceptors in the fetal lamb appear to be sensitive to hypoxia (43), and perfusion of the carotid sinus of the anesthetized dog with deoxygenated blood causes a rise in vasopressin secretion (44). When vasopressin is administered to normoxic fetal lambs, the cardiovascular response is similar to that seen with hypoxia (20). Included in this response is vasoconstriction in peripheral structures (musculoskeletal system and skin), which does not occur as an α-adrenergic effect. However, in blocking studies using AVP antagonists, they failed to show any vasodilation of the musculoskeletal vasculature, although there was an increase in blood flow to the liver and gut, and also to the placenta (42).

β-Endorphin and probably other endogenous opioids also participate in the response to hypoxia (45). The blockade of its receptors with naloxone further increases the hypertensive response by increasing the vasoconstriction in the kidneys and musculoskeletal tissues.

The possibility that the renin-angiotensin system may be involved in the fetal hypoxic response has been studied by infusing angiotensin II into normoxic sheep fetuses (46). However, the majority of the resultant cardiovascular responses are opposite to those that occur with hypoxia and it is, therefore, unlikely that angiotensin II has a major role in the cardiovascular response to hypoxia.

In summary, the cardiovascular adaptation by hypoxia/asphyxia appears to be initiated by increased autonomic activity with subsequent humoral contributions. This increased activity includes the vagus nerve, sympathetic nerves, and catecholamine secretion from the adrenal medulla and is modulated by endogenous opioid production. Vasopressin has an important additive effect to this response. Other agents may also be involved.

REFERENCES

1. Dawes GS. Foetal and neonatal physiology. Chicago: Year Book, 1968.
2. Edelstone DI, Merick RE, Caritis SN, Mueller-Heubach E. Umbilical venous blood flow and its distribution before and during autonomic blockade in fetal lambs. Am J Obstet Gynecol 1980;138:703–707.
3. Rudolph AM. Congenital diseases of the heart. Chicago: Year Book, 1974.
4. Reed KL, Meijbuom EJ, Sahn DJ, Scagnelli SA, Valdes-Cruz LM, Shenicer L. Cardiac Doppler flow velocities in human fetuses. Circulation 1989; 73:41–46.
5. Kenny JF, Plappert T, Doubilet P, Saltzman DH, Cartier M, Zollars L, Leatherman GF, Sutton MG. Changes in intracardiac blood flow velocities and right and left ventricular stroke volumes with gestational age in the normal human fetus: a prospective Doppler echocardiographic study. Circulation 1986; 74:1208–1216.
6. Kitterman JA, Phibbs RH, Tooley WH. Aortic blood pressure in normal newborn infants during the first 12 hours of life. Pediatrics 1969; 44:959–968.
7. Schifferli PY, Caldeyro-Barcia R. Effects of atropine and beta-adrenergic drugs on the heart rate of the human fetus. In Boreus L, ed. Fetal pharmacology. New York: Raven Press, 1973, pp 259–279.
8. Mendez-Bauer C, Poseiro JJ, Arellano-Hernandez G, et al. Effects of atropine on the heart rate of the human fetus during labor. Am J Obstet Gynecol 1963; 85:1033–1053.
9. Harris JL, Krueger TR, Parer JT. Effect of parasympathetic and β-adrenergic blockade on the umbilical circulation in the unanesthetized fetal sheep. Gynecol Obstet Invest 1979; 10:306–310.
10. Parer JT, Laros RK, Heilbron DC, Krueger TR. The roles of β-adrenergic activity in beat-to-beat fetal heart rate variability (FHRV). Physiological Sciences 8:327–329. Kovach AGB, Monose E, Rubanyi G, eds.: Cardiovascular physiology. New York: Pergamon Press, 1981.
11. Dalton KR, Dawes GS, Patrick JE. The autonomic nervous system and fetal heart rate variability. Am J Obstet Gynecol 1983; 146:456–462.
12. Reuss ML, Parer JT, Harris JL, Krueger JR. Hemodynamic effects of α-adrenergic blockade during hypoxia in fetal sheep. Am J Obstet Gynecol 1982; 142:410–415.
13. Cohn HE, Sacks EJ, Heymann MA, Rudolph AM. Cardiovascular responses to hypoxemia and acidemia in fetal lambs. Am J Obstet Gynecol 1974; 120:817–824.
14. Itskovitz J, Rudolph AM. Denervation of arterial chemoreceptors and baroreceptors in fetal lambs in utero. Am J Physiol 1982; 242:H916–H920.
15. Parer JT, Krueger TR, Harris JL. Fetal oxygen con-

sumption and mechanisms of heart rate response during artificially produced late decelerations of fetal heart rate in sheep. Am J Obstet Gynecol 1980; 136:478–482.

16. Shinebourne EA, Vapaavouri EK, Williams RL, et al. Development of baroreflex activity in unanesthetized fetal and neonatal lambs. Circ Res 1972; 31:710–718.

17. Faber JJ, Green TJ, Thornburg KL. Arterial blood pressure in the unanesthetized fetal lamb after changes in fetal blood volume and haematocrit. Q J Exp Physiol 1974; 59:241–255.

18. Itskovitz J, LaGamma EF, Rudolph AM. Baroreflex control of the circulation in chronically instrumented fetal lambs. Circ Res 1983; 52:589–596.

19. Nijhuis JG, Prechtl HFR, Martin CB Jr, Bots RSGM. Are there behavioural states in the human fetus? Early Hum Dev 1982; 6:177–195.

20. Iwamoto HS, Rudolph AM, Keil LC, Heymann MA. Hemodynamic responses of the sheep fetus to vasopressin infusion. Circ Res 1979; 44:430–436.

21. Anderson PA, Glick KL, Killiam AP, Mainwaring RD. The effect of heart rate on in utero left ventricular output in the fetal sheep. J Physiol 1986; 372:557–573.

22. Kenny J, Plappert T, Doubilet P, Salzman D, Sutton MG. Effects of heart rate on ventricular size, stroke volume, and output in the normal human fetus: a prospective Doppler echocardiographic study. Circulation 1987; 76:52–58.

23. McCallum WD. Thermodilution measurement of human umbilical blood flow at delivery. Am J Obstet Gynecol 1977; 127:491–496.

24. Gill RW, Trudinger BJ, Garret WT, et al. Fetal umbilical venous flow measured in utero by pulsed Doppler and β-mode ultrasound; I. Normal pregnancies. Am J Obstet Gynecol 1981; 139:720–725.

25. Lotgering FK, Gilbert RD, Longo LD. Exercise responses in pregnant sheep: oxygen consumption, uterine blood flow and blood volume. J Appl Physiol 1983; 55:834–841.

26. Lotgering FK, Gilbert RD, Longo LD. Exercise responses in pregnant sheep: blood gases, temperatures, and fetal cardiovascular system. J Appl Physiol 1983; 55:842–850.

27. Peeters LLH, Sheldon RE, Jones MD, et al. Blood flow to fetal organs as a function of arterial oxygen content. Am J Obstet Gynecol 1979; 135:637–646.

28. Court DJ, Parer JT, Block BSB, Llanos AI. Effects of beta-adrenergic blockade on blood flow distribution during hypoxemia in fetal sheep. J Dev Physiol 1984; 6:349–358.

29. Mann LI. Effects in sheep of hypoxia on levels of lactate, pyruvate and glucose in blood of mothers and fetuses. Pediatr Res 1970; 4:46–54.

30. Parer JT. The effect of acute maternal hypoxia on fetal oxygenation and the umbilical circulation in the sheep. Eur J Obstet Gynaecol Reprod Biol 1980; 10:125–136.

31. Jones MD Jr, Sheldon RE, Peeters LL, et al. Fetal cerebral oxygen consumption at different levels of oxygenation. J Appl Physiol 1977; 43:1080–1084.

32. Fisher DJ, Heymann MA, Rudolph AM. Fetal myocardial oxygen and carbohydrate consumption during acutely induced hypoxemia. Am J Physiol 1982; 242:H657–H661.

33. Yaffe H, Parer JT, Llanos A, Block B. Cardiorespiratory responses to graded reductions of uterine blood flow in the sheep fetus. J Dev Physiol 1987; 9:325–336.

33a. Field IR, Parer JT, Auslender RA, Cheek DB, Baker W, Johnston J. Cerebral oxygen consumption during asphyxia in fetal sheep. J Dev Physiol (in press) 1990.

34. Parer JT. The effect of atropine on heart rate and oxygen consumption of the hypoxic fetus. Am J Obstet Gynecol 1984; 148:1118–1122.

35. Parer JT. The influence of β-adrenergic activity on fetal heart rate and the umbilical circulation during hypoxia in fetal sheep. AM J Obstet Gynecol 1983; 147:592–597.

36. Iwamoto HS, Rudolph AM, Mirkin BL, Keil LC. Circulatory and humoral responses of the sympathectomized fetal sheep to hypoxemia. Am J Physiol 1983; 245:H767–H772.

37. Comline RS, Silver M: The release of adrenaline and noradrenaline from the adrenal glands of the foetal sheep. J Physiol (Lond) 1961; 156:424–444.

38. Parer JT, Krueger TR, Harris JL, Reuss ML. Autonomic influences in umbilical circulation during hypoxia in fetal sheep. Proceedings of the Quilligan Symposium, San Diego, 1978.

39. Court DJ, Parer JT. Unpublished observations.

40. Berman W, Goodlin RC, Heymann MA, Rudolph AM. Relationships between pressure and flow in the umbilical and uterine circulations of the sheep. Circ Res 1976; 38:262–266.

41. Rosenberg AA, Jones MD, Traystman RJ, Simmons MA, Molteni RA. Response of cerebral blood flow to changes in Pco$_2$ in fetal, newborn and adult sheep. Am J Physiol 1982; 242:H862–H866.

42. Perez R, Espinoza M, Riquelme R, Parer JT, Llanos AJ. Arginine vasopressin mediates cardiovascular responses to hypoxemia in fetal sheep. Am J Physiol 1989; 256:R1011–1018.

43. Itskovitz J, LaGamma EF, Bristow J, Rudolph AM. Role of arterial chemoreflex in fetal circulatory response to acute hypoxemia. Proceedings of the Society for Gynecologic Investigation. Washington, DC, 1983, p 126.

44. Share L, Levy MN. Effect of carotid chemoreceptor stimulation on plasma antidiuretic hormone titer. Am J Physiol 1966; 210:157–161.

45. Espinoza M, Riquelme R, Germain AM, Tevah J, Parer JT, Llanos AJ. Role of endogenous opioids in the cardiovascular responses to asphyxia in fetal sheep. Am J Physiol 1989; 256:1063–1068.

46. Iwamoto HS, Rudolph AM. Effects of angiotensin II on the blood flow and its distribution in fetal lambs. Circ Res 1981; 48:183–189.

8

Body Composition in Pregnancy

Robert N. Girandola, Nazareth Khodiguian, Raul Artal Mittelmark, and Robert A. Wiswell

Body composition evaluation of humans, in vivo, generally involves the quantification of storage fat and fat-free weight. The human body is composed of a number of tissues and organs, all of which are part of the fat-free weight. Although many of these tissues may vary among individuals in terms of size, the greatest differences occur in the skeletal muscle and skeleton. It has been shown that fat-free weight (or lean body weight (LBW) which will be discussed later) is affected by race (1, 2), age (3–5), sex (6–8), and stature (9). Finally, it is well established that LBW can be markedly affected by physical training in both sexes (10).

If LBW is so variable then it must follow that body fat is also quite variable, and it is. The percentage of body fat in men has been found to range from low values of 3–5% to extremely high values, above 40%, in obese individuals. Values for women have also been found to vary, perhaps even more so, from lows of 6–10% to highs of 40–50%, and possibly higher.

Why is it so important to measure and quantify body composition? A report by Buskirk (11) stated the reasons extremely well:

1. "As a tool in characterizing populations or specific segments of a population;
2. As a tool in studying gender and ethnic differences;
3. As a tool in describing normal or abnormal growth, development, maturation, and aging;
4. To follow changes in status as occur in pregnancy and lactation;
5. To provide bases of reference for dietary and nutritional counseling;
6. To provide bases of reference for drug and other therapeutic administrations;
7. As a tool in physical fitness appraisal;
8. As a guide to athletes who are preparing for competition or engaged in competition."

The relationship between obesity and various degenerative diseases such as coronary heart disease, hypertension, and diabetes has been well established (Surgeon General's report, 1988). The incidence of obesity in the United States is anywhere from 25–40% of the adult population. To make matters worse, it appears that the incidence of obesity in young children is also on the rise.

For many years, individuals have been evaluated for "obesity" or "physique" by measuring their height and weight, with "criterion" values being supplied by the Metropolitan Life Insurance Company. Although height-weight tables are reasonably good for evaluating overweightness, it is well established that the overweight person is not necessarily the obese (too much fat) person (12). Many organizations that had utilized height-weight tables for years have now adopted some form of body composition evaluation. These include the military and emergency service organizations, such as police, firefighters, and lifeguards, among others.

METHODS OF MEASURING BODY COMPOSITION

There are several methods that can be utilized to measure body composition in the living organism, some of which are highly practical and some of which are limited, due to economics, to a very few research or clinical institutes (Table 8.1). Because all of these methods are indirect or predictive, there are errors associated with the techniques. These "errors" (or variations) are caused by the errors of measurement (associated with the specific technique) and biological variation of the subject.

Densitometry

Densitometry is generally considered the "gold standard" or criterion method to eval-

99

Table 8.1. Comparison of the Methods Discussed for the Assessment of Components of Body Composition[a]

Method	Validity	Reliability	Cost	Applicability for Pregnant Subjects
Hydrodensitometry	2	2	3	1
Total body water (TBW)				
D_2O, ^3H_2O	1	1	2	5
BIA	3	2	2	1
TOBEC	3	2	4	2
Neutron activation analysis				
(NAA)	1	1	5	?
Total body potassium (TBK)	1	1	5	2
Creatinine excretion (Cr)	3	3	2	2
3-Methylhistidine excretion				
(3-MH)	2	2	2	2
Dual photon absorptiometry				
(DPA)	1	2	4	5

[a]Rating System: 1 = superior, 5 = poor. Abbrevations: BIA = body impedance analyzer; TOBEC = total body electrical conductivity.
From Buskirk ER. Body composition analysis: the past, present and future. Res Quart 1987; 58:1–10.

uate body composition. This method has been in use for more than 50 years and probably most of the data available on body composition have been collected by this technique. Body density is measured by weighing an individual on land and then in water during a maximal lung expiration (Fig. 8.1). With the calculation of residual lung volume, body density can be calculated. Percentage of fat is calculated by one of a number of formulas, the most common of which is that by Brozek et al. (13). The prediction of fat from density is based upon the constancy of the LBW, which has been stated as 1.10 g/ml. However, Lohman (14) has estimated the LBW to be 1.08 in young children (10 years) and Schutte, et al. (2) have stated that the LBW of blacks is 1.13. Thus, using present prediction formulas for percentage of fat one would overestimate fat in children and underestimate fat in blacks.

Total Body Water (TBW)

The body water makes up the single largest component of the body. Data from Widdowson and Dickerson (15) and Forbes (16) indicate that TBW ranges from 69–73% of the LBW. Basically this technique attempts to quantify the TBW and from this estimate LBW. Although there are several techniques available to measure TBW perhaps the most common method is to utilize an isotope dilution, commonly deuterium oxide. The subject ingests a known quantity of the isotope and waits a period of time for equilibration to occur. Measurement of the diluted tracer can be made through the blood, urine, or saliva. Unfortunately, this technique is highly dependent upon normal hydration of the subject.

Gamma Radiometry

The measurement of potassium is also an important method of body composition evaluation. Potassium is an intracellular cation. There is a naturally occurring ^{40}K in the body with a fairly constant percentage (0.012) that emits a characteristic gamma ray. This method requires a shielded room (to shield out other contaminating radiation) and a sensitive gamma ray detector. Essentially this method predicts LBW. Unfortunately, the instrumentation is extremely expensive and not likely to be found in other than a handful of specialized laboratories.

Computerized Tomography

This method is a modern radiographic method used to determine regional body composition. While this technique is promising to identify regional fat deposits its wide-

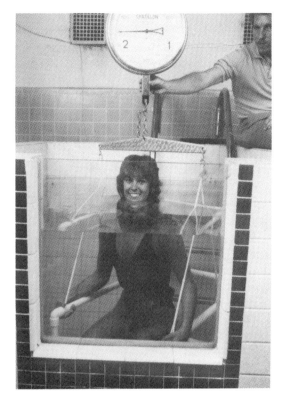

Figure 8.1. The hydrostatic weighing procedure. The subject is submerged and weighed after maximal expiration. The data are corrected for residual lung volume (O_2 washout method).

spread use is limited. First, the instrument is extremely expensive and likely to be found only in specialized clinical facilities (i.e., cancer centers) and second, the exposure to ionizing radiation would limit its use for whole body or repeated measures.

Bioelectrical Impedance

This technique makes use of the fact that the body fluids are excellent conductors of electrical current (Fig. 8.2). In living organisms, electrical conduction is related to the water and electrolyte distribution in the biological conductor. Because the LBW contains most of the body water, conductivity will be greatest in this type of tissue. This technique has received a great deal of publicity recently. Several studies have indicated very good relationships to densitometry with standard errors that are in the 2–4% range. The reason why the method is so desirable stems from

its low cost, portability, and reliability (17–19).

Anthropometry

Anthropometric methods make use of either skinfold fat and/or various body circumferences or bone diameters to predict body composition. These methods have been in use for over 20 years. Skinfold fat measures are made by the use of a device called a skinfold caliper that measures a double layer of fat and skin between two pincers with an analog scale to read the value in mm. Forbes (16) has shown that skinfold fat makes up approximately 42% of total fat in adults. There are literally hundreds of prediction formulas available to quantify total body fat from a series of skinfold measures. Although many of these have been validated against more accurate methods (densitometry), the fact that there are so many is an indication that many of them may be population specific. Another problem associated with the skinfold method is that experimenters must be well trained in the method. Skinfolds have not been recommended for evaluating body composition changes (20) or for measuring the obese (16).

Behnke and Wilmore (10) elaborate on the use of circumferences and skeletal diameters to predict body composition. Circumferences are made using cloth or metal tape at specific landmarks. Diameters are measured by the use of an anthropometer (a ruler with a slid-

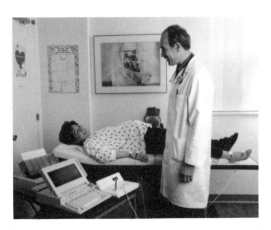

Figure 8.2. Body composition assessment by the bioelectrical impedance method (pictured a Bio-Analogics® system).

ing scale and arm attached). Again, whereas these methods have been validated, they have not been used extensively by others.

Body Mass Index (BMI)

The use of height and weight in a specific ratio has also been used to evaluate obesity in subjects. The BMI is a measure of an individual's weight divided by his or her height squared $(BMI = W (kg)/H^2(m^2))$. Normal ranges for BMI in men and women would be 19–27 (16). Jackson, et al. (22) have shown that BMI may be a reasonably good predictor of body fat. However, our data indicate that the validity coefficients (compared to densitometry) were .52–.69, for males and females, respectively, and standard errors of approximately 4.5% fat.

BODY WEIGHT AND BODY COMPOSITION CHANGES

As stated earlier, the variability of the storage fat as well as the LBW is great indeed. Some of these changes may take years but they do in fact occur. Those individuals suffering from morbid obesity may have body weights approaching (and exceeding) 500 lb, the majority of which is fat. Some young athletes, through a program of heavy resistive exercises, have added as much as 50 lb of lean weight over a period of several years. Weight gain (as well as weight loss) occurs as a result of a positive or negative caloric balance. The caloric equivalent of a pound of weight (most of which would be fat) is usually accepted to be 3500. However, the exact caloric equivalents are as follows:

Fat = 4100 kcal/lb
Carbohydrate = 1800 kcal/lb
Protein = 1800 kcal/lb

Typically, weight gain and/or loss, is made up of a combination of the former, as well as water. Therefore, the actual caloric equivalent of tissue weight changes cannot be predicted with great accuracy until one knows what type of tissue is actually metabolized or gained. During weight loss, individuals will invariably lose both fat as well as fat-free weight, in various combinations. In addition, the combination of tissues will vary over time,

with a greater proportion of fat being lost during the latter stages of a dietary and/or exercise intervention program. A program of endurance-type exercise appears to increase the proportion of fat tissue that is lost when compared to simply a dietary restriction. This is probably due to the increased secretion of lipolytic hormones, such as epinephrine and growth hormone, during exercise (23, 24).

The use of body composition evaluation to identify tissue changes after weight loss is extremely valuable, both to the clinician as well as to the patient, for motivational reasons. Certain techniques may not accurately predict body composition changes, due to large variability in the measurement or for biological reasons. Wilmore et al. (20) have stated that the use of skinfolds alone to identify body composition changes is not accurate enough. Because there may be hydration differences during the weight loss, techniques that predict total body water may also be contraindicated. A combination of techniques would appear to be ideal, such as densitometry, anthropometry, and impedance.

The composition of weight gain is also somewhat variable. It appears that weight gain as a result of a positive caloric balance combined with a program of physical exercise results in a greater proportion of fat-free weight being accumulated. However, there are great differences in composition gained between individuals, some of which may simply be related to hereditary factors. Similar to the methodological problems discussed previously, it is imperative that before and after measurements be made under the most exacting conditions. That is, subjects should be measured at the same time of day, in a fasted state, and assurances (as well as possible) that they are "normally" hydrated.

BODY COMPOSITION DURING PREGNANCY

The measurement of body composition during pregnancy, similar to other weight-gain situations, has been considered to be a valuable addition to the clinical care and evaluation of the patient during gestation. The health risks of obesity have been cited previously. However, for the obese pregnant woman there is the additional risk of gestational diabetes. Twenty-five percent of infants born to these mothers are hypoglycemic and hyperinsulinemic.

The average weight gain after a typical 40-week pregnancy amounts to approximately 12.5 kg, about a 20% increase in body weight for most women (average weight = 60 kg) (16). Most of this weight gain (68%) occurs during the last 20 weeks of pregnancy. The composition of this weight gain is of great interest; however, the ability to separate the fetomaternal unit in vivo through traditional methods of body composition evaluation have been sketchy at best. It is known that about 40% of the total gain is represented by the fetus plus placenta and amniotic fluid (16). The remaining 60%, therefore, is the mother's body weight change.

Tissue Changes in the Mother

There is evidence that some of the weight gains of the pregnant female are due to increases in mammary, uterine, kidney, and heart tissues. In addition, there is an increase in plasma volume and other fluid volumes (mostly extracellular fluid) (21, 25). Obviously, fat stores also increase somewhat, but there has been a difficulty in quantifying this change.

Because the full-term (40 weeks) fetus, placenta, and amniotic fluid constitute 40% of the mother's weight gain, it is imperative to know their composition when attempting to estimate the pregnant female's body composition. Obviously, the proportion of fetal weight varies throughout the course of the gestation period. A pregnant woman may only gain about 1 kg during the first 13 weeks. At term, the fat content of the fetus has been estimated at approximately 14% of body weight (15). It would appear from the data of Widdowson and Dickerson (15) that the proportion of fat accumulation in the fetus follows the same pattern that fat-free weight does. Therefore, in terms of percentage of body fat, it would appear that this value is somewhat similar throughout the gestational period.

In addition to the fat percentage, the total water weight of the fetus, placenta, and amniotic fluid amounts to 3.8 kg of a total 4.7 kg (81%). In fact, it has been estimated that 60% of the total weight gain of the fetomaternal unit is water (21). One other factor that confounds body composition measurement techniques is the fact that the density of the fat-free body of the newborn is less than that which is accepted for the adult (1.10 g/ml). Thus, techniques that measure body composition by densitometry or by total body water may not give the most accurate estimation of fat percentage during the latter period of gestation.

Several researchers have attempted to monitor body composition changes in pregnant women during the gestational period. Seitchik et al. (26), utilizing densitometry as the method of evaluation, found an increase in estimated percentage of fat from 31.2 to 33.8 for 21 women from early pregnancy to the 37th through 40th week. They also found that those women who gained more than 8.5 kg of weight had a greater fat accumulation. McCartney et al. (27) found an increase in body fat amounting to 8% during pregnancy, based upon densitometry. Forsum et al. (29), utilizing ^{18}O-labeled water and total body potassium, reported that the majority of fat gain in pregnancy is observed during the first trimester (Table 8.2).

METHODOLOGICAL QUESTIONS

In the area of exercise physiology we have always been concerned with body weight as a factor that affects performance. More recently, we have partitioned the body into components in order to evaluate more, elaborately, the role of body composition on performance and, more importantly, on health and disease. Increase in adiposity influences performance negatively and increases one's risk of life-threatening diseases. Lean weight, on the other hand, is related to strength and is not specifically related to disease. The challenge, therefore, has been for exercise physiologists to measure body composition accurately and to relate these results to associative changes in function and/or disease.

There are several methods that can and

Table 8.2. Maternal Body Weight (MBW), Total Body Water (TBW), Total Body Potassium (TBK), Total Body Fat (TBF), and Resting Metabolic Rate (RMR) in Healthy Swedish Women Before, During, and After Pregnancy[a,b]

	MBW		TBW		TBK		TBF		RMR	
	kg	%	kg	%	mmol	%	kg	%	kcal/min	%
Prepregnancy	61.0 ± 9.9		33.0 ± 4.3		2397 ± 327		17.2 ± 6.9		0.936 ± 0.124	
Gestational weeks 16–18	63.7 ± 9.7[c]	104.7 ± 3.6	32.5 ± 3.7	99.1 ± 8.5	2224 ± 298[d]	93.5 ± 11.6	20.7 ± 6.0[c]	128.3 ± 28.7	1.000 ± 0.157	107.8 ± 17
Gestational week 30	70.2 ± 9.9[c]	115.6 ± 4.6	36.7 ± 3.7[c]	112.3 ± 11.6	2290 ± 330[d]	95.8 ± 9.0	22.6 ± 6.9[c]	141.3 ± 39.5	1.147 ± 0.143[c]	1240 ± 18
Gestational week 36	72.7 ± 10.3[c]	119.8 ± 5.1	38.7 ± 4.4[c]	118.4 ± 13.3	2507 ± 307	105.8 ± 14.4	22.3 ± 7.1[c]	139.2 ± 39.6	1.223 ± 0.124[c]	132.5 ± 18.9
5-10 days postpartum	67.6 ± 10.8[c]	111.1 ± 5.7	34.2 ± 3.7[e]	104.3 ± 12.9[e]	2366 ± 294[e]	99.0 ± 10.8[e]	22.9 ± 7.8[c,e]	142.9 ± 40.8[e]	1.063 ± 0.169[e,d]	114.1 ± 23.8[f]
6 months postpartum	61.9 ± 10.9[f]	101.7 ± 5.8[f]	31.4 ± 4.0[d,f]	95.6 ± 7.3[f]	2240 ± 252[d,f]	95.1 ± 8.3[f]	20.4 ± 7.9[f,g]	123.2 ± 28.9[f]	0.984 ± 0.103[d,f]	108.6 ± 16.8[f]

[a] From Forsum E, Sadurskis A, Wager J. Resting metabolic rate and body composition of healthy Swedish women during pregnancy. Am J Clin Nutr 1988;47:942–947.
[b] $\bar{x}$ ± SD; n = 22 except where otherwise indicated; % = percent of value obtained before pregnancy.
[c] Significantly different from prepregnancy value ($p < 0.001$).
[d] Significantly different from prepregnancy value ($0.05 > p > 0.01$).
[e] n = 21.
[f] Significantly different from prepregnancy value ($0.01 > p > 0.001$).
[g] n = 20.

have been used to evaluate percentage of fat and fat-free weight (FFW). These methods, as well as the validity, reliability, cost, and criterion potential are summarized in Table 8.1 (11). It is unfortunate, but many of these methodologies are not usable for the pregnant subject. Others that are usable are potentially not valid. This is a major dilemma for the clinician and research scientist who are trying to understand the effects of pregnancy on body composition components.

The question of validity of body composition measurement has remained unanswered over the years. Hydrostatic weighing provides a reliable estimation of density and has been used as the criterion measure for the estimation of fat for more than 50 years. Underwater weighing provides an accurate method for estimating body density but the conversion from body density (volume) to percentage of body fat is open to controversy. The assumptions that are made concerning body composition assessment from density using hydrostatic weighing are:

1. Densities of individual tissues composing the lean tissue are constant within and between individuals;
2. Density of lean and fat weight are constant;
3. Individual tissues composing the lean tissue are constant relative to their proportional contribution.

It is obvious that pregnancy can cause maternal changes that would violate these assumptions. The fact that FFW of the developing fetus is less than the average density of 1.10 g/ml suggests that an underestimation of maternal FFW could result. Furthermore, the assumption that 73.2% of the FFW is water can be challenged in pregnancy due to the large and significant increase in fluid retention that occurs in mid to late gestation.

Because of the violations of basic assumption required for evaluation of the percentage of fat that occurs during pregnancy, it may be that the criterion measure (hydrostatic weighing) is not a valid index of body composition over this time period. Equations have been reported to adjust the hydrostatic density to the increased fluid retention (Tables

8.3 and 8.4) (28). In the study of van Raaij et al. (28), new equations were developed that supposedly take into account the alterations in density and composition of the maternal fat-free mass throughout pregnancy, but validation of these procedures has not been reported.

The problem of the validity of hydrostatic weighing is of particular concern when attempting to use other methodologies, such as bioelectrical impedance or ultrasound techniques in measuring FFW, in that these methods have been developed using regression from hydrostatic weighing technique. Utilizing bioelectrical impedance, we have observed the changes in body weight and body fat during pregnancy (Figs. 8.3 and 8.4). Our data indicate that the measurements of

Table 8.3. Usual and New Equations for Estimating Body Fat Mass From Body Density and Body Weight[a,b]

General equation

$$W_{FM} = \frac{W_B}{100} \times \frac{\left(\dfrac{100}{D_B} - \dfrac{100}{D_{FFM}}\right)}{\left(\dfrac{1}{D_{FM}} - \dfrac{1}{D_{FFM}}\right)}$$

Usual (Siri's) equation $W_{FM} = \dfrac{W_B}{100} \times \left(\dfrac{495}{D_B} - 450\right)$

New pregnancy equations
 No edema or leg edema only

10-wk gestation $W_{FM} = \dfrac{W_B}{100} \times \left(\dfrac{496.4}{D_B} - 451.6\right)$

20-wk gestation $W_{FM} = \dfrac{W_B}{100} \times \left(\dfrac{502.2}{D_B} - 458.0\right)$

30-wk gestation $W_{FM} = \dfrac{W_B}{100} \times \left(\dfrac{510.8}{D_B} - 467.5\right)$

40-wk gestation $W_{FM} = \dfrac{W_B}{100} \times \left(\dfrac{522.5}{D_B} - 480.5\right)$

[a]Reproduced from VanRaaij J, Peek MEM, Vermaat-Miedema SH, et al. Am J Clin Nutr 1988;48:24–29.
[b]V_B, V_{FM}, V_{FFM}: volume of body, fat mass, and fat-free mass ($\times 10^{-3}$ m³): W_B, W_{FM}, W_{FFM}: Weight of body, fat mass, and fat-free mass (kg): D_B, D_{FM}, D_{FFM}: density of body, fat mass, and fat-free mass.
Derivation: $V_B = V_{FM} + V_{FFM}$; so

$$\frac{W_B}{D_B} = \frac{W_{FM}}{D_{FM}} + \frac{W_{FFM}}{D_{FFM}} = \frac{W_{FM}}{D_{FM}} + \frac{(W_B - W_{FM})}{D_{FFM}}$$

$$= W_{FM}\left(\frac{1}{D_{FM}} - \frac{1}{D_{FFM}}\right) + \frac{W_B}{D_{FFM}}$$

Table 8.4.   Usual and New Equations for Estimating Body Fat Mass From Total Body Water and Body Weight[a]

General equation[b]	$W_{FM} = W_B - \dfrac{TBW}{WATER\%_{FFM}}$
Usual equation[c]	$W_{FM} = W_B - \dfrac{TBW}{0.724}$

New pregnancy equations
  No edema or leg edema only

10-wk gestation	$W_{FM} = W_B - \dfrac{TBW}{0.725}$
20-wk gestation	$W_{FM} = W_B - \dfrac{TBW}{0.732}$
30-wk gestation	$W_{FM} = W_B - \dfrac{TBW}{0.740}$
40-wk gestation	$W_{FM} = W_B - \dfrac{TBW}{0.750}$

[a] Reproduced from Van Raaij J, Peek MEM, Vermaat-Miedema SH, et al. Am J Clin Nutr 1988; 44:24–29. W_B, W_{FM}, W_{FFM}: weight of body, fat mass and fat-free mass (kg); TBW: total body water (kg); WATER$\%_{FFM}$: water content fat-free mass ($\times 10^2\%$).
[b] Derivation: $W_B = W_{FM} + W_{FFM}$, $W_{FFM} = TBW/WATER\%_{FFM}$.
[c] Assumed water content of fat-free mass 72.4%.

percentage of body fat obtained by bioelectrical impedance were significantly lower than the measurements obtained by either densitometry or skinfold techniques and may be reflective of the increase in total body water that occurs progressively throughout pregnancy. Unfortunately, what may be happening is that the hydrostatic procedure may actually be in error and, thus, precludes the new methodology from obtaining a higher degree of precision. Due to the nature of validation, we have no way of verifying which methods are correct nor can we actually suggest that any method would provide reasonable results.

As an example of question of validity we will use the impedance methodology. The basic assumption of the use of impedance is that (a) impedance is an accurate means of assessing total body water, and (b) that lean weight is 72.3% H_2O. In hyperhydrative states, such as the fluid retention of pregnancy, the impedance device will accurately assess TBW. Unfortunately, the conversion of TBW to FFW will be in error. The higher water content will indicate a much greater FFW than actually exists. The overestimation of FFW may or may not cause an error in the evaluation of fat. Although more research is required to resolve these methodological problems, we have no valid measuring tools to provide the criterion measure at this time.

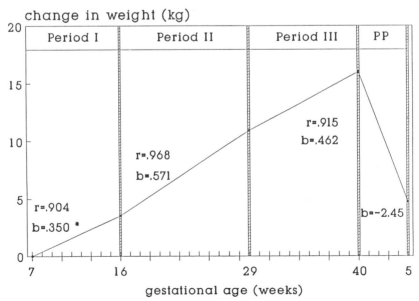

Figure 8.3.   Changes in body weight through gestation in a large obstetrical population (R. Artal and N. Khodiguian, unpublished observations).

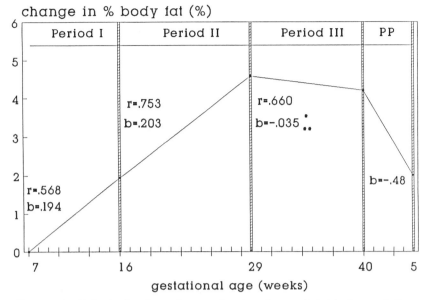

Figure 8.4. Changes in % body fat through gestation in a large obstetrical population as measured by bioelectrical impedance (R. Artal and N. Khodiguian, unpublished observation).

REFERENCES

1. Nagamine S, Suzuki S. Anthropometry and body composition of Japanese young men and women. Hum Biol 1964; 36:8–15.
2. Schutte JE, Townsend EJ, Hugg JH, et al. Density of lean body mass is greater in Blacks than in Whites. J Appl Physiol 1984; 56:1647–1649.
3. Cohn SH, Vaswani A, Zanzi I, et al. Effect of aging on bone mass in adult women. Am J Physiol 1976; 230:143–148.
4. Flynn MA, Woodruff C, Chase G. Total body potassium in normal children. Pediatr Res 1972; 6:239–245.
5. Novak LI. Aging, total body potassium, fat-free mass, and cell mass in males and females between ages 18 and 85 years. J Gerontol 1972; 27:438–443.
6. Borisov BK, Marei AN. Weight parameters of adult human skeleton. Health Physics 1974; 27:224–229.
7. Cohn SH, Vartsky D, Yasumura S, et al. Compartmental body composition based on total-body nitrogen, potassium, and calcium. Am J Physiol 1980; 239:E524–E530.
8. Forbes GB. Stature and lean body mass. Am J Clin Nutr 1974; 27:595–602.
9. Bouchard C, Savard R, Despres JP, et al. Body composition in adopted and biological siblings. Hum Biol 1985; 57:61–75.
10. Behnke AR, Wilmore JH. Evaluation and regulation of body build and composition. Englewood Cliffs, NJ: Prentice Hall, 1974.
11. Buskirk ER. Body composition analysis: the past, present and future. Res Quart 1987; 58:1–10.
12. Harrison GG. Height-weight tables. Ann Intern Med 1985; 103:989–994.
13. Brozek J, Grande F, Anderson JT, et al. Densitometric analysis of body composition: revision of some quantitative assumptions. Ann NY Acad Sci 1963; 110:113–140.
14. Lohman TG. Applicability of body composition techniques and constants for children and youths. In Exercise and sport sciences reviews. New York: MacMillan, vol. 14, 1986; p 325–357.
15. Widdowson EM, Dickerson JWT. Chemical composition of the body. In Comar CL, Bronner F, eds. Mineral metabolism. New York: Academic Press, vol. 2, Part A, 1964, pp 2–247.
16. Forbes GB. Methods for determining composition of the human body. Pediatrics 1962; 29:477–494.
17. Lukaski HC, Bolonchuk WW, Hall CA, et al. Estimation of fat free mass in humans using the bioelectrical impedance method: a validation study. J Appl Physiol 1986; 60:1327–1332.
18. Hodgdon JA, Fitzgerald PI. Validity of impedance predictions at various levels of fatness. Hum Biol 1987; 59:281–298.
19. Guo S, Roche AF, Chumlea WC, et al. Body composition predictions from bioelectric impedance. Hum Biol 1987; 59:221–233.
20. Wilmore JH, Royce J, Girandola RN, et al. Body composition changes with a 10-week program of jogging. Med Sci Sports 1970; 2:113–117.
21. Forbes GB. Human body composition: growth, aging, nutrition and activity. New York: Springer-Verlag, 1987.
22. Jackson AS, Pollock ML, Graves JE, et al. Reliability and validity of bioelectrical impedance in determining body composition. J Appl Physiol 1988; 64:529–534.
23. Oscai LB, Spirakis CN, Wolff CA, et al. Effects of exercise and of food restriction on adipose tissue cellularity. J Lipid Res 1972; 13:588–592.
24. Zuti WB, Golding LA. Comparing diet and exercise as weight reduction tools. Phys Sportsmed 1976; 4:49–53.
25. Hytten FE, Chamberlain G, eds. Clinical physiology in obstetrics. Oxford: Blackwell Scientific, 1980.
26. Seitchik J, Alper C, Szutka A. Changes in body

composition during pregnancy. Ann NY Acad Sci 1963; 110:821–829.

27. McCartney CP, Pottinger RE, Harrod JP. Alterations in body composition during pregnancy. Am J Obstet Gynecol 1959; 77:1038–1053.

28. vanRaaij JMA, Peek MEM, Vermaat-miedema SH, Schonk CM, Hautvast JGAJ. New equations for estimating body fat mass in pregnancy for body den-

sity or total body water. Am J Clin Nutr 1988; 48:24–29.

29. Forsum E, Sadurskis A, Wager J. Resting metabolic rate and body composition of healthy Swedish women during pregnancy. Am J Clin Nutr 1988; 47:942–947.

30. U.S. Department of Health and Human Services. The Surgeon General's Report on Nutrition and Health. PHS. 1988; no. 88–50211.

Nutritional Needs of Physically Active Pregnant Women

Gail Butterfield and Janet C. King

During pregnancy, the mother's diet supplies the nutrients needed by the fetus for development. If the nutrient supply from the diet is deficient, fetal growth may slow and an infant with a high risk of morbidity and mortality may be born (1). The dramatic detrimental effect of severe maternal food restriction on fetal growth was demonstrated in western Holland during the winter months of 1944–1945 when, as a result of a food embargo, the population had its average daily food ration reduced from 1800 to 600 kcal/day (2). The famine lasted 28 weeks, and some women were affected during the last two trimesters of pregnancy. In these women, the average birth weight fell 327 g, or 9%, compared to the prefamine mean value. Also, the incidence of stillbirths and neonatal mortality increased.

Today, situations still exist where a poor maternal diet reduces fetal growth. Among low income women in developing countries, the food supply is limited, and infants born to these underfed women weigh an average of 300 g less at birth than infants born to well-fed mothers. However, maternal malnutrition also exists among more affluent women who either are advised to or choose to limit their food intake. For example, the average birth weight of all infants born in Motherwell, Scotland, between 1938 and 1977 was 400 g less than in Aberdeen, Scotland, because all pregnant women in Motherwell at that time were advised to restrict their food intake (3). Fetal growth retardation is very likely if the maternal food supply and, therefore, dietary energy supply is restricted.

Heavy maternal physical activity can expend the available maternal energy and possibly deprive the fetus of needed energy for growth. For example, the birth weights of infants born to women in developing countries during the months of heavy agricultural labor are lower than those born at other times of the year (4).

However, there is some evidence under circumstances of marginal energy intake that physiological adaptations can occur that conserve energy for fetal growth (5, 6). Such adaptations have not been evaluated where high intensity exercise is performed for short periods each day, as is done by some women in more affluent societies where exercise has a recreational rather than an economic motivation. Reported energy intakes in professional and recreational women athletes are low in comparison to theoretical need (7–9), suggesting that there may be a physiological adaptation to conserve energy stimulated by exercise that is already in place (10). One report in pregnant runners showed energy intake to be no different from that of sedentary pregnant controls (11). The ability of the system to adapt to both exercise and low energy intake when both are continued into pregnancy is untested. The birth weight of babies born to women who continued recreational exercise during pregnancy has been shown by some to be decreased (12).

At this time, the nutritional needs of physically active pregnant women are undefined. Therefore, inferences must be drawn from knowledge of the nutritional requirements of pregnant, sedentary women and of nonpregnant, active women. Before discussing the nutritional needs of active pregnant women in this chapter, we will first review those of pregnant sedentary women and those of active nonpregnant women.

NUTRIENT REQUIREMENTS OF PREGNANT SEDENTARY WOMEN

Nutritional advice given to pregnant women varies between and within cultures. Some cultures recommend nutritious foods for the pregnant woman, such as leafy greens, fruits, and milk. Others forbid foods that clearly make an important nutrient contribution to the diet. For example, one African tribe forbids eggs and milk during pregnancy (13). Within Westernized cultures, nutritional advice seems to change with generations. Presently, pregnant women are advised to eat to appetite, gain approximately 25 lb, salt their food to taste, and breast-feed their infants. This prescription is exactly the opposite of what their mothers were told.

It is becoming evident from a historical and cultural review of food practices during pregnancy that there are many different, acceptable ways of providing the nutrients needed for fetal growth. This diversity of practice is an important issue to keep in mind when counseling pregnant women about their dietary habits. It is not necessary that all women consume meat, milk, vegetables, and bread. But, it is important that they select carefully from a wide variety of foods to provide the calories and nutrients needed for the fetus and themselves.

Energy

Total caloric intake appears to be the most important nutritional factor affecting infant birth weight. It has been estimated that a typical pregnancy requires about 85,000 additional calories, or approximately 300 extra calories per day above that needed in the nonpregnant state (14). About one-third of these calories are thought to be accounted for by maternal fat gain. The remainder is primarily the energy needed for metabolism by the new tissue gained.

If energy intake is sufficient, estimates for increased metabolic needs seem to hold (5), although actual fat accumulation is somewhat less than theoretical (5). If energy intake is marginal or inadequate, metabolic adaptations occur that conserve energy for fetal growth. Maternal fat accretion is diminished (5) and basal energy needs remain constant or actually decline in early pregnancy rather than increasing across the entire pregnancy (6). The resultant fetus is only slightly smaller

(by about 300 g) than one born to a well-nourished woman.

Total weight gain during an adequately nourished pregnancy averages between 10 and 12 kg (14). However, individual energy intakes and weight gains vary widely. Maternal pregravid weight and daily energy expenditure are two factors that influence appetite, energy intake, and weight gain.

Women who begin pregnancy weighing 15% or more below the suggested weight for their height deliver low birth weight infants more frequently and have a greater risk of developing preeclampsia and preterm labor (15). Intensive nutritional counseling and provision of supplemental calories in the form of high quality foods has been successful in improving their weight gain and in increasing infant birth weight (16). Therefore, underweight women should be encouraged to increase their energy intake and to gain between 12 and 15 kg.

Obese women (greater than 20% above standard weight for height) more frequently deliver large infants (greater than 4.0 kg). These women also are prone to develop glucose intolerance or hypertension during gestation. Food restriction and weight reduction are not recommended during pregnancy, however. Past studies of food restriction in obese pregnant women indicate that maternal fat losses are very low. For example, a 500-kcal restriction daily during the last 10 weeks of pregnancy caused less than a 0.5-kg maternal fat loss (17). This small fat loss does not warrant the discomfort of a restricted food intake during pregnancy when appetite is increased and the woman is prone to hypoglycemia.

A gradual, progressive weight gain of 9–11 kg is ideal for obese pregnant women. This goal is best attained through individual diet assessment and counseling with emphasis on foods rich in nutrients but low in fat. Breast-feeding should be encouraged, and, after weaning, a comprehensive program of exercise and diet for weight reduction should be suggested. Occasionally, a very obese woman loses weight during pregnancy without conscious dieting. The mechanism for this weight loss is unknown, but infant birth weight is not affected negatively.

In all pregnant women, a weight gain of less than 1.0 kg per month during the last two trimesters is considered to be insufficient (18). A low rate of weight gain may lead to delivery of a low birth weight infant. In obese women, a low weight gain does not seem to be as detrimental as in an underweight woman (19). Possibly, lower weight gains are better tolerated by obese women because some of the energy needed for pregnancy can be provided by maternal stores. Or, the metabolic adjustments associated with obesity may alter the use of energy for fetal growth.

Identification of excessive weight gain can be difficult in pregnant women. Individual variability leads to a wide range of weight gains compatible with appropriate birth weights. What is excessive for one woman may not be for another. Also, in pregnancy, excessive weight gain may result from accumulation of body water as well as body fat, and it is difficult to distinguish the two types of tissue gain. Sometimes the pattern of weight gain is helpful in assessing the composition of tissue gain. Water may be accumulated more rapidly than fat.

Excessive fat gain during pregnancy does not appear to cause preeclampsia, as thought previously. But, unless the woman in underweight or carrying twins or triplets, gaining more than 16–18 kg can lead to postpartum obesity and a source of anxiety for some women. If weight gain is high, food restriction should not be initiated in the third trimester when fetal growth is maximal and most sensitive to growth retardation. Instead, reduced intakes of fats and sweets and increased exercise can help normalize the rate of weight gain until term.

It is insufficient to consider only the total energy intake when counseling pregnant women; the source of calories should also be reviewed. Nutrient density, the quantity of protein, vitamins, and minerals per 100 calories is a measure of diet quality. The recommended additional calories for pregnancy, 300 kcal/day during the 2nd and 3rd trimesters (20), can easily be provided by many different foods. Depending on the food choice, additional nutrients may also be provided or the food may only provide "empty calories." A pint of low-fat milk or a peanut butter sandwich on whole grain bread each provide about 300 kcal, as do six small cookies or a 12-oz can of soda and 10 french-fried potatoes. The milk or sandwich have a much higher nutrient density than the cookies or soda with french fries. The iron density of common foods is compared in Table 9.1. This information may be helpful in counseling pregnant women to select foods with a high iron density.

Protein

An additional 10 g protein, or a total of 60 g, is recommended for pregnancy (20). But, protein-rich foods are plentiful in the United States, and *nonpregnant* women often select diets that provide more than the amount recommended for pregnancy. If this is true, no further increase in protein intake is needed for pregnancy. Protein-containing foods are excellent sources of many vitamins and minerals essential for fetal growth and development, such as iron, vitamin B_6, and zinc. There is, however, no evidence that high protein diets, greater than 100 g/day, are beneficial during pregnancy, and at least one study has suggested that "excessive amounts" may be harmful (21). An intake of 60–100 g protein per day, or 12% of the calories as protein calories, should be appropriate for pregnancy. Some animal protein sources, such as red meat, whole milk, and cheese are high in saturated fats. These foods should be limited and consumption of chicken, fish, nonfat milk, and vegetable protein sources, such as beans, encouraged.

Vegetarian Diets

Within the past 10 years, diets that exclude some or all animal protein sources have become quite popular. These diets can provide adequate nutrition for pregnant women, but more care in food selection is needed. Diets that include dairy products and/or eggs easily provide the nutrients needed for pregnancy. But, if all animal protein sources are avoided,

Table 9.1.   Iron Density of Some Foods

Food	Serving Size	Iron	
		mg/serving	mg/100 kcal
Dairy products			
Milk			
Whole	1 cup	0.1	0.1
Nonfat	1 cup	0.1	0.1
Yogurt, plain	8 oz	0.2	0.1
Cheese, cheddar	1 oz	0.2	0.2
Meat and meat alternatives			
Hamburger	3 oz	2.6	1.1
Beef stew	1 cup	2.9	1.3
Chili	1 cup	4.3	1.3
Chicken			
Thigh	1 medium	1.2	1.0
Breast	½	1.3	0.8
Eggs	1 whole	1.0	1.2
Fish sticks	4 sticks	0.4	0.2
Salmon	1 average steak	1.5	0.7
Sardines	3 oz	2.4	1.4
Tuna, in water	3 oz	1.6	1.2
Lamb, leg	3 oz	1.9	1.2
Lentils, cooked	½ cup	2.1	1.9
Liver, calf	3 oz	12.1	5.5
Macaroni and cheese	1 cup	1.8	0.4
Oysters	6	8.6	7.8
Peanut butter	1 tbsp	0.3	0.3
Pork chop	1 medium	1.6	1.5
Frankfurter	1 average	0.7	0.5
Liverwurst	1 oz	1.5	1.8
Tofu	1 2-inch cube	2.3	2.7
Turkey			
Dark	3 oz	2.0	1.2
Light	3 oz	1.0	0.7
Vitamin C-rich fruits and vegetables			
Grapefruit	½ raw	0.4	1.0
Lemonade	1 cup	0.1	0.1
Cantaloupe	½ melon	0.6	1.2
Orange juice	¾ cup	0.4	0.5
Green peppers	½ cup	0.5	3.3
Dark leafy green vegetables			
Broccoli	½ cup	0.6	3.0
Romaine lettuce	1 cup	0.8	8.0
Spinach	½ cup cooked	2.0	10.0
Swiss chard	½ cup cooked	1.3	8.7
Other fruits and vegetables			
Apricots, canned	4 halves	0.4	0.4
Banana	1 medium	0.8	0.8
Cabbage, cooked	½ cup	0.2	1.3
Carrots, boiled	½ cup	0.4	2.0
Corn, sweet	½ cup	0.4	0.6
Peas, canned	½ cup	1.6	2.1
Potatoes			
Baked	1 large	1.1	0.8
French-fried	20 each	0.8	0.4
Sprouts, alfalfa	1 cup	1.4	3.5
Raisins	½ cup	1.3	1.3
Breads and cereals			
Whole wheat bread	1 slice	0.8	1.2

Food	Serving Size	Iron	
		mg/serving	mg/100 kcal
White			
Enriched	1 slice	0.6	0.9
Unenriched	1 slice	0.2	0.3
Cereals			
Bran flakes	1 cup	12.4	12.4
Corn flakes	1 cup	0.6	0.6
Puffed rice	1 cup	0.3	0.5
Oatmeal	½ cup	0.7	1.1
Grits	½ cup	0.2	0.3
Other foods			
Cracker, graham	1 cracker	0.2	0.4
Doughnut, cake	1 average	0.6	0.4
Noodles, enriched	⅔ cup cooked	0.9	0.9
Popcorn	1 cup w/oil	0.2	0.5
Wheat germ	1 oz	2.5	2.1

vitamin B_{12} intakes will be inadequate and zinc, iron, calcium, vitamin D, and riboflavin intakes may be low. Also, due to the low fat and high bulk of vegetarian food sources, pregnant women may have difficulty consuming sufficient energy. Vitamin and mineral supplements may be recommended when the dietary assessment shows that intakes are inadequate. Use of vegetable oils and fats should be encouraged if the rate of weight gain is low as a result of insufficient energy intakes. Vegetable protein foods should be combined to ensure adequate protein quality at each meal. Guidelines for patient education have been prepared [22].

Iron

Additional iron is needed during pregnancy for expansion of maternal red blood cell volume and for fetal erythropoiesis and tissue gain. About 800 mg iron are gained during the last half of pregnancy; this is about 5–6 mg daily [23]. Because most women cannot provide this iron without depletion of their own stores, a daily oral supplement providing 30 mg elemental iron is recommended [20] for all pregnant women. A reduction in mean corpuscular volume along with a fall in hemoglobin and hematocrit is indicative of iron depletion during pregnancy. Women with such iron depletion should be given therapeutic doses of iron.

Food selection not only influences the amount of iron ingested (Table 9.1), but it also influences the amount of iron that will be absorbed. Some foods enhance iron absorption in the gut, whereas others inhibit it. Animal protein, or the "meat factor," and ascorbic acid enhance iron absorption [20]. Tea binds iron in the gut and reduces its absorption. Tea should be avoided at meals when good iron sources are consumed. Also, iron absorption will be reduced if iron pills are taken with tea or milk. Cast iron pans may provide significant amounts of iron, particularly if acidic foods, such as spaghetti sauce, are cooked in the pans.

Calcium

A daily allowance of 1200 mg calcium is recommended to provide the 30 g of calcium gained during pregnancy without maternal skeletal demineralization [20]. Although rare, neonatal hypocalcemia has been reported when maternal calcium and/or vitamin D intakes were inadequate [24].

A quart of cow's milk would provide most of the calcium and vitamin D recommended for pregnancy and a significant amount of protein. But, many ethnic groups, including people of Asian, Black, and Middle Eastern descent, are lactase deficient and are unable to digest the lactose in milk. These people may experience abdominal cramping, bloating, flatulence, and diarrhea when milk is consumed. Low lactose dairy products are cheese and yogurt. These foods may be substituted for milk. Other calcium-rich foods include salmon or sardines, fortified soymilk, ground sesame seeds, and leafy green vegetables.

Sodium

The increase in total body water by pregnant women also causes an increase in total body sodium. The net gain is about 22 g sodium (14). This gain occurs even though there is an increase in the glomerular filtration rate and in natriuretic hormones.

In the past, salt was forbidden to pregnant women, and diuretics were used whenever edema occurred. It was then thought that high sodium intakes caused toxemia and that the condition could be treated effectively with sodium restriction and diuretics (25). Now it appears that sodium restriction does not prevent toxemia, nor is it an effective way to treat toxemia. Diuretics are discouraged during pregnancy because they can cause electrolyte imbalances, hyperglycemia, hyperuricemia and other problems, and women are told to "salt to taste." High salt diets are not condoned, however, because they may precipitate hypertension in susceptible individuals. A diet composed primarily of natural foods can be safely salted "to taste"; processed foods are already seasoned with salt and should be used in moderation without further salting.

Other Nutrients

The dietary need for folic acid is increased during pregnancy for support of tissue synthesis (20). Foods rich in folic acid include eggs, leafy vegetables, oranges, legumes, whole grain cereals, and wheat germ.

Refinement of grains removes many nutrients in the germ and bran. Of particular concern are zinc, vitamin B_6, magnesium, and vitamin E because these nutrients are not replaced during the enrichment process. To assure an adequate intake of these nutrients for increased metabolic needs of pregnancy, whole grain cereals should be used. Whole grains also are excellent sources of fiber.

WOMEN AT NUTRITIONAL RISK DURING PREGNANCY

Women who may be at risk for nutritional problems are listed in Table 9.2. In general, women at risk are those who have economic, social, or medical problems that may lead to nutritional problems. Women with these problems often develop malnutrition because they do not consume enough food or because they make poor food choices. Asking a woman what she usually eats and then estimating her intake during the previous 24 hours will identify nutritional problems due to insufficient amounts of food or poor food choices. Presence of a poor weight gain pattern, obesity or underweight, or anemia is documentation of poor dietary habits and malnutrition. These women need in-depth nutritional counseling and follow-up.

NUTRITIONAL ADVICE FOR PREGNANT WOMEN

Nutritional counseling for pregnant women should emphasize the use of a wide variety of foods. A low-fat diet composed of lean animal foods, nonfat dairy products, and limited amounts of added fat is recommended for the average women. Soft drinks, alcoholic beverages, pastries, and candy have a low nutrient density and should be limited in the diet along with high fat, salty snacks such as potato chips. Total food intake should be increased to provide about 300 additional cal-

Table 9.2.   Nutritional Risks During Pregnancy

1. Pregravid weight 15% below or 20% above suggested weight for height
2. Insufficient or excessive rate of weight gain
3. Age of less than 15 years or more than 35 years
4. Presence of social, cultural, religious, psychological, or economic factors that limit or affect adequacy of nutrition
5. History of a low birth weight baby or other obstetric problems
6. Chronic disease, such as diabetes, thyroid disorders, or sickle cell disease
7. Presence of twins or triplets
8. Pica
9. Abnormal laboratory values, such as low hemoglobin level, abnormal blood glucose level, albuminuria, and ketonuria

ories daily. A supplement providing 30 mg iron is suggested as is the use of iodized salt. A prenatal vitamin-mineral supplement may be provided, but probably is not necessary if nutrient dense foods are routinely selected.

NUTRIENT REQUIREMENTS OF ACTIVE NONPREGNANT WOMEN

At present, there is little specific information regarding nutrient needs of active women. In general, careful review of the available literature (26) suggests that the needs of the athlete differ little from those of the sedentary individual, with the exception of those nutrients lost during an exercise bout (energy, water, and electrolytes) and those nutrients necessary for release of the energy expended. The general dietary advice for the physically active woman is similar to that of the nonactive pregnant women, i.e., to eat to appetite from a wide variety of foods, and to give special attention to those foods that replace the components lost during a training event.

Energy

As with the pregnant woman, energy is the most important nutrient for the athlete. Without adequate energy intake to cover that expended in all daily activities, both training and routine maintenance, lean tissue mass, the predominant component of which is muscle, is lost (27). In addition, fat stores cannot be maintained. Recommendations for energy intakes, as set by the National Research Council (20), assume only a small proportion of light activity daily in addition to sedentary maintenance activities; the suggestion is made to increase intakes if activity is heavier.

However, reported energy intakes of many active women seem to fall far short of the theoretical totals derived from their maintenance and activity requirements. In some cases, such as ballet dancers (9) and gymnasts (7), these low energy intakes are designed to maintain body weight (and body fat) well below the mean for age and height. In other cases, such as recreational runners, these lower than expected intakes are associated with maintenance of normal body weight (8). In women running 25 miles per week (considered moderately active), energy intakes were only 200 kcal/day higher than those reported by sedentary women. The theoretical discrepancy between energy intake and output in these women was 650 kcal/day. Investigation of energy balance in such women (Butterfield et al., Energy balance in women runners. Manuscript in preparation) shows no difference in basal energy needs as compared to sedentary controls, nor any difference in thermic response to a meal. Study of activity patterns show that the active women do not decrease time spent at other high energy-expending activities as shown in individuals placed on an energy-restricted diet (28). Physically active women may have an increased efficiency of energy utilization, as implicated in some obese individuals (29).

Composition of the food used to replace energy utilized in activities is also important. Complex carbohydrates are recommended in amounts to cover the energy expended at the activity because a high carbohydrate diet best replaces the critical fuel (muscle glycogen) lost during the exercise bout (30). Complex carbohydrates, such as whole grains, breads, pastas, and whole grain pastries, have the added benefit of providing matching amounts of the vitamins, niacin, and thiamin, required for energy release. The recommendation for these vitamins is proportional to energy intake (20). Fat, although providing energy in a very concentrated form, is ineffective at replacing the glycogen stores, and as such is discouraged as a major fuel replacement source.

Protein

Protein is used both as a muscle fuel and as a substrate for gluconeogenesis at rest and during exercise. This utilization of protein may increase with training (31). However, the effect of these uses of protein on long-term total body protein (after days or weeks of exercise) in the athlete is not clear. Some investigators suggest 1.5–2.0 g dietary protein/kg body weight to maximize protein accumulation and to avoid the transient signs of protein insufficiency that may accompany initiation of an exercise program [i.e., decreased hemoglobin levels (32), or transient negative nitrogen balance (33)]. Recent investigations indicate that male endurance athletes previously trained at relatively high intensities (65–75% of $V_{O_{2max}}$) require 0.92 g protein/kg body weight to maintain protein mass (34). However, others have found accumulation of body protein in individuals initiating a moderate exercise program on protein intakes as low as 0.57 g/kg body weight provided energy intake was adequate for the added exercise (35) and that 2 g protein/kg body weight is inadequate to maintain protein mass in individuals running at 65% of $V_{O_{2max}}$ when energy intake is inadequate (36). In any event, as stated previously, the average protein intake in the United States is high and generally exceeds 1.5 g/kg body weight in women who exercise. Any increased need for protein with exercise would not warrant an increase in protein intake over that usually consumed, provided energy intake is adequate.

In fact, a further increase in protein intake may have deleterious effects. Increased dietary protein has been shown to increase calcium and water excretion. Over the long-term, urinary calcium losses may contribute to bone demineralization and the development of osteoporosis (37). More immediately, the increase in water loss necessary to remove the by-products of protein degradation could contribute to an already potential dehydration state. In addition, high protein intakes have recently been implicated in the deterioration of kidney function in chronic renal failure (38).

Iron

Iron is a functional component of several of the elements necessary for oxygen transport (hemoglobin, myoglobin) and energy release (cytochromes). As these elements increase with training, one might expect the requirement for iron to increase. Such thinking, as well as reports of significant decreases in hemoglobin levels with training (39, 40), has led many coaches to recommend iron supplements to their athletes, both male and female. However, the low iron intakes associated with low energy intakes in women athletes are implicated as the primary cause for reduced iron stores (40, 41). Vegetarian athletes are particularly at risk due to the lack of highly available iron (heme iron) in their diets (42). In cases where iron status is low, as determined by hematological and iron indices, iron supplementation is effective in reversing these abnormalities (43). Iron supplementation in active women with previously adequate hemoglobin levels has shown no consistent improvement in parameters of iron status or performance after supplementation. Recommendation is made that both hematological and dietary parameters be monitored in physically active women, and that effort be made to ensure adequate dietary intake before initiating supplementation (41).

Calcium

Exercise has a beneficial effect on bone density in men (45) and women (46), both young and old. The greater bone density of active individuals implies that calcium retention is higher in the active individual than it is in the inactive and that, perhaps, calcium utilization is improved by activity. Diminished bone density found in amenorrheic athletes is thought to be consequent to low estrogen secretion and not subject to dietary manipulation. There are also reports of increased bone density in postmenopausal women who have initiated an exercise program while consuming their usual intake of calcium (46). Thus, the need for calcium in the athlete is probably not greater than that of a sedentary individual. However, the high protein diets of many athletes, may, as indicated previously, increase calcium excretion.

Water

For every 580 kcal of energy used during an exercise bout, 1 liter of water may be lost in removing that heat from the body. This loss of body water leads to a decrease in circulating blood volume, which in turn, decreases the ability to further remove heat. Over a training session, as much as 3 or 4% of the body water may be lost, equivalent to about 6 lb in a 150-lb person. Such a decrease may hamper performance. Replacement of the water lost during an exercise bout as well as that required for removal of the waste products of protein degradation is necessary to ensure continued ability to train and perform. Unfortunately, in the chronically exercising individual, the thirst mechanism alone does not seem to be sufficient to ensure complete rehydration; rather, only about 50% of that water lost over the day will be replaced, leaving the athlete chronically dehydrated, and with diminished blood volume (47). Maintenance of a pre-exercise weight log, with return to the previous day's pre-exercise weight as goal is a useful tool in ensuring appropriate rehydration (48). A daily intake of 10–12 glasses of water or other fluids is not unreasonable for the training athlete. During workouts of longer than one-half hour, periodic fluid consumption is recommended. Fluid and electrolyte replacement drinks are as effective as water (but no more so) for replenishing fluids lost during exercise, and may assist in replacing electrolytes so that the thirst mechanism is more effective (49).

A number of electrolytes are lost in association with water. (See Table 9.3 for primary components of sweat.) Of primary concern are sodium and potassium. Replenishing these electrolytes is mandatory for continued performance, and can be accomplished by careful dietary choices.

Sodium

Although the loss of sodium in sweat is significant, several factors in the active individual compensate for that loss so that sodium is not a critical concern for most athletes. First, with training, sweat sodium

Table 9.3. Electrolyte Composition of Sweat (g/liter)[a]

Sodium	0.8–1.4
Chloride	1.0–1.75
Potassium	0.25–1.0
Magnesium	0.0004–0.004
Calcium	0.02–0.16

[a]Adapted from Consolazio CF, Johnson RE, and Pecora LJ. Physiological measurements of metabolic function in man. New York: McGraw-Hill, 1963.

content decreases slightly from 1.0 g/liter to around 0.8 g/liter, diminishing the overall losses. In addition, the kidney conserves sodium when extracellular levels start to drop; this adaptive mechanism compensates for much of the loss of sodium in sweat. Many common foods naturally contain a significant amount of sodium so that the average intake may be as high as 5 or 6 g/day. With such high intakes and the ability to conserve body sodium, losses in sweat seldom become critical. Salt intake should be monitored when exercising in the heat for extended periods of time (more than 2 hours). Under such circumstances, fluid and electrolyte replacement drinks may ensure short-term needs, and salting food to taste and eating salty foods should be adequate to replace the increased losses (50). Salt tablets are unnecessary.

Potassium

The question of potassium replacement is controversial. Potassium content of sweat (0.25–1.0 g/liter) is low in comparison to usual intakes (6–8 g), and highly variable. However, potassium losses in sweat during exercise in the heat may be as high as 6 g/day (51). Overt signs of potassium deficiency in athletes have not been reported, although the possibility of a subclinical deficiency leading to muscle necrosis has been suggested (52). Potassium is normally an intracellular cation; when extracellular potassium increases above a threshold level, the kidney excretes it. Because potassium is stored with glycogen, it is released when glycogen is burned, increasing the blood potassium levels during and immediately after an exercise bout. This transient increase may trigger the kidney's excretory mechanisms. Thus, significant amounts of potassium may be excreted postexercise, with replenishment required to accompany replacement of the glycogen stores. Negative potassium balances have been reported in active individuals given 2–4 g of potassium/day (53). However, tissue potassium levels have been maintained in individuals exercising repeatedly for 4 days while consuming less than 1 g of potassium/day (54). In any event, thoughtful inclusions in the diet of high potassium foods such as citrus fruits, cantaloupes, bananas, and nuts may help avoid any potential depletion.

Other Nutrients of Concern

Nutrient supplements often recommended for athletes include riboflavin, vitamin C, and vitamin E. Because riboflavin is necessary for the release of energy from foods, as are niacin and thiamin, one might expect the increased energy release that accompanies physical activity to create a need for riboflavin. Recent work on riboflavin requirements show an increased need in women *initiating* a moderate exercise program (55), but no improvement in riboflavin status or performance in trained swimmers given a 60-mg riboflavin/day supplement (56). In any event, the magnitude of any increased need is small and could be easily provided by foods rich in riboflavin such as milk, yogurt, and whole wheat breads.

The answer to the question of need for the vitamins C and E is not so clear. Both of these vitamins act as antioxidants; in association with the increased flow of oxygen through the tissues with physical activity, there is an increase in tissue oxidative damage (57). It is not known if this increased need for detoxification of oxygen radicals increases the need for the antioxidant nutrients, vitamins C and E. In rats fed a vitamin E-deficient diet, red blood cell hemolysis, a sign of vitamin E deficiency, appeared more slowly in exercising animals than in sedentary ones (58). The need for vitamin C is even more controversial. Scientific evidence suggests there is no increase in need with exercise but lay publications continue to suggest supplementation. Studies of the effect of vitamin C supplementation on performance suggest that supplementation has little effect in individuals previously ingesting adequate amounts of vitamin C. In a group of individuals consuming a diet containing only that vitamin C found in foods (about 350 mg/day), serum levels of the vitamin were consistently higher in the active individuals than in the sedentary ones (59). In general, any increased need of athletes for these nutrients can probably by fulfilled by consuming a diet of a variety of foods from all of the food groups.

NUTRIENT RECOMMENDATIONS FOR ACTIVE PREGNANT WOMEN

As stated previously, nutritional needs of the physically active pregnant woman have not been studied. However, based on our knowledge of the nutritional needs for pregnancy and for heavy activity, some general recommendations can be made.

Energy

The recommended additional energy for pregnancy, 300 cal/day, provides for only the increased basal metabolic needs. Energy needs for physical activity are greater in the pregnant than nonpregnant state because of the increased body weight; more energy is required to move the heavier body. At present, recommendations for energy intake during pregnancy include no addition for the increased energy cost of activity because it is assumed that pregnant women decrease their level of activity during pregnancy (20).

However, surveys of the activity patterns of pregnant women do not show that they become more sedentary (60). Instead, they tend to maintain the same pattern of activity throughout pregnancy, and the energy required for activities involving the movement of the body, i.e., walking, is greater late in pregnancy than in midpregnancy (61). These data suggest that physically active pregnant women need more than 300 additional calories per day.

The energy needs of the physically active pregnant woman will vary with the amount of activity she performs. Therefore, it is impossible to make a general recommendation.

To estimate total energy needs for the woman who participates in significant strenuous activity, an amount of energy equivalent to that expended during the strenuous activities must be added to the maintenance need (see Table 9.4 for list of energy expenditures for women performing various strenuous activities). If the rate of weight gain begins to fall below normal at any stage of pregnancy (Fig. 9.1), additional calories should be recommended. At all times, the physically

Table 9.4. Approximate Energy Expenditure at Various Strenuous Activities[a]

Activity	Energy Expended (kcal/kg/hr)
Walking, on level, without load	
2 mph	2.6
2.5 mph	2.9
3 mph	3.3
Walking, uphill, 2 mph	
10% grade	5.4
20% grade	8.3
Running	
Cross country (3–4 mph)	9.7
Track (10 mph)	16.7
Cycling	
5.5 mph	3.4
10 mph	6.5
racing	10.1
Dancing	
Waltz	5.0
Square	8.0
Aerobic	10.0
Swimming	
Leisurely	4.5
Fast crawl	9.3
Breast or back stroke	9.6

[a] Adapted from Briggs GM, Calloway DH. Nutrition and physical fitness, ed. 11. Philadelphia: WB Saunders, 1984; Astrand P, Rodahl K. Textbook of work physiology, ed. 2. New York: McGraw-Hill, 1977; and Brooks G, Faheg T. Exercise physiology. New York: John Wiley & Sons, 1984.

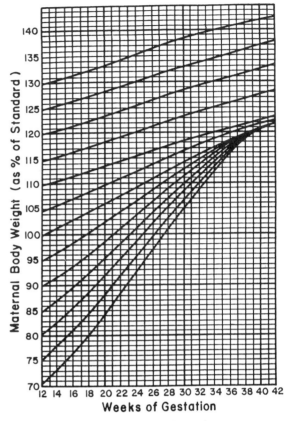

Figure 9.1. Weight gain chart for pregnant women. (From Rosso P. A new chart to monitor weight gain during pregnancy. Am J Clin Nutr 1985;41:644–652.)

active pregnant woman should be encouraged to eat to appetite. A diet high in complex carbohydrates is advised since carbohydrate best replaces muscle glycogen lost during exercise and will minimize the threat of ketosis (see description of shifts in fuel utilization with pregnancy in Chapter 6).

Protein

Pregnancy increases the need for protein and, some feel that physical activity may do so as well. However, the usual dietary intake of protein in the United States is above the requirement for pregnancy and probably provides the additional needs for both pregnancy and exercise. It may be useful to base the protein recommendation for physically active pregnant women on energy intakes to assure that a high energy, high carbohydrate, low protein diet is not consumed. As stated previously, a diet providing 12% of the energy as protein should be adequate. This

means that a woman consuming 2300 kcal/day should ingest 69 g protein, whereas a woman consuming 3000 kcal/day should ingest 90 g protein.

Iron

The iron needs of the trained pregnant woman maintaining her level of physical fitness are similar to those of sedentary pregnant women because additional iron does not appear to be required by the trained woman. Both sedentary and physically active pregnant women need to accumulate about 800 mg iron in the last half of pregnancy (23). To prevent depletion of maternal iron stores, this need is best provided by a 30-mg iron supplement. A woman with low iron stores contemplating pregnancy should increase her iron intake before getting pregnant.

Water

Water retention is normal during pregnancy, but the amount retained varies from 7–12 liters (14). Administration of diuretics is associated with a reduction in birth weight (62). This expansion of the total body water is an important determinant of pregnancy outcome, and it should not be impaired.

The physically active pregnant woman probably has an increased need for water to support expansion of total body water and to maintain normal body temperature (see earlier in this chapter). Consumption of 8–12 cups of water daily is probably prudent to maintain normal hydration and expansion of total body water under circumstances of exercise.

Sodium

Additional sodium is needed for expansion of the extracellular fluid volume in the sedentary pregnant woman (14). This additional need coupled with increased sodium losses during exercise may place the physically active pregnant woman at risk for sodium depletion if her exercise is vigorous and if her sodium intake is low. Most pregnant women in the United States consume at least twice as much sodium as is needed. Thus, it is quite unlikely that sodium depletion will develop in the physically active pregnant woman. Pregnant, as well as nonpregnant, women participating in prolonged exercise in the heat should be advised to consume salty foods and to salt their foods to taste after the exercise bout. Fluid and electrolyte replacement drinks may be especially useful for rehydration during a workout (49).

SUMMARY

Based on current knowledge, energy seems to be the major nutritional concern for physically active pregnant women. If energy needs are met, it seems likely that the other nutritional needs will be satisfied as long as a wide variety of foods is consumed. Maternal appetite may be the best indicator of total energy needs, and all women should be urged to eat to appetite. This advice, however, does not mean that food intake should not be controlled. The rate of maternal weight gain

is the best clinical measure of the adequacy of maternal energy intake. Weight gain of physically active pregnant women should be monitored monthly throughout pregnancy. If the rate of gain deviates from the ranges around the normal curve (Fig. 9.1) at any time, daily energy intakes should be estimated using a 24-hour recall of all food eaten, and the intake adjusted appropriately.

REFERENCES

1. Bergner L, Susser MW. Low birthweight and prenatal nutrition: an interpretive review. Pediatrics 1970; 46:946.
2. Rosso O, Cramoy C. Nutrition and pregnancy. In Winick M, ed. Human Nutrition. A comprehensive treatise. New York: Plenum Press, 1979; vol 1.
3. Kerr JF, Campbell-Brown BM, Johnstone FD. Dieting in pregnancy. A study of the effect of a high protein, low carbohydrate diet on birthweight in an obstetric population. In Sutherland HW, Stowers JM, eds. Carbohydrate metabolism in pregnancy and the newborn. New York: Springer-Verlag, 1978, pp 518–534.
4. Prentice AW, Whitehead RG, Roberts SB, Paul AA. Long-term energy balance in child-bearing Gambian women. Am J Clin Nutr 1981; 34:2790.
5. Durnin JVGA. Energy requirements of pregnancy: an integration of the longitudinal data from the five-country study. Lancet 1987; 2:1131.
6. Lawrence M, Lawrence F, Coward WA, Cole TJ, Whitehead RG. Energy requirements of pregnancy in the Gambia. Lancet 1987; 2:1072.
7. Ledoux M, Brisson G, Peronnet F. Nutritional status of adolescent female gymnasts. Med Sci Sports Exerc 1982; 14:145.
8. Mulligan K, Butterfield GE. Discrepancies between energy intake and expenditure in physically active women. Br J Nutr (submitted for publication). 1989.
9. Novak LP, Magill LA, Schultz JF. Maximal oxygen intake and body composition of female dancers. Eur J Appl Physiol 1978; 39:277.
10. Brownell KD, Steen SN, Wilmore JH. Weight regulation practices in athletes: analysis of metabolic and health effects. Med Sci Sports Exerc 1987; 19:546–556.
11. Slavin J, Lee V, Lutter JM. Nutrient intakes of women who exercise while pregnant. XIII Int'l Congress of Nutrition, Brighton, U.K., 18–23 August, 1985, p 28.
12. Clapp JF, Dickstein S. Endurance exercise and pregnancy outcome. Med Sci Sports Exerc 1984; 16:556.
13. Root BA, King JS. Maternal nutrition. In Creasy RK, Resnik R, eds. Maternal fetal medicine. Philadelphia: WB Saunders, 1984, p 181.
14. Hytten FE, Chamberlain G, eds. Clinical physiology in obstetrics. Oxford: Blackwell, 1980.
15. Hunscher HA, Tompkins WT. The influence of maternal nutrition on the immediate and long-term outcome of pregnancy. Clin Obstet Gynecol 1970; 13:130.
16. Primrose T, Higgens A. A study of human antepartum nutrition. J Reprod Med 1971; 7:257.
17. Campbell DM. Dietary restriction in obesity and its

effects on neonatal outcome. In Campbell DM, Gillmer MDG, eds. Nutrition in pregnancy. London: Royal College of Obstetrics and Gynaecologists, 1982; p 243.

18. Pitkin RM. Obstetrics and gynecology. In: Schneider HA, Anderson CE, Coursin DB, eds. Nutritional support of medical practice. Hagerstown, MD: Harper & Row, 1977; p 407–421.

19. Garrow JS. Treat obesity seriously. A Clinical Manual. Edinburgh: Churchill Livingstone, 1981, pp 174–177.

20. National Research Council. Recommended dietary allowances, ed 10. Washington, DC: National Academy of Sciences, 1989.

21. Rush D, Stein Z, Susser M. A randomized controlled trial of prenatal nutritional supplementation in New York City. Pediatrics 1980; 65:683.

22. California Department of Health. Nutrition during Pregnancy and Lactation: For Professional Use. Sacramento, CA, 1975.

23. Lind T. Iron supplementation during pregnancy. In Campbell DM, Gillmer MDG, ed. Nutrition in pregnancy. London: Royal College of Obstetricians and Gynaecologists, 1982, pp 181.

24. Pitkin RM, Calcium metabolism in pregnancy: a review. Am J Obstet Gynecol 1975; 121:724.

25. Committee on Maternal Nutrition, Food and Nutrition Board, National Research Council. Maternal Nutrition and the Course of Pregnancy. Washington, DC: National Academy of Sciences, 1970.

26. American Dietetic Association, Position of the American Dietetic Association: Nutrition for physical fitness and athletic performance for adults. J Am Dietet Assoc 1987; 87:933–939.

27. Calloway DH, Spector H. Nitrogen balance as related to caloric and protein intake in active young men. Am J Clin Nutr 1954; 2:405.

28. Troup JDG. Measurements of the sagittal mobility of the lumbar spine and hips. Arch Phys Med 1968; 9:308.

29. Pittet PH, Chappuis PH, Acheson K, De Techtermann F, Jéquier E. Thermic effect of glucose in obese studied by direct and indirect calorimetry. Br J Nutr 1976; 35:281.

30. Costill DL, Miller JM. Nutrition for endurance sport: carbohydrate and fluid balance. Int J Sports Med 1980; 1:2–14.

31. Young VR, Torun B. Physical activity. Impact of protein and amino acid metabolism and implications for nutritional requirement. Nutrition in Health and Disease and International Development. In Symposia from XIIth International Congress of Nutrition, 1981, pp 59–85.

32. Yoshimura H, Inoue T, Yamada T, Shiraki K. Anemia during hard physical training (sports anemia) and its causal mechanism with special reference to protein nutrition. World Rev Nutr Diet 1980; 35:1.

33. Gontzea I, Sutrescu P, Dumitreche S. The influence of adaptation to physical effort on nitrogen balance in men. Nutr Rep Int 1975; 11:231.

34. Meredith CN, Zachin MJ, Frontera WR, Evans WJ. Dietary protein requirements and body protein metabolism in endurance-trained men. J Appl Physiol 1989; 66:2850.

35. Butterfield GE, Calloway DH. Physical activity improves protein utilization in young men. Br J Nutr 1984; 51:171.

36. Butterfield GE. Whole body protein utilization in humans. Med Sci Sports Exerc 1987; 19:S157–S165.

37. Anonymous: High protein diets and bone homeostasis. Nutr Rev 1981; 39:11.

38. Brenner BM, Meyer TW, Hostetter TH. Dietary protein intake and the progressive nature of kidney disease: the role of hemodynamically medicated glomerular injury in the pathogenesis of progressive glomerular sclerosis in aging, renal ablation, and intrinsic renal disease. N Engl J Med 1982; 307:652–659.

39. Lind T. Iron supplementation during pregnancy. In Campbell DM, Gillmer MDG, ed. Nutrition in pregnancy. London, Royal College of Obstetricians and Gynaecologists, 1982, pp 181.

40. Nagy L, King JC. Energy expenditure of pregnant women at rest or walking self-paced. Am J Clin Nutr 38:369, 1983.

41. National Research Council. Recommended Dietary Allowances, ed 9. Washington DC, National Academy of Sciences, 1980.

42. Novak LP, Magill LA, Schultz JE. Maximal oxygen intake and body composition of female dancers. Eur J Appl Physiol 39:277, 1978.

43. Oyster N, Morton M, Linnell S. Physical activity and osteoporosis in post-menopausal women. Med Sci Sports Exerc 16:44, 1984.

44. Pitkin RM. Obstetrics and gynecology. In: Schneider HA, Anderson CE, Coursin DB, eds. Nutritional Support of Medical Practice. Hagerstown, MD: Harper & Row, 1977, pp 407–421.

45. Pitkin RM. Calcium metabolism in pregnancy: a review. Am J Obstet Gynecol 121:724, 1975.

46. Pittet PH, Chappuis PH, Acheson K, De Techtermann F, Jéquier E. Thermic effect of glucose in obese studied by directg and indirect calorimetry. Br J Nutr 35:281, 1976.

47. Prentice AW, Whitehead RG, Roberts SB, Paul AA. Long-term energy balance in child-bearing Gambian women. Am J Clin Nutr 34:2790, 1981.

48. Block A, Ikeda J. Eat to Compete, a Workbook on Proper Eating Habits for Teenage Athletes. Cooperative Extension, Berkeley: University of California, 1982.

49. Nose H, Mack GW, Shi X, Nadel ER. Shift in body fluid compartments after dehydration in humans. J Appl Physiol 1988; 65:318–324.

50. Fink WJ. Fluid intake for maximizing athletic performance. In Haskell W, Scala T, Whittam J, eds. Nutrition and athletic performance. Palo Alto, CA: Bull Publishing, 1982, p 52–63.

51. Cade TR, Spooner GR, Schlien EM, Pickering MJ, Dean RC. Effect of fluid, electrolyte and glucose replacement during exercise on performance, body temperature, rate of sweat loss, and compositional changes of extracellular fluid. J Sports Med Phys Fitness 1972; 12:150.

52. Knochel JP: Rhabdomyolysis and effects of potassium deficiency on muscle structure and function. Cardiovasc Med 1978; 3:247.

53. Lane HW, Roessler GS, Nelson EW, Cerda IJ. Effect of physical activity on human potassium metabolism in a hot and humid environment. Am J Clin Nutr 1978; 31:838.

54. Costill DI., Cate R, Fink WJ. Dietary potassium and heavy exercise: effects on muscle water and electrolytes. Am J Clin Nutr 1982; 36:266.

55. Belko AZ, Ovarzanek E, Kalkway HJ, Rotler MA, Bogusy DA, Miller D, Hass JD, Roe DA. Effects of

exercise on riboflavin requirements of young women. Am J Clin Nutr 1983; 39:509.

56. Fremblay A, Boilard F, Breton MF, Bessette H, Roberge AC. The effects of riboflavin supplementation on the nutritional status and performance of elite swimmers. Nutr Res 1981; 4:201.

57. Davies KJA, Quintanilha AT, Brooks GA, Packer I. Free radicals and tissue damage produced by exercise. Biochem Biophys Res Commun 1982; 107:1198.

58. Aikawa K, Quintanilha AT, DeLumen BO, Brooks GA, Packer L. Effect of exercise endurance training

of rodents on vitamin E tissue levels and red blood cell hemolysis. Biosci Rep 1984; 4:253.

59. Fishbaine B, Butterfield G. Ascorbic acid status of running and sedentary men. Int J Vitam Nutr Res 1984; 54:243.

60. Blackburn MW, Calloway DH. Energy expenditure and consumption of mature, pregnant and lactating women. J Am Dietet Assoc 1976; 69:29.

61. Nagy L, King JC. Energy expenditure of pregnant women at rest or walking self-paced. Am J Clin Nutr 1983; 38:369.

10

Orthopedic Injuries in Pregnancy

Ronald P. Karzel, Jr. and Marc J. Friedman

Physiological changes occurring during pregnancy affect the musculoskeletal system and may increase the chance of orthopedic injuries. One such change is the soft tissue swelling that is frequently noted during pregnancy. A study by Robertson (1) showed that 83% of pregnant women reported swelling during some stage of their pregnancy. The majority had continued swelling only during the last 8 weeks of pregnancy. Soft tissue swelling may decrease the available space in relatively constrained anatomic areas. This may result in nerve compression syndromes, or, less commonly, in compartment syndromes. A second important change during pregnancy is increased ligamentous laxity, which is thought to be due to the influence of estrogen and relaxin. Loosening of ligamentous support may lead to an increased chance of sprains. Ligamentous laxity is probably also the major cause of sacroiliac problems that are the primary cause of low back pain in pregnant women. The increase in weight occurring during the later stages of pregnancy also significantly increases stresses across weight bearing joints. Activities such as stair climbing result in a force of three to five times body weight across joints such as the hip or knee. Thus, a woman whose weight increases 20% during pregnancy may increase the forces on her joints by 100%. Such large forces may cause increased discomfort in normal joints and may cause increased damage in joints that already have some underlying arthritis or previous instability. As pregnancy progresses, the gravid uterus displaces anteriorly and superiorly, shifting the woman's center of gravity. To compensate for this increased anterior force, the lumbar spine must assume a lordotic posture. Lordosis is also increased by the increased forward inclination of the pelvis that occurs from the normal 55°. The result of these changes is increased stress on the lumbosacral spine and sacroiliac joints. A secondary change is a more unstable weight distribution with resultant instability of balance. The pregnant woman is thus more likely to fall and is also putting abnormal stresses on many of her muscles and joints in an effort to counteract this new distribution of body mass. Clearly, therefore, the changes occurring during pregnancy can significantly affect the musculoskeletal system and may limit the pregnant woman's ability to participate in her previous athletic activities. In this chapter, we will first discuss specific regions of the musculoskeletal system and common injuries that may occur in these regions secondary to the pregnant state. We will then mention specific sporting activities and the effects of pregnancy on the performance of these activities.

NERVE COMPRESSION SYNDROMES

Carpal Tunnel Syndrome

The median nerve is an important nerve supply to the hand, innervating the thenar muscles of the thumb that allow opposition of the thumb to the fingers (Fig. 10.1). It also supplies sensory branches to the thumb, index, and middle fingers. The median nerve travels through the carpal tunnel at the level of the wrist. This space is bounded by the carpal bones below and a rigid fibrous ligament above (Fig. 10.2). Running through this space with the nerve are the flexor tendons to the fingers. Space in the carpal tunnel is therefore limited, and with significant soft tissue swelling, the nerve can be compressed. This problem is known as carpal tunnel syndrome.

This syndrome commonly arises during the last trimester of pregnancy. The patient presents with complaints of numbness and tingling of the thumb, index, and middle fingers and may be aware of clumsiness when using

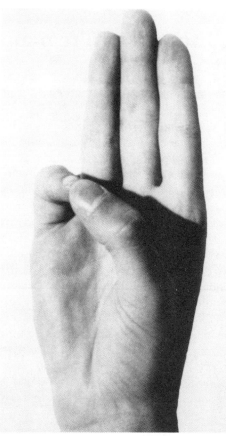

Figure 10.1. Opposition of the thumb requires an intact median nerve.

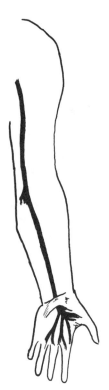

Figure 10.2. Median nerve through carpal tunnel at wrist.

the hand, secondary to loss of thumb function. Particularly characteristic is pain that is bothersome at night and often awakens her from sleep.

Examination reveals tenderness over the median nerve at the wrist. A positive Tinel's sign may be present, which is pain radiating to the thumb, middle, and index fingers with palpation of the median nerve. Weakness and atrophy of the thenar muscles may be apparent, although this is usually a relatively late sign. Another diagnostic test is Phalen's test, which is performed by hyperflexing the wrist and holding it in this position for a period of 30–45 seconds. If this position reproduces the symptoms of numbness in the thumb, index, and middle fingers, this is considered to be a positive test. When in doubt, the diagnosis can be confirmed using electromyographic and nerve conduction testing.

Treatment in pregnancy is usually nonoperative. This involves placing the patient in a neutral wrist extension splint for sleeping at night and avoiding the hyperflexion posture, which tends to diminish the space available in the carpal tunnel (Fig. 10.3). Ice packs applied to the area two to three times a day may help limit the inflammation, as anti-inflammatory medication is usually not prescribed during pregnancy. In cases that are resistant to the previous treatment, one or two injections of Xylocaine (lidocaine) and steroid preparation into the space around the nerve can often dramatically relieve the symptoms.

This problem is very common during pregnancy and will usually resolve completely after the completion of pregnancy. A study by Gould and Wissinger (2) found evidence of median nerve symptoms in 21 of 100 consecutive obstetric OB admissions. Of the 21,

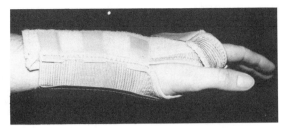

Figure 10.3. Patient in a neutral wrist extension splint.

18 became asymptomatic shortly after delivery and remained asymptomatic 3 months after delivery. In those cases that persist after pregnancy, further work-up can be performed followed by surgical decompression of the carpal tunnel.

Other Nerve Compression Syndromes

The ulnar nerve travels to the hand through Guyon's canal at the wrist and may also be compressed in a manner similar to that described for the median nerve (Fig. 10.4). These patients have numbness and tingling of the fourth and fifth fingers, and they have weakness of their interosseous muscles. Treatment is the same as that outlined for carpal tunnel syndrome.

The ulnar nerve may also be compressed

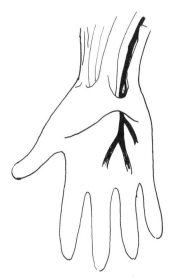

Figure 10.4. Ulnar nerve passing through Guyon's canal at wrist.

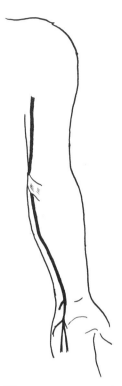

Figure 10.5. Ulnar nerve can become compressed where it passes behind medial epicondyle.

at the medial aspect of the elbow, posterior to the medial epicondyle (Fig. 10.5). This is often due to incorrect sleeping posture with the head resting over the area of the elbow. These cases usually respond well to conservative treatment using a posterior splint for immobilization of the elbow, ice packs, and/or possible injection.

In the leg, a similar situation arises in the tarsal tunnel. This is a thick fibrous layer of tissue that surrounds the flexor tendons to the foot and the posterior tibial nerve, artery, and vein lying just posterior to the medial malleolus (Fig. 10.6). In some cases, with increased edema and/or trauma, the tibial nerve can be compressed and produce numbness and tingling in the medial aspect of the foot with some weakness of the flexor muscles of the toes. Examination will show a positive Tinel's sign over the posterior tibial nerve, with decreased sensation along the medial arch and foot. Treatment minimizes

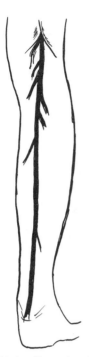

Figure 10.6.   Posterior tibial nerve.

ankle motion, using ice packs to the area and possible injections around the nerve.

Injury can also occur to the peroneal nerves, which are vulnerable as they wrap around the neck of the fibula near the area of the knee joint. This important nerve supplies the muscles that dorsiflex the ankle and prevent foot drop. A recent case report documented bilateral peroneal nerve palsy which followed the use of the squatting position for a prolonged period of time during delivery (3). Women who use the squatting position during delivery should be counseled to arise from the squatting position and move about whenever possible to prevent prolonged pressure on the nerve.

BACK PAIN

Separate studies by Berg et al. (4) and Mantel and associates (5) have documented an approximately 50% incidence of backache during pregnancy. Lumbosacral pain is more common in patients with increased age or parity. Most of these cases are considered to be secondary to sacroiliac strain. The pelvis normally tends to rotate about a fulcrum situated at the second sacral segment. The strong sacroiliac ligaments resist this forward rotation. During pregnancy, the tendency for rotation is increased as the lumbar lordosis increases and the center of gravity shifts anteriorly. In addition, the ligaments become increasingly lax, allowing increased excursion and placing additional strain upon the ligaments at their attachment to the ilium.

Patients complain of low back pain that is persistent and usually not severe. The pain may radiate to one or both buttocks, but does not usually radiate down the leg in a sciatic distribution. Pain is often unilateral, and is aggravated by walking and relieved by rest. Characteristically, there is no night pain.

On examination, spasm of the paraspinal muscles may be present. Patrick's test is commonly used to determine if sacroiliac dysfunction is present. This is performed with the patient supine by placing one heel on the opposite knee and simultaneously externally rotating the crossed-over leg at the hip. A painful reaction indicates sacroiliac dysfunction providing that the hip joint is otherwise normal. Pain may also be present with manual compression or distraction of the pelvis. Most women with this condition respond well to decreased activity and possibly bed rest. However, the study by Berg et al. (4) demonstrated that approximately 9% of the patients had a more severe course. These women were unable to continue their work because of severe low back pain. These women were more likely to have physically strenuous occupations and previous low back pain. These women also had a prolonged duration of symptoms after the end of their pregnancy, although the symptoms eventually resolved.

A related condition is osteitis condensans ilii. The patient complains of back and pelvic pain, similar to that with sacroiliac dysfunction. On x-ray examination, these patients show increased condensation of bone in the articular portion of the ilium without a corresponding change in the sacroiliac joint or the sacrum (Fig. 10.7). However, x-ray diagnosis during pregnancy is usually unnecessary. The bony condensation seen in the ilium may be secondary to increased traction

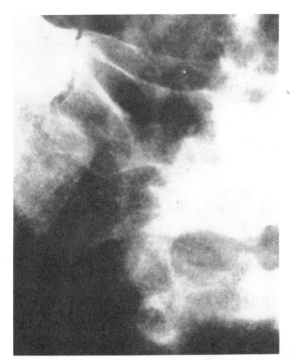

Figure 10.7. Condensations of the auricular portion of the ilium in osteitis condensans.

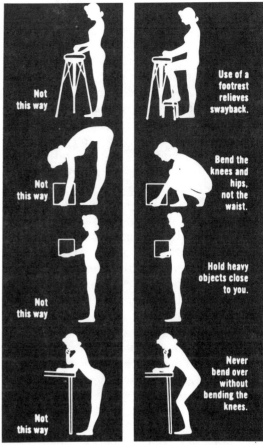

Use of a footrest relieves swayback.

Bend the knees and hips, not the waist.

Hold heavy objects close to you.

Never bend over without bending the knees.

Not this way

Figure 10.8. Use of proper body mechanics may help diminish back pain during pregnancy.

on the articular processes of the ilium from the sacroiliac ligaments.

Treatment is similar for both conditions. Reducing the lumbosacral angle will usually decrease the pain. This may be accomplished by postural exercises with abdominal strengthening, a firm mattress or bed board, weight reduction, and a specialized lumbosacral corset. Instruction in proper sitting and lifting mechanics may be helpful (Fig. 10.8). Occasionally, an injection of lidocaine and steroid into the sacroiliac joint may result in pain relief. Most of these problems resolve with the termination of pregnancy, but may recur with subsequent pregnancies.

In contrast to sacroiliac problems as a cause of low back pain during pregnancy, true lumbar disc herniation is rare. A 1983 study has documented the incidence to be approximately 1/10,000 pregnancies (6). Patients with disc herniation usually present with leg pain in addition to the back pain. They will have pain and limitation with straight leg raising. They may have neurological deficits including a dermatomal sensory loss, a decrease in deep tendon reflexes, or decreased muscle strength. If a diagnosis of lumbar disc herniation is suspected clinically, the diagnosis can be confirmed using magnetic resonance imaging, which is safe and accurate (7). Both myelography and spinal CT scanning result in relatively large radiation doses to the fetus and are contraindicated. If neurological symptoms are present, then electromyography (EMG) may confirm the presence of nerve root compression. Most patients with this problem can be treated conservatively until the termination of pregnancy. All five patients in LaBan's series underwent cesarean sections to prevent exacerbation of the disc herniation that might be expected with straining during a vaginal delivery. Surgical intervention can then be undertaken as necessary after the patient has recovered from the effects of pregnancy.

Meralgia paresthetica can occur during

pregnancy and should be differentiated from radicular pain (6). This syndrome is commonly produced by entrapment of the lateral femoral cutaneous nerve at the level of the inguinal ligament. However, in the pregnant patient, the entrapment is more likely to occur in the retroperitoneal space as the nerve is stretched over the increasing sacral promontory due to the increased sacral angulation. Symptoms include burning and numbness over the anterolateral aspect of the thigh, which is usually severe and sharply demarcated. This syndrome may also respond to the previously mentioned maneuvers that decrease sacral tilt. Occasionally, a steroid injection into the area of the sacroiliac joint may provide relief of this syndrome.

Spondylolisthesis is a forward slipping of the L5 vertebra on the sacrum, secondary to a defect in the pars interarticularis. If the slip is severe, it may interfere with the ability of the woman to have a vaginal delivery. In a woman with a previous spondylolisthesis who becomes pregnant, these has previously been concern that the slip could progress. However, a study by Saraste (8) found that there was no increase in low back symptoms or in the degree of slip in women who had spondylolisthesis and were followed during pregnancy.

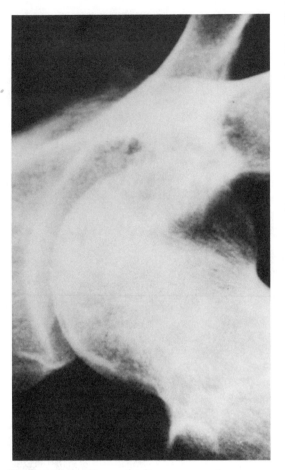

Figure 10.9. X-ray findings—avascular necrosis—femoral head.

HIP PAIN

Hip pain in a pregnant woman may be related to low back pain with sciatic adiation. However, if hip pain is persister and is not in conjunction with localized back pain, the possibility of avascular necrosis of the femoral head must be considered. Cheng et al. (9) reported seven cases of avascular necrosis of the femoral head that were related to pregnancy. They believed that higher adrenal cortical activity during pregnancy combined with the increased mechanical stress due to weight gain may have been important factors in the etiology. X-ray findings show early lucency with segmental collapse of the femoral head (Fig. 10.9). Magnetic resonance imaging is helpful in making this diagnosis without exposing the patient to x-ray. During pregnancy, the patient should be treated with decreased weight bearing on the hip, using

a walker or crutches. Surgical intervention may be necessary after delivery.

PUBIC PAIN

Symphysitis

Loosening of ligaments that occurs during pregnancy may also lead to symphysitis, which is an irritation of the pubic symphysis caused by increased motion at the joint. This may often be associated with sacroiliac back pain (4).

Women with symphysitis complain of pain and/or tenderness over the symphysis. This pain is usually worsened with exercise, straining or walking up stairs. Pain and tenderness are reproduced by pressure over the symphysis. Mild cases usually respond to rest and ice. A pelvic belt that compresses the pelvis and minimizes motion in the sacroiliac joint and symphysis may be helpful.

In contrast to these partial symphyseal separations, complete symphyseal dislocations may occur. This usually occurs at the time of delivery, with an incidence of approximately one in 600 (10). The relaxation of the ligaments during pregnancy commonly allows a physiological separation of approximately 3–7 mm of the symphysis. This is usually clinically insignificant. However, complete separation may result in a gaping pubic defect with tenderness, crepitus, and difficulty with ambulation. In these cases, the symphysis will usually be separated greater than 10 mm. All these cases were treated conservatively. The patients were placed in pelvic girdles to reduce the diastasis after 24–48 hours of bed rest. They were allowed to ambulate using a walker. The long-term outlook for these patients has been excellent. This complication is more likely to occur if the second stage of labor is rapid, with rapid fetal descent (10).

Osteitis Pubis

Osteitis pubis is a painful condition that may occur during pregnancy. It is characterized by bony resorption about the symphysis, followed by spontaneous reossification with resolution of symptoms. Predisposing factors may be the softening of pelvic ligaments that occurs during pregnancy.

The typical history is of a gradual onset of pain about the symphysis pubis. This progresses over the period of a few days to excruciating pain around the pubis, the pubic rami, and radiating along the adductor aspects of both thighs. The pain is increased by any movement of the extremities, especially abduction of the legs, which stretches the adductor muscles. The attachment sites of the adductors to the pubis are particularly tender. There is no sign of swelling, redness, or warmth that would suggest infection. Frequently injection of a local anesthetic into the attachment of the adductors relieves the pain. The patient is often disabled and bedridden. She may seek a position of maximum comfort, which is one of hip flexion and adduction. The pain is intense for a period varying

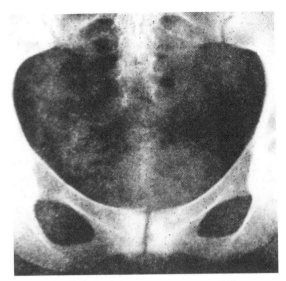

Figure 10.10. Widening appearance of the symphyseal gap in osteitis pubis.

from days to weeks and then gradually subsides over an indefinite period up to several years in length. X-rays in the early days or weeks are negative. As the disease progresses, the bone adjacent to the symphysis undergoes spotty demineralization, which intensifies until the symphyseal gap appears to be widened (Fig. 10.10). Characteristically, the opposing aspects of the pubic bodies are moth-eaten, rarified and cup-shaped. The rami are diffusely osteopenic. Gradually, over many months, reossification occurs with restoration of bony architecture.

The patient is usually placed in absolute bed rest with lower extremities flexed and adducted over a pillow. Ice is applied to the inflamed area. Narcotics may occasionally be necessary.

Pubic Stress Fracture

Stress fractures of the pubis have been reported both in the late stages of pregnancy and subsequent to difficult vaginal deliveries (11). These present with localized pubic tenderness. Often, fracture callus will be seen when the x-ray is taken, indicating a previously undiagnosed fracture. There is no displacement of the bones. A period of bed rest followed by partial weight bearing ambulation is usually sufficient to allow complete healing of the problem.

KNEE AND LOWER LEG PAIN

Chondromalacia Patella

A common cause of knee pain in women is a disorder of normal patellofemoral motion that is commonly known as chondromalacia of the patella. Predisposing factors to chondromalacia patella are increased ligament laxity, increased femoral torsion, and a wider pelvis. All of these factors combine to produce increased lateral motion of the knee cap during flexion-extension maneuvers. Patients with this problem complain of an anterior aching pain in the knee that increases with flexion of the knee or prolonged sitting. A characteristic complaint is discomfort in the knees while sitting in a movie with their knees maximally flexed. During pregnancy, these symptoms are often increased due to the increased weight that increases the load across the patellofemoral joint, the increased ligamentous laxity, and increased swelling about the knee.

Treatment is usually conservative and consists of strengthening the quadriceps muscles to allow the kneecap to track correctly. This is usually done isometrically using straight leg lifts and quad setting exercises. In addition, ice packs about the anterior knee two to three times a day may be helpful in reducing symptoms. A patellar restraining brace prevents lateral motion of the patella and may also be helpful (Fig. 10.11).

If these measures are unsuccessful, one or two intraarticular injections of lidocaine and steroid immediately beneath the patella can dramatically relieve the symptomatology. In most cases, if this is an entirely new symptom complex associated with pregnancy, it goes into remission after pregnancy. The problem may be exacerbated once the child begins crawling at which time the woman again begins squatting and kneeling to pick the child up, thus exacerbating the preexisting condition.

Edema

As previously noted, a large percentage of pregnant women develop significant amounts of lower leg edema. The tight fascial envelopes surrounding the lower leg muscles are

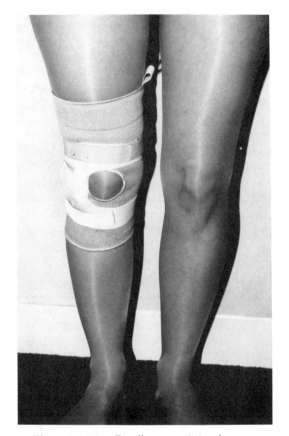

Figure 10.11.   Patellar restraining brace.

relatively unyielding to stretch. There have been reports of pregnant women who develop reversible compartment syndromes in their lower legs due to a combination of the edema of pregnancy and increased size of muscles in the lower leg compartment with exercise (12). This is manifested as anterolateral leg pain that recurs reproduceably after a set amount of activity. With rest, the pain and aching gradually subside. This problem can generally be treated in pregnancy by decreasing activity. When symptoms occur secondary to this compartment syndrome, it is not advisable to elevate the legs higher than heart level. This will actually decrease blood flow to the muscles and may further exacerbate the compartment syndrome. The syndrome usually resolves after the end of pregnancy. If the symptoms persist, surgical division of the tight fascial structures will allow return to competition without pain.

Women with significant dependent edema

from pregnancy may also develop joint effusions and secondary aching pain in the lower legs. The joint effusions should be treated in the same way as the lower leg edema, in general. Aspiration of the joints is not helpful, as the fluid will merely reaccumulate. Instead, elevation, support stockings, and in severe cases, appropriate diuretic therapy may be helpful in reducing the joint symptoms.

MISCELLANEOUS INJURIES

As the abdominal musculature is stretched during pregnancy, a weakening of the seam of central fibrous tissue between the rectus abdominae may occur and lead to diastasis. This may be present in up to 30% of pregnant women (13). Although no treatment is needed for mild separations, if the separation exceeds approximately 7 cm, the patient should be counseled to modify abdominal strengthening exercises to prevent further separation. Generally, this means avoiding leg lifts or full bent leg sit-ups. The diastasis usually decreases after delivery.

In addition to the stress fractures previously mentioned around the pubis, stress fractures have also been reported in the ribs, long bones, and feet of pregnant women (14, 15). The ligamentous laxity of pregnancy may predispose to the development of stress fractures. These are generally treated with rest and will heal rapidly. Casting is often difficult in the pregnant woman due to the tendency to develop swelling.

SPORTS INJURIES

There is little specific information available about the incidence of sports injuries during pregnancy. Anecdotal reports suggest that there are few problems in the highly trained, well-conditioned athletes who maintain their endurance activities into the second trimester (16, 17). Reports have focused on the possibly harmful effects to the fetus of water skiing, scuba diving, mountain climbing, and contact sports (18–20). However, possible harmful effect of sports activities on the mother are not well documented.

The previous discussion about the physiological changes that occur during pregnancy and the common orthopedic injuries that may result suggests some possible guidelines for determining sports participation. During the first trimester, few unusual orthopedic injuries secondary to the pregnancy would be expected. However, as maternal size increases and the center of gravity shifts during the second trimester of pregnancy, the chance for orthopedic injury is increased. Sports in which balance and coordination are important, such as ice skating and skiing, and those that also carry a significant risk of falling, would obviously be increasingly risky after this point. As previously mentioned, even small increases in weight may result in large increases in force across the joints. At the same time, the change in center of gravity results in increased stress on ligaments and muscles, and increased ligamentous laxity predisposes to sprains. It would, therefore, seem prudent at this point to reduce weight bearing sports in favor of lower impact activities. For the woman who wishes to continue jogging, the recommendation would be use of a soft running surface and well-cushioned shoes to lower the impact across her joints. Likewise, the woman should be careful to run only on level ground to reduce the chance of falling or causing joint sprains. Avoiding running on hills will help to decrease the chance of developing chondromalacia. Whenever possible, it may be wise to encourage the patient to switch to lower impact, more stable activities, such as brisk walking, cycling, or low impact aerobics. A stationary bicycle will generally be safer than a standard bicycle. The seat of the bicycle should be adjusted as high as possible to prevent extreme flexion of the knees that may contribute to chondromalacia. Riding with a more upright posture and use of a padded seat may help prevent coccydynia, which is increased in frequency during pregnancy, secondary to ligamentous laxity. Swimming provides a good aerobic exercise in a nonweight bearing environment. Care should be taken to prevent hypo- or hyperthermia while engaging in this exercise. For the dedicated athlete who wishes to continue with her weight bearing exercises, consideration should be given to decreasing the mileage or the frequency of these exercises to help prevent stress fractures and overuse syndromes. Often the regular regimen can be varied using non-weight bearing exercises alternating with the regular weight bearing exercises.

Pregnant women may also benefit from the use of machines such as treadmills or the commercially available Stair Master (Tri-Tech, Inc., Tulsa, OK), which allow exercise at controlled aerobic rates with little risk of sprains. Weight training may be continued during pregnancy, but only light weights with decreased repetitions should be used. Care should be taken to breathe properly during those exercises and avoid the Valsalva maneuver. Overhead lifting of heavy weights, rowing exercises, and squatting-type exercises should be eliminated to prevent injury to the lower back. Racquet sports may generally be continued through pregnancy, but care should be taken to prevent sprains due to sudden acceleration or deceleration on the court. The pregnant woman should also be aware that her increased size and shift in center of gravity predisposes her to falling with sudden changes of direction in racquet sports. For this reason, doubles play may be preferable to singles play in the later stages of pregnancy.

In summary, the physiological changes occurring during pregnancy may lead to an increased chance of orthopedic injury. The increased susceptibility to orthopedic injury needs to be considered when counseling women about the respective benefits and hazards of sporting activities during pregnancy. Knowledge of these potential injuries should help the physician design a program of activity that will satisfy the woman and prevent unnecessary injury to the mother or to the fetus.

REFERENCES

1. Robertson EG. The natural history of edema during pregnancy. J Obstet Gynecol Br Commonw 1971; 78:49–54.
2. Gould JS, Wissinger HA. Carpal tunnel syndrome in pregnancy. South Med J 1978; 71:144–145.
3. Reif ME. Bilateral common peroneal nerve palsy secondary to prolonged squatting in natural childbirth. Birth 1988; 15:100–102.
4. Berg G, Hammer M, Moeller-Nielsen J. Low back pain during pregnancy. Obstet Gynecol 1988; 71:71–75.
5. Mantle MJ, Greenwood RM, Currey HL. Backache in pregnancy. Rheumatol Rehabil 1977; 16:95–101.
6. LaBan MM, Perrin JCS, Latimer FR. Pregnancy and the herniated lumbar disc. Arch Phys Med Rehabil 1983; 64:319–321.
7. Weinreb JC, Wolbarsht LB, Cohen JM, et al. Prevalence of lumbosacral intervertebral disk abnormalities on MR images in pregnant and asymptomatic nonpregnant women. Radiology 1989; 170:125–128.
8. Saraste H. Spondylosis and pregnancy—a risk analysis. Acta Obstet Gynecol Scand 1986; 65:727–729.
9. Cheng N, Burssens A, Mulier JC. Pregnancy and post-pregnancy avascular necrosis of the femoral head. Arch Orthop Trauma Surg 1982; 100:199–210.
10. Taylor RN, Sonson RD. Separation of the pubic symphysis. An underrecognized peripartum complication. J Reprod Med 1986; 31:203–206.
11. Mikawa Y, Watanabe R, Yamano Y, et al. Stress fracture of the body of pubis in a pregnant woman. A case report. Arch Orthop Trauma Surg 1988; 107:193–194.
12. Hammond DS, Ryan AJ. Leg pain in a pregnant runner. Phys Sports Med 1982; 10:8.
13. Mullinax KN, Dale E. Some considerations of exercise during pregnancy. Clin Sports Med 1986; 5:559–570.
14. Moran JJM. Stress fractures in pregnancy. Am J Obstet Gynecol 1988; 158:1274–1277.
15. Even-Tov I, Yedwab GA, Persitz E, et al. Stress fractures of ribs in late pregnancy. Int Surg 1979; 64:85–87.
16. Jarrett JC, Spellacy WN. Jogging during pregnancy: an improved outcome? Obstet Gynecol 1983; 61:705–709.
17. Cohen CG, Prior JC, Vigna Y, et al. Intense exercise during the first two trimesters of unapparent pregnancy. Phys Sports Med 1989; 17:87–94.
18. Newhall JF. Scuba diving during pregnancy, a brief review. Am J Obstet Gynecol 1981; 140:893–894.
19. Gensburg RS, Wojcik WG, Mihta SD. Vaginally induced pneumoperitoneum during pregnancy. Am J Radiol 1988; 150:595–596.
20. Diddle AW. Interrelationship of pregnancy and athletic performance. J Tenn Med Assoc 1984; 77:265–269.

11

Biomechanics Related to Exercise in Pregnancy

Jill L. McNitt-Gray

The purpose of this chapter is to provide a biomechanical basis for exercise prescription in pregnancy. Biomechanical analysis of human movement examines the geometry of human movements (kinematics) and the internal and external forces and torques responsible for the observed motion (kinetics). Results from biomechanical studies are used to improve body function and reduce injury by providing a quantitative means for assessing interactions between the human body and the environment. By using newtonian mechanics, cinematography, electromyography, and the assistance of various means of instrumentation, the external forces acting on the body can be measured and the internal forces and torques produced by the muscles and soft tissues may be estimated (1). These data may then be incorporated with research findings from engineering and medical disciplines to study the physiological effects of mechanical loads, such as those experienced during exercise and/or pregnancy.

Few biomechanical analyses of the changes in mechanical loading experienced by pregnant women exist in the literature (2). Thus several analyses, although not based on pregnant populations, have been provided to as-sist in identifying activities that minimize the potential of injury and provide the most benefit to pregnant women.

INCREASES IN BODY WEIGHT DURING PREGNANCY

During pregnancy, the total body mass (TBM) of the pregnant woman increases as the fetus develops, producing an increase in total body weight (BW) (3). The additional weight gained during pregnancy increases the load placed on the structures of the musculoskeletal system even while performing daily activities (4, 5) (Fig. 11.1). The weight gain during pregnancy was found on average to be 109 newtons (std = 48N) (3, 5). During the first trimester, the average weight gain was reported as 11.1 newtons, whereas the average weight gain during the second and third trimesters was found to be 48 and 50 newtons, respectively (3). The rate of weight gain during the last trimester was found to be highly variable between patients. In addition, 50% of the patients with toxemia were found to experience twice the average weight gain of normal patients some time during the pregnancy (3).

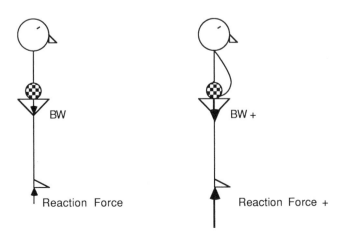

Figure 11.1. Free body diagrams of a nonpregnant and pregnant women during stance.

CHANGES IN REACTION FORCES DURING PREGNANCY

The acceleration of the body mass during daily or recreational activities may also increase the magnitude of the forces applied during contact with supporting surfaces (reaction forces) (1) (Fig. 11.2). Vertical reaction forces during stance, under static conditions (Fig. 11.2, a = 0), are equal in magnitude and opposite in direction to body weight. Vertical reaction force applied to the feet during dynamic activities, such as walking, running, and jumping, reach larger magnitudes ranging from two to five times body weight (6–8). The magnitudes of the horizontal forces in the anterior-posterior and medial-lateral directions also increase during dynamic activity (6–8).

Based on data obtained from nonpregnant subject populations, activities involving high velocity impacts tend to produce reaction forces of the highest magnitude and frequency (6–8). The amplitude and frequency characteristics of these reaction forces may also vary depending on the techniques used to complete the task. Low frequency forces (less than 2 Hz) are associated more with muscle control, whereas the high frequency forces are associated with transient forces experienced during impact (6–8).

MODIFICATIONS IN CENTER OF MASS DURING PREGNANCY

During pregnancy, the addition of body mass also produces greater internal forces and joint torques as a result of a change in the location of the total body center of mass (TBCM). The TBCM is a theoretical point representing the point in space where the force due to body weight (BW) effectively acts (1). The location of the TBCM may be altered as a result of a redistribution of body mass or by changes in the geometric arrangement of segments during the performance of the task (1). By monitoring the location of TBCM during activities performed by a pregnant woman, the effect of the TBM on the mechanics of daily activities may be determined.

The distribution of the body mass gained during pregnancy is spread over the entire body; however, the majority of the mass is retained in the trunk region (2). Based on a weight gain of 109 newtons, 45% is related to the conceptus, 10% is associated with uterine growth, 12% is due to breast growth, 15% is protein retention, and the remaining 18% is interstitial water (3). Further redistribution of mass may occur due to fluid accumulation in the legs after prolonged standing. The mass centered in the trunk region, however,

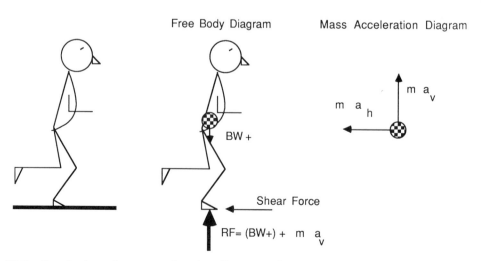

Figure 11.2.   Free body and mass acceleration diagrams of pregnant women during dynamic activity.

is expected to have the greatest influence on the mechanical loading experienced during pregnancy.

Geometric constraints imposed by an enlarged uterus may also influence the mechanical loading experienced during the last two trimesters. During the first 12 weeks of gestation, the growing uterus remains confined to the pelvis (1). At 20 weeks' gestation, the uterus reaches umbilical level and begins to protrude from the pelvis limiting the range of hip joint motion (1). This reduction in joint range of motion at the hip is expected to contribute to changes in the joint kinematics and subsequent kinetics of controlling the additional mass acquired in the trunk region (1).

EFFECT OF PHYSICAL CHANGES ON MECHANICAL LOADING

The biomechanical analysis by Ellis et al. (4) on women rising from a chair in pregnant and nonpregnant states provides the best example of the increases in loading in response to the increases in mass and modifications of center of mass associated with pregnancy. The kinematic data indicate that pregnant women prior to giving birth were unable to move their trunk forward to the same degree when rising from a chair as they were able to do after giving birth (Fig. 11.3). This reduction in hip flexion effectively repositions the center of mass farther from the axis of rotation and thus, requires greater muscular effort to rise from a chair.

The kinematic data when combined with the electromyographic data (EMG) and force records revealed that women rising from a chair when pregnant experienced a 33% increase in tibiofemoral joint force, an 23% increase in tangential tibiofemoral force, a 83% increase in patellofemoral force, a 100% increase in the activity of the quadriceps muscles, and a 35% increase in the activity of the hamstring muscles over the forces and activity levels measured after delivery. The increased muscular effort needed to accomplish this relatively simple task suggests that pregnant women may benefit from strength training of the lower extremity muscles.

One way to reduce the muscular effort of the lower extremity muscles is to utilize the upper extremity muscles when rising from a chair (4, 9). By using the arms, pregnant women were able to reduce the tibiofemoral force by 20% and the patellofemoral force by 57% (4). In addition, rising from a chair with the aid of arms reduced the activity of the quadriceps and the hamstrings by 57% and 40%, respectively (4). Rising from a chair with the aid of arms before and after giving birth produced no significant differences in patellofemoral force or quadriceps activity (4). Thus, utilization of the upper extremities may be useful in reducing the additional loads applied to the lower extremities during pregnancy. If techniques incorporating the use of the upper extremity muscles are adopted, strength training of the upper extremities may benefit pregnant women.

Another way to reduce the internal forces experienced in pregnancy is to modify the environment so that higher loading conditions may be avoided. In the case of chair

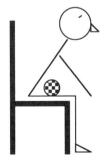 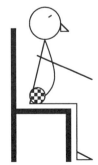

Figure 11.3. Kinematics of woman rising from a chair without the aid of arms before and after delivery.

rising, seat height has been shown to influence the magnitude of the knee joint torques required to complete the task (9). The results obtained by Rodosky, et al. (9) indicate that the hip torques reached the largest magnitudes independent of seat height; knee torques, however, were nearly halved when rising from a chair with a high seat position (115% of the knee height of the subject) as compared to sitting in a chair with a low seat position (65% of the knee height of the subject) (9). Thus, pregnant women may realize a reduction in load by sitting in a chair with a high seat (9) and rising from the chair with the assistance of the arms (4).

The results from these biomechanical studies indicate that pregnant women need to become more aware of environmental conditions that produce high internal loads. Further, pregnant women need to be educated about techniques that reduce the potential of injury (10). Improvement of upper and lower extremity muscle strength may also assist in keeping the additional loads applied within the limits of the musculoskeletal system.

STABILITY DURING PREGNANCY

During stance, the TBCM location continually oscillates over the base of support (the feet). The degree of posture sway is usually assessed by monitoring the change in location of the center of pressure (CP) when standing on a force platform. The CP is the point of application of the net reaction force applied by the support surface. As the TBCM sways forward over the base of support (the feet), the CP shifts forward, neutralizing the torque created by the BW.

Even with modifications in TBM and TBCM positions, pregnant women are able to maintain balance and preserve equilibrium by making compensatory posture adjustments. The degree of posture sway demonstrated by pregnant women has not been reported in the literature. The influence of externally applied loads, however, has been evaluated and published in the motor control and biomechanics literature (6, 7).

When a nonpregnant person is carrying a back pack, the additional load applied to the posterior of the trunk produces a compensatory forward lean of the trunk and a posterior lean of the legs resulting in an increase in hip flexion (11) (Fig. 11.4). The posture adjustment is necessary in order to keep the CM of the system over the base of support. This modified posture, although stable, deviates from the ideal standing posture.

Ideally, the mass of the segments supported by a joint must be evenly distributed so that the weight of the segments does not produce a torque about the joint axis. If the posture selected deviates from the ideal alignment of the segments, additional internal muscle forces will be necessary to maintain the compensatory position.

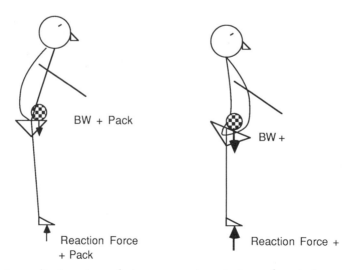

Figure 11.4.   Posture adjustments made in response to anterior and posterior applications of load.

When supporting a back pack, the CM of the system (body + pack) is positioned within the base of support, however, the mass of the head, arms, trunk, and pack (HAT + pack) is not balanced over the hip joint. In order for this posture to be maintained, internal forces must be produced by the hip extensor muscles to control the flexion torque created by the mass supported by the hip joint (11).

To produce internal forces, muscles are activated creating pulling force on the bones at the points of insertion (1). The resultant force produced by the muscle contributes to rotation of the segments and stabilization of the joints. As shown in Figure 11.5, the resultant muscle force vector comprises two components: a rotary component and a stabilization component. The rotary component, oriented perpendicular to the long axis of the segment, creates a torque contributing to the rotation of the segment about the joint axis. The stabilizing component, oriented parallel to the long axis of the segment, assists the ligaments in stabilizing the joint. When carrying a back pack, sufficient force must be developed by the hip extensors to produce a torque by the rotary component in order to off set the flexion torque produced by the weight of the HAT and back pack. Data based on load carrying indicate that no matter how the mass is distributed within the pack or along the back, the appropriate posture adjustments are made automatically to keep the CM of the system (BW + pack) within the base of support (11). The closer the additional mass is located to the normal position of the TBCM, the smaller the posture adjustments made in response to the applied load (11).

Posture adjustment when carrying a fetus in the anterior pelvic region has been observed to produce an anterior tilt of the pelvis (Fig. 11.4), an increase in kyphosis, and modifications in lordosis (2). Recent quantitative investigations, however, suggest that a variety of posture adjustment strategies are used to compensate for the anteriorly applied load during pregnancy.

Pregnant women may adjust their posture to maintain stability either by increasing the lumbar curve (12, 13) or by decreasing the

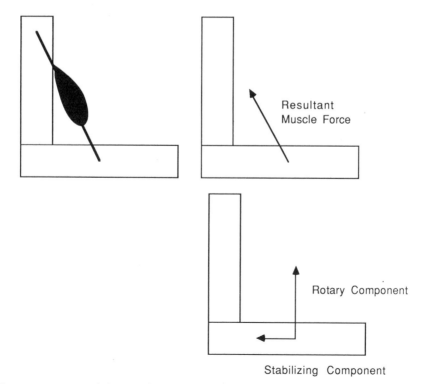

Figure 11.5.   The components of the resultant muscle force contributing to rotation and stabilization of the joints.

lumbar curve (13, 14). Moore and associates (13) propose that the flattening of the lumbar spine may be due to reduced iliopsoas muscle activity. As the fetal mass positioned anterior to the hip joint axis grows, the flexion torque created by the weight will also increase. Thus, the flexion torque created by the iliopsoas is no longer needed (13). The addition of mass associated with the fetus may also be nullified by a compensatory posterior shift of the mass of the upper trunk. This posterior shift of upper body mass is evident in those subjects demonstrating an increase in lumbar curvature (13).

The posture adjustments made by pregnant women to compensate for the anteriorly applied weight may contribute to low back pain (10). Each individual must be assessed to determine the most appropriate compensatory posture to neutralize the additional mass acquired during pregnancy so that pain may be reduced (10).

Pain in the low back region may also be reduced by improving the strength and control of the muscles attached to the spine and pelvis (10). Anterior pelvic tilt may be reduced by activating the abdominals and the hamstring muscle groups and relaxing and/or stretching of the erector spinae and hip flexors (Fig. 11.6). When activated, the hamstrings and abdominals produce forces that create an internal torque opposing the torque created by the mass positioned anterior to the joint axis. During the advanced stages of pregnancy, the abdominals are lengthened, which may reduce their effectiveness in reducing anterior pelvic tilt (10).

In this case, the hamstrings must produce additional force to compensate for the loss in force supplied by the abdominals. Thus, patients experiencing low back pain originating from anterior pelvic tilt may find relief by increasing the strength of the hamstring muscles and using them to reduce anterior tilt of the pelvis. Similarly, low back pain originating from posterior pelvic tilt may be relieved by activating the erector spinae and the hip flexors (iliopsoas and rectus femoris) and stretching the hamstrings and the abdominals (15). Flexibility exercises, however, should be used with caution by pregnant women. Laxity of the ligaments and joints may be sufficiently altered by the hormonal changes associated with pregnancy (10, 16, 17).

INFLUENCES OF HORMONAL CHANGES ON MECHANICS

During pregnancy, the level of the hormone relaxin rises (18). This increase in relaxin has been associated with increases in laxity of the pelvic joints (19). Recent evidence indicates that peripheral joints, such as the feet, teeth, fingers, and knees, also experience increases in joint laxity during pregnancy (2, 19, 20). The loosening of the connective tissue, in combination with the changes in mechanical loading, may produce serious mechanical consequences to the pregnant woman.

Both mechanical loading and/or ligament laxity brought on by relaxin have been associated with the high incidence of low back pain among pregnant women (21). Back pain has been associated with posture adjust-

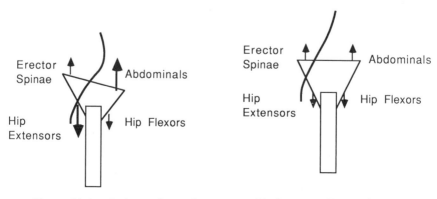

Figure 11.6.   Actions of muscles responsible for controlling pelvic tilt.

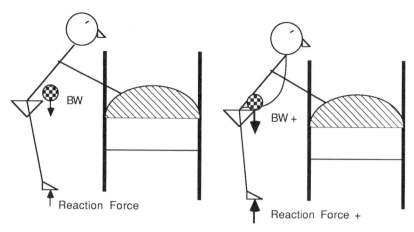

Figure 11.7.   Free body diagrams of nonpregnant and pregnant women making beds.

ments in response to increases in body weight, changes in TBCM, strenuous work requiring forward bending, twisting, and lifting, or even daily activities, such as standing, sitting, walking, and making beds (Fig. 11.7) (21–23). Women suffering from back pain before pregnancy also tend to experience more back pain during pregnancy (21).

If back pain is mechanically induced, knowledge of preferred methods of posture adjustment and lifting may prove useful in identifying techniques that minimize the risk of injury. For example, lifting techniques that emphasize the use of the legs and keep the center of mass of the object close to the body throughout the lift have been shown to minimize the magnitude of the forces transmitted to the structures of the low back of nonpregnant individuals (24, 25). Thus, lifting objects between the knees, as shown in Figure 11.8, may prevent or assist in reducing the low back pain experienced by pregnant women.

Back pain associated with the changes in hormonal levels during pregnancy, however, may be more difficult to prevent. The relaxing of the ligaments associated with the hormonal changes leads to increases in the mobility of the joints. Ligament laxity in the pelvis region has been linked with the sacroiliac dysfunction (26) and the changes in the pubis symphysis (26, 27) observed in pregnant women. Pain from the symphysis has been strongly associated with sacroiliac joint dysfunction, particularly during the later stages of pregnancy (26). Pregnant women with sacroiliac joint dysfunction tend to have more unilateral pain in the pelvis when walking (26). Relief from pelvic joint mobility may be achieved using a trochanteric belt; however, reliance on an external device may produce atrophy of the muscles responsible for maintaining pelvic stability (10). Thus, training of the muscles stabilizing the pelvic joints may be helpful in reducing pain due to ligament laxity.

Ligament laxity observed in the foot region

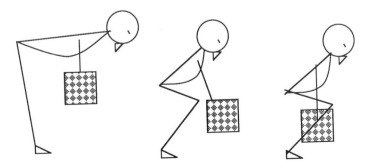

Figure 11.8   Three lifting techniques performed by pregnant women.

may also be related to pain experienced in the back and lower extremities of the pregnant woman (17, 20). Increased pronation of the foot, joint laxity of the first metatarsophalangeal joint, and mobility of the midtarsal joint observed in pregnant women may influence the mechanical loading experienced by the lower extremities and back (20). The changes in foot mobility may also effect the posture adjustment strategies observed during pregnancy (20).

The degree of ligament laxity observed in the joints of the feet and pelvis may also be dependent on the impulsive characteristics of the mechanical loads experienced during pregnancy. Under normal conditions, bone and soft tissue adapt in response to the mechanical loads experienced (28). The structural adaptation of the tissues is also largely dependent on the magnitude, direction, and duration of the forces applied (28). Thus, participation in one type of dynamic activity may produce beneficial loading.

REFERENCES

1. Miller DI, Nelson RC. Biomechanics of sport. Philadelphia: Lea & Febiger, 1973.
2. Danforth DN. Pregnancy and labor. Am J Phys Med 1967; 46:653–658.
3. Chesley LC. Weight changes and water balance in normal and toxic pregnancy. Am J Obstet Gynecol 1944; 48:565–593.
4. Ellis MI, Seedhom BB, Wright V. Forces in women 36 weeks pregnant and four weeks after delivery. Engineering Med 1985; 14(2):95–99.
5. Paisley JE, Mellion MB. Exercise during pregnancy. Austral J Phys 1988; 38:143–150.
6. Hay JG. A bibliography of biomechanics literature, 4th ed. 1981.
7. Hay JG. A bibliography of biomechanics literature, 5th ed. 1987.
8. Nigg BM. Biomechanics, load analysis, and sport injuries in the lower extremities. Sports Med 1985; 2:367–379.
9. Rodosky MW, Andriacchi TP, Andersson GBJ. The influence of chair height on lower limb mechanics during rising. J Orthop Res 1989; 7:266–271.
10. Gleeson PB, Pausl JA. Obstetrical physical therapy. Phys Ther 1988; 68:1699–1702.
11. Hellebrandt FA, Fries EC, Larsen EM, Kelso LEA. The influence of the army pack on postural stability and stance mechanics. Am J Phys 1943; 645–655.
12. Bullock JE, Gwendolen JA, Bullock MI. The relationship of low back pain to postural changes during pregnancy. Austr J Physiother 1987; 33:11–17.
13. Moore K, Dumas GA, Reid JG, Stevenson JM. A longitudinal study of the mechanical changes in posture associated with pregnancy: A preliminary report. Proceedings: Fifth Biennial Conference and Symposium 1988; 114–115.
14. Snijders JG, Hoest HT. Change in form of spine as a consequence of pregnancy. In Digest of the 11th International Conference on Medical and Biological Engineering. Ottawa, 1976.
15. Day JW, Smit GL, Lehmann T. Effect of pelvic tilt on standing posture. Phys Ther 1984; 64:510–516.
16. Abramson D, Robert SM, Wilson PD. Relaxation of the pelvic joints in pregnancy. Surg Gynecol Obstet 1934; 58:595–613.
17. Alvarez R, Stokes IAF, Asprino DE, Trevino S, Braun T. Dimensional changes of the feet in pregnancy. J Bone Joint Surg 1988; 70A:271–274.
18. Tipton CM, Vailas AC, Matthes RD. Experimental studies on the influences of physical activity on ligaments, tendons and joints: A brief review. Acta Med Scand 1986; Suppl 711:157–168.
19. Calganeri M, Bird HA, Wright V. Changes in joint laxity occurring during pregnancy. Ann Rheum Dis 1982; 41:126–128.
20. Block RA, Hess LA, Timpano EV, Serlo C. Physiological changes in foot in pregnancy. J Am Podiatr Med Assoc 1985; 75:297–299.
21. Berg G, Hammer M, Moller-Neison J, Linden U, Thorblad J. Low back pain during pregnancy. Obstet Gynecol 1988; 71:71–74.
22. Fast A, Shapiro D, Duommun EJ, Friedmann LW, Bouklas T, Floman Y. Low back pain in pregnancy. Spine 1987; 12:368–371.
23. Mantle MJ, Greenwood RM, Currey HLF. Backache in pregnancy. Rheumatol Rehabil 1977; 16:95–101.
24. Hansson T, Bigos S, Wortley M, Spengler D. Load on the lumbar spine during isometric strength testing. Spine 1984; 9:720–724.
25. Szlachter BN, Quagliarello J, Jewelewicz R, Osathanondh R, Spellacy WN, Weiss G. Relaxin in normal and pathogenic pregnancies. Obstet Gynecol 1982; 59(2):167–170.
26. DonTigny RL. Function and pathomechanics of the sacroiliac joint. Phys Ther 1985; 65(1):35–41.
27. Mikawa Y, Watanabe R, Yamano Y, Miyake S. Stress fracture of the body of pubis in a pregnant woman. Arch Orthop Trauma Surg 1988; 107:193–194.
28. Troup JDG. Measurements of the sagittal mobility of the lumbar spine and hips. Arch Phys Med 1968; 9:308.

Acknowledgements—The author would like to thank Sharon Wentzel and Dawn Irvine for their assistance with the literature search, Carolyn Barbieri for providing the graphics, and Patty Sanchez for typing the reference list.

12

Exercise Physiology

Robert A. Wiswell

Exercise physiology is the study of the functional changes that occur, within an organism, as a result of acute or chronic exposure to exertion. Acute exercise is a physiological stressor, and as such, requires a major homeostatic adjustment in all organ functions if the exercise is to be continued. Very heavy exercise may require the body to increase its energy output by 20-fold. It may require up to an 8-fold increase in cardiac output. The exercise may stimulate a major increase in endocrine activity and an increased neuromotor recruitment. As well, the body has to adjust to accelerated heat production by modifying its normal mechanisms of thermoregulation. Fluid and electrolyte balance will be disturbed and fuel sources may become depleted. Fortunately, the body adjusts quite well to this stress and, in fact, over time is able to perform at much higher levels without similar fatigue.

The magnitude of the adjustment to chronic stress (or exercise) is dependent on several factors, such as: *(a)* the age, sex, and body size of the individual; *(b)* the type of exercise, intensity of training, duration of the activity, the muscles involved, and the body position; *(c)* the environment in which the exercise is performed (high altitude, heat, cold, underwater, in a polluted environment, etc.); as well as *(d)* the health and nutritional status of the individual.

In general, it is believed that the chronic adaptations in physiological function that accrue as a result of physical training are beneficial to the individual and may even affect mortality and morbidity. As a result, exercise patterns in the United States over the past years have changed dramatically, showing a renewed interest in vigorous physical activity. Consequently, more and more people are participating in long-distance running and marathons. Millions of people are enrolling in organized aerobic and anaerobic exercise programs. New weight-training devices are available, and emphasis is being placed on strength training and power lifting. Academically, there has been a interest in studying special groups such as elite athletes, women, children, and older people.

With the interest in encouraging the participation of women in sport, and with the pressure exerted by the female athletes themselves demanding a right to exercise, several questions have arisen about performance capability, influence of menstrual cycling during participation, and possible risks involved for women while exercising. New and greater opportunities became available for women to compete. As a result, several studies have been conducted to assess the fitness potential of these now competing women (1–8).

Several authors have provided information as to the possible role of exercise on maturation in young girls (2, 9, 10) and on menstrual irregularities in women who engage in rigorous physical training (11–16). As a result, a growing amount of literature is now available to assist the physician, therapist, and exercise physiologist in understanding the effects and importance of exercise for women.

Pregnant women are joining this fitness revolution as well, and want to maintain their activity levels. If previously sedentary, they may want to begin participating in vigorous exercise throughout the duration of their pregnancy, and are in need of relevant information to direct their exercise programs. Statements have been made about the exercise potential for childbearing women but the scientific literature is limited. The special needs of pregnancy may vary and, on one extreme, bed rest may be recommended for some pa-

complicated pregnancies; in the me, we have examples of pregnant women running a marathon the day before delivery. In the past, attempts have been made to tailor exercise programs for pregnant women from research studies conducted on normal nonpregnant females. In general, recommendations were conservative but, even so, did not have a scientific basis (prescription concepts are detailed in Chapters 20, 28, and the Appendix). Fox (17) provides some very specific statements about exercise in pregnancy to support the concept that exercise is nct harmful. He reports that complications of pregnancy are fewer in athletes, that performance returns to prepregnancy levels within 2 years, that pregnancy does not adversely affect athletic participation and that serious injuries to the breasts or the external and internal reproductive organs is very rare in female athletes. While these statements may have some research support, the academic community is not willing to accept them without considerably more research.

Exercise during pregnancy is probably beneficial to most women. On the other hand, exercise in some may actually be detrimental to both mother and fetus; therefore, recommendation for exercise, as such, should be individualized. It must be emphasized that the same generalizations about individual response to exercise can also be made about work. Work in this context may require as much energy as expended during moderate exercise and may be considered harmful or beneficial depending on the individual and the situation.

In this chapter, information will be presented about basic physiological responses to exercise with special reference to pregnant women. As well, a brief introduction to the nomenclature of the field will be presented. This chapter will present physiological information about exercise response in general and will not include information about sports injuries or health effects. More detailed information on exercise physiology is beyond the scope of this book; ample literature is available for the interested reader (17–19).

MEASUREMENT OF AEROBIC FITNESS

Before the application of science to physical fitness assessment, work capacity was mea-sured in terms of running times, pounds lifted, distance covered, etc. With more sophisticated methodologies, these performance measurements were replaced with laboratory measures. Fitness is now assessed using parameters such as oxygen-pulse, ventilatory equivalents, respiratory exchange ratios, lactic acid production, and maximal oxygen consumption. These terms will be elucidated later in this chapter. Suffice it to say, at this time, with the greater sophistication in evaluation, a more in-depth understanding of exercise physiology is required to interpret this new information.

It has been suggested that an individual's capacity for exercise is limited by the combined ability of the respiratory and cardiovascular systems to meet the increased oxygen demand of the muscles. Assessment of cardiorespiratory function can be made at rest but, generally speaking, is more definitive when appraised under exertional stress. Higher levels of stress up to maximal exertion seemingly allow a more reliable, valid measure of the adaptive capacities of an individual.

Of the many noninvasive measures of fitness, maximal oxygen consumption is regarded by exercise physiologists as the best single measurement of physical working capacity (20, 21). Maximal oxygen consumption is highly related to maximal cardiac output and is an excellent discriminatory measure of an individual's prior exercise history (22, 23). In some instances, however, it is not advisable for the subject to perform at maximal exercise. For these individuals, submaximal tests may give some indication of exercise tolerance but the interpretation of submaximal tests is difficult and often misleading.

Maximal Oxygen Uptake

Maximal oxygen consumption ($\dot{V}_{O_2max}$) is defined as the maximal rate at which oxygen can be utilized by the body. It relates to the power or capacity of the aerobic system (17). There are two very important equations that help describe the significant systems that influence and/or regulate the uptake of O_2. The first, the Fick equation, suggests that the two most important parameters in determining V_{O_2} are cardiac output and the arteriovenous (A-V) oxygen difference.

$$\dot{V}_{O_2} = \text{Cardiac output (Q)} \times \text{A-V } O_2 \text{ difference}$$

Thus, there is a circulatory component to oxygen uptake (oxygen delivery) and an extraction component (oxygen utilization). The circulatory component is influenced by myocardial contractility, venous return, blood volume, oxygen carrying capacity, and peripheral resistance. It can also be influenced by intrinsic factors as well as neurogenic factors that may influence heart rate. Oxygen extraction, on the other hand, is related to cellular metabolic function and is regulated by enzyme activity and production, as well as fuel availability.

Pregnancy is known to have a major impact on the circulatory system. The blood volume is increased, blood pressure may either increase or decrease, and there are significant changes in both resting and exercise heart rate. The literature related to the oxygen extraction side of the equation suggests that during pregnancy there is a significant decrease in A-V O_2 difference that has been attributed to the increase in blood volume and cardiac output rather than to any specific changes occurring at the cellular level (24).

It would be simple to calculate V_{O_2} if the inspired ventilatory volume was equal to the expiratory volume. However, this is only the case when the respiratory exchange ratio equals one and when the primary fuel for cellular metabolism is carbohydrate. To account for this problem of substrate utilization, adjustments have to be made to the expired oxygen concentration (25).

$$\dot{V}_{O_2} = VE_{STPD} \times \frac{\%N_{2EXP}}{79.04} \times \frac{20.93}{100}$$
$$- VE_{STPD} \times \frac{\%O_{2EXP}}{100}$$

where

VE_{STPD} = expired ventilatory volume corrected to standard temperature and pressure dry;

$\%N_{2EXP}$ = the percentage expired nitrogen concentration;

20.93 = the assumed inspired oxygen concentration;

79.04 = the assumed ambient/inspired nitrogen concentration;

$\%O_{2EXP}$ = the percentage of expired oxygen.

This equation reveals that, in addition to those already mentioned parameters of circulation and extraction, one must consider ventilatory function as an important contributor to exercise tolerance and maximal capacity. Normally, respiratory function is not considered a major limiting factor to exercise performance, but during pregnancy, when limits to diaphragmatic excursion occur and, when coupled with significant change in maternal hemodynamics, maximal and/or submaximal ventilation may be reduced or influenced.

For most individuals, oxygen uptake increases linearly with increasing workloads until a plateau is reached; at this point, more work can be applied without further increases in $\dot{V}_{O_2}$ (Fig. 12.1). Thus, a further definition of $\dot{V}_{O_2max}$ would be the point during incrementally increasing work in which further increases in workload do not elicit an increase in oxygen consumption. The usual criteria employed to ascertain whether or not maximal oxygen uptake has been achieved are:

1. The subject's having reached a plateau (less than 150-ml increase) or decrease in $\dot{V}_{O_2}$ with increasing work load (26);

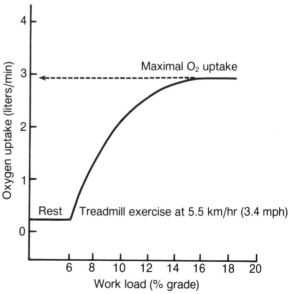

Figure 12.1. The plateau in oxygen uptake with increasing work load at maximal oxygen consumption. (From Lamb DR. Physiology of exercise: responses and adaptations. New York: MacMillan, 1978.)

2. The respiratory exchange ratio having reached a level greater than 1.1 (21);
3. The pulse rate reaching the age-adjusted maximal level; maximal heart rate can be estimated by subtracting one's age from 220; this figure may slightly underestimate the actual HR_{max}; or by subtracting one-half age from 210, which gives a less conservative estimate (27);
4. Plasma lactate concentrations in excess of 10.0 mM (21);
5. The subject's inability to maintain the work load.

Unfortunately, during clinical practice, most of the subjects are not of sufficient physical condition to achieve a "true" $\dot{V}_{O_2max}$ and stop exercise before a plateauing of $\dot{V}_{O_2}$ due to a variety of symptoms that generally includes shortness of breath and/or leg fatigue. In these subjects, the test is called a "symptom limited $\dot{V}_{O_2max}$ test" or peak $\dot{V}_{O_2}$ and only approximates the subject's actual aerobic capacity. Table 12.1 presents standards for $\dot{V}_{O_2max}$ (values in $ml\cdot kg^{-1}\cdot min^{-1}$).

If one uses these standards, it becomes obvious that pregnancy is a detriment to fitness or aerobic capacity simply because of the increase in body weight. However, this increased weight may also serve as a stimulus to improve oxygen uptake (29). In effect, the system may adjust to the increase in weight by improving its aerobic capacity.

Drinkwater (30) suggests that when comparing subpopulations with regard to aerobic capacity the method in which it is expressed becomes important. If the question relates to the ability of performing a specific task, $\dot{V}_{O_2max}$ expressed in liters per minute is appropriate. If the goal is to compare individuals with

regard to endurance capacity, $\dot{V}_{O_2max}$ should be expressed in $ml\cdot kg^{-1}\cdot min^{-1}$.

The problem associated with the selection of the method of expressing $\dot{V}_{O_2}$ also becomes a problem when addressing the issue of expressing the metabolic cost of an activity and has led to some major confusion within the field. In the next section, we will try to present some information related to the methods of expressing resting and exercise energy expenditure. This may be helpful in trying to compare scientific studies related to energy expenditure and oxygen uptake.

Prediction of Maximal Oxygen Consumption

Due to a general concern in clinical practice of performing maximal testing on pregnant subjects, several indirect methods have been employed to predict maximal aerobic power. A quote from Wyndham (31) provides a short summary of the general consensus of the research community about the use of predicted $\dot{V}_{O_2max}$:

Exercise physiologists have tried to develop a test using submaximal effort which will give a reliable and accurate estimate of an individual's true maximal oxygen intake. Success in this field of research has been as elusive as that for the philosopher's stone. In consequence there are almost as many submaximal tests of maximal oxygen consumption as there are exercise physiologists (31, p 736).

In one of the earliest studies, performed in nonpregnant women, Astrand and Rhyming (32), using a submaximal step test or a submaximal work load on a bicycle ergometer, reported an accuracy of ±9.5% in women in predicting $\dot{V}_{O_2max}$. Work loads were set at approximately 50% of V_{O_2max} with an average heart rate of 138 bpm for women. Wyndham et al. (33) suggested the need to fit appropriate curves to the data to test their "goodness of fit" rather than to extrapolate to maximal heart rate as Astrand and Rhyming (32) had done. By curve fitting, Wyndham et al. (33) were able to reduce the coefficient of variation in prediction to 4.3%. Issekutz et al. (34) reported that respiratory exchange ration (R) or the change in R from .75 could be used to predict maximal oxygen consump-

Table 12.1. Aerobic Capacity Standards of Women[a]

Age	Maximal Oxygen Consumption ($ml\cdot kg^{-1}\cdot min^{-1}$)				
	Low	Fair	Average	Good	High
20–29	28	29–34	35–40	41–46	47
30–39	27	28–33	34–38	39–45	46
40–49	25	26–31	32–37	38–43	44
50–65	21	22–28	29–34	35–40	41

[a]Adapted from Katch FI, McArdle WD. Nutrition, weight control and exercise. Philadelphia: Lea & Febiger, 1983, p 291.

tion accurately. They reported an accuracy of ± 10% when using change in R.

In the early 1970s, it became quite popular to use multiple regression technique in the development of prediction equations. Mastropaolo (35) used stepwise regression to predict $\dot{V}_{O_2max}$ and reported a multiple correlation of 0.93 with a standard error of the estimate of .172 liters per minute. He used steady state R, work rate, VE, diastolic blood pressure, and expired oxygen concentration obtained at 600 kpm/min on a bicycle ergometer as variables in the equation. Hermiston and Faulkner (36) similarly reported the use of multiple stepwise regression in predicting maximal oxygen consumption. A multiple correlation of 0.90 was reported using lean body mass, heart rate, F_{ECO_2}, and tidal volume as the predicting variables.

More recently, several studies have addressed the issue of improvement in aerobic capacity as a result of conditioning in pregnancy (37–39) and have employed prediction of $\dot{V}_{O_2max}$ as the major dependent measure. The usefulness of prediction equations in estimating maximal aerobic capacity in pregnancy may be questioned, however.

There are several basic assumptions that have been reported as a justification to account for the expected accuracy of predicting maximal oxygen consumption. They are:

1. Heart rate and oxygen consumption are linearly related up to maximal levels;
2. Heart rate and oxygen consumption reach asymptomatic maximal values at a common high level of work;
3. Individual variation about population means is small;
4. Maximal heart rate occurs at approximately the same rate of work as maximal oxygen consumption (31).

The validity of these assumptions, however, is open to question, particularly with regard to pregnant women. We have reported that resting, submaximal heart rates, and maximal heart rate may be influenced by pregnancy (Fig. 12.2). While estimated work capacity may be used to indicate the effectiveness of training, its use in evaluating maximal aerobic power is questionable.

Relative Versus Absolute Work

It is common practice to report the cardiorespiratory responses to exercise as a function of absolute work intensity or as a function of relative work intensity, expressed as a percentage of the individual maximal oxygen uptake. Clausen (40) suggests that heart

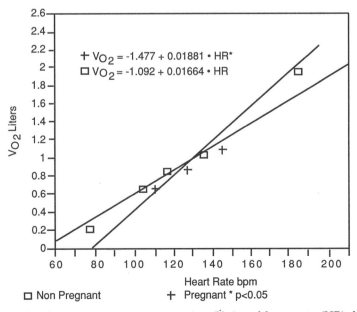

Figure 12.2.   Relationship between oxygen consumption ($\dot{V}_{O_2}$) and heart rate (HR) during exercise.

rate and arterial pressure responses are closely related to the relative work load while cardiac output is more a function of absolute work load (41).

As one improves his or her physical fitness, the metabolic and circulatory response to the same (absolute) work load may be reduced (e.g., lower ventilation) while when expressed relative to the $\dot{V}_{O_2max}$, the fit and unfit may have a similar response. There are several metabolic parameters that demonstrate significant changes during exercise in pregnancy; yet if these changes are not viewed in light of the reduced fitness of the individual, one may misinterpret the results. Some of the apparent differences between male and female response to exercise reported in the literature are the result of using the same absolute work load in the protocol, which penalizes women because they are usually at a higher percentage of $\dot{V}_{O_2max}$. If $\dot{V}_{O_2max}$ changes during pregnancy, this may confound determining changes at submaximal workloads.

Energy Expenditure

Energy expenditure refers to the total calories required to complete a given task. It is usually estimated from the amount of oxygen consumed during the activity (17). Measuring oxygen consumption can be useful as an index of energy liberation and, thus, fuel catabolism. The specific use of oxygen during exercise is that of a hydrogen acceptor. The source of the excessive hydrogen pool is derived from substrate catabolism (ATP, CP, CHO, fats, and proteins). For every liter of oxygen utilized by the body, approximately 5 kcal of energy would have been liberated from the substrate pool. During the high-energy demands of exercise, oxygen uptake goes up as much as 15 times, increasing caloric expenditure from 1 kcal/min at rest to as much as 15 kcal/min during high-intensity exercise. To obtain the rough caloric expenditure of an activity, one simply multiplies the oxygen uptake in liters by 5 kcal.

Oxygen uptake can be expressed in liters per minute or in terms of one's body weight. In some instances, it is presented in relationship to one's body surface area. The expression of metabolic cost in liters gives one an indication of the energy requirement of the task. Expressing the metabolic cost in $ml·kg^{-1}·min^{-1}$, gives an indication of one's efficiency in utilizing oxygen based upon his orf her own body weight. A normal exercise task, such as casual walking, may require 20 $ml·kg^{-1}·min^{-1}$ in relative terms. In a 50-kg woman, the oxygen uptake would be 1 liter·min^{-1}, and the same activity in a 60-kg woman would be 1.2 liters·min^{-1}.

Another means of expressing energy cost of activity rather than the absolute oxygen cost is to express energy requirements in METs. One MET is equivalent to 3.5 $ml·kg^{-1}·min^{-1}$, which in most people approximates their metabolic rate while sitting quietly. A 3-MET activity would be an activity that raises the resting metabolic rate 3 times. The 1-liter oxygen consumption per minute during a 1-mile walk could be expressed as a 3–4-MET activity. The use of METs allows one to obtain a relative scale of work intensity and is used for exercise prescription.

The advantage or disadvantage of one system over another is solely based upon the preference and background of the investigator. It is unfortunate that there is no uniform method of expressing energy requirements of exercise (Table 12.2).

It is a common trend in exercise prescription to suggest that individuals should be involved in an exercise program that elevates energy expenditure 150–300 kcal/day. In simple terms, one estimates the caloric cost of walking a mile to be approximately 80–120 kcal (depending on weight). Therefore, the exercise program of choice seems to be one that would be equivalent in energy expenditure terms to between 1.5 and 3 miles of walking or running per day. It must be noted that these values have not been standardized for pregnant women. The oxygen cost of any weight bearing exercise is greater during pregnancy due to the increase in body weight and reduced efficiency of oxygen utilization. It is interesting to note that the question of speed is relatively unimportant in terms of energy expenditure, although it is believed that faster work rates lead to slightly (6–10%) greater caloric expenditures. This caloric difference is not, however, of major physiological significance. An excellent review of the

Table 12.2.   Methods of Classifying Energy Requirements of a Task

Activity[a]		Weight in Kilograms			
		50	65	80	95
Caloric cost: kcal·min					
Sitting quietly		1.1	1.4	1.7	2.0
Walking		4.0	5.2	6.4	7.4
Running—5 mph		6.8	8.8	10.5	12.9
Running—6.6 mph		9.7	12.5	15.4	18.3
O_2 cost: liters·min^{-1}					
Sitting quietly		.22	.28	.34	.40
Walking		.80	1.04	1.28	1.48
Running—5 mph		1.36	1.76	2.10	2.58
Running—6.6 mph		1.94	2.50	3.08	3.66
O_2 cost: ml·kg^{-1}·min^{-1}					
Sitting quietly		4.4	4.3	4.2	4.2
Walking		16.0	16.0	16.0	15.6
Running—5 mph		27.2	27.1	26.2	27.2
Running—6.6 mph		38.8	38.5	38.5	38.5
Metabolic Equivalent: METs; O_2 cost = liters/min / caloric cost = kcal/min					
Sitting	1 MET	.18/0.9	.23/1.2	.28/1.4	.33/1.6
Walking	3-4 METs	.70/3.5	.91/4.5	1.12/5.6	1.33/6.6
Run—5 mph	6-7 METs	1.20/6.2	1.59/7.9	1.96/9.8	2.33/11.6
Run—6 mph	10-11 METs	1.92/9.6	2.50/12.5	3.08/15.4	3.65/18.3

[a] Interpretation:

Caloric cost—A 65-kg person would expend approximately 5.2 kcal per minute while walking.

O_2 cost —An 80-kg person would have an oxygen uptake of approximately .34 liters per minute while sitting quietly. In relationship to his body weight, this would represent 4.2 ml·kg^{-1}·min^{-1}.

METs   —Running at 5 mph is a 6–7 MET activity. It requires approximately 1.2 liters of oxygen per minute in a 50-kg person and represents a caloric expenditure of 6.2 kcal/min.

caloric cost of various activities was reported by Passmore and Durnin (42).

Mechanical Efficiency

Based upon the scientific literature, one may assume that the oxygen cost of performing a given amount of work is the same between individuals. However, although the oxygen cost of an activity is work load-dependent, there are several factors that may influence the absolute amount of oxygen consumed. The economical use of oxygen by an individual is termed metabolic efficiency. Biomechanical factors can affect efficiency as well as the type of activity and type or size of the muscles involved. Several different mathematical equations of mechanical efficiency have been applied to address the question of differences in O_2 cost between activities. With regard to these models, efficiency is defined as the ratio of useful work output to energy expended (43). In most machines, efficiency is lost due to friction between parts. In this example, the extra amount of energy required to overcome frictional factors serves to reduce the machine's efficiency. The human is less efficient than most machines in the use of its energy sources. As a result, the human uses a disproportionate amount of fuel and generates an excessive amount of heat when performing physical work. Table 12.3 is an example of how mechanical efficiency is determined in individuals who are doing bicycle exercise.

The determination of work efficiency on the treadmill is considerably more difficult due to problems imposed in calculating the amount of distance (both horizontal and vertical) transversed during the exercise task. An excellent review of the methods and

Table 12.3.   An Example of Mechanical Efficiency Determinations Using a Bicycle Ergometer[a]

Work Output	Energy Expenditure

Work = Force × Distance

Bicycle resistance	= 4 kg	Steady-level $\dot{V}_{O_2}$ = 1.2 liters	
Wheel circumference	= 2 meters	Caloric cost	= 1.2 × 4.83[b]
			= 5.79 kcal
Revolutions per min	= 60 rpm	(caloric cost × 426.8 converts to work units—kg)	
Work = 4 kg × (60 × 2) = 480 kg		Work = 5.79 × 426.8 = 2474 kg	

$$\text{Efficiency} = \frac{\text{Work Output}}{\text{Energy Expenditure}} = \frac{480 \text{ kg}}{2474 \text{ kg}} = 19.4\%$$

[a] Adapted from Fox EL, Mathews DK. The physiological basis of physical education and athletics. Philadelphia: WB Saunders, 1981.
[b] Assumes an R = .83

mathematical procedures is provided by Fox and Mathews (43).

Donovan and Brooks (44) reported efficiencies for horizontal walking of 19.6–35.2%. Gaesser and Brooks (45) reported 20.6–43% efficiency for cycling. Pendergast et al. (46) found much lower efficiencies in swimming freestyle (2.9–7.4% in men; 2.7–9.4 in women). In general, tasks requiring larger muscle groups result in better efficiency than those using smaller muscles. However, one must be cautious when comparing the efficiencies reported between studies because of the different equations used and the fact that some authors report gross rather than net efficiencies.

Girandola et al. (9) reported efficiency difference between pre- and postpubescent girls. The younger girls were less efficient having higher $\dot{V}_{O_2}$ for similar work loads. The differences were attributed to shorter limb length causing more strides for the same running pace or a possible deficiency in motor development that may have resulted in more extraneous movement during the run. A final possibility was that the taller, older girls may have been able to walk at the speed used for comparison, whereas the younger girls may have been running. Running has been reported to be less efficient than walking and could help explain this disparity (47).

The literature relating to efficiency difference during pregnancy is contradictory. Knuttgen and Emerson (48) reported a lower O_2 cost of treadmill walking at 14 weeks postpartum compared to prepartum values. This difference was attributed to maternal weight gain, and was consistent with several earlier studies (49, 50). Knuttgen and Emerson (48) also reported that the O_2 cost of cycling was not significantly different in this study, implying no effect of pregnancy on efficiency. Seitchik (51) studied the oxygen requirement of a submaximal bicycle task in 195 pregnant women and concluded that pregnancy did not significantly incease oxygen cost of exercise. Edwards et al. (52) reported a significant increase in resting metabolism but no difference in submaximal oxygen uptake (50 W bicycle exercise). Pernoll et al. (29) contradict this by reporting significantly greater exercise $\dot{V}_{O_2}$ in mild nonweight bearing steady-state exercise that occurred from the 27th week of gestation and continued through delivery. They also reported a significant reduction in efficiency.

Ueland et al. (53) also support the finding that oxygen cost of exercise is greater in pregnancy. An explanation of the decreased efficiency is related to the increase in ventilation induced by pregnancy. The hyperventilation of pregnancy both at rest and at various levels of submaximal exercise increases the O_2 cost of breathing and, therefore, would reduce the efficiency of O_2 delivery to the working muscles. However, this ventilatory inefficiency accounts for less than 20% of the observed changes (53). Cardiac output is also greater in pregnancy, indicating a slightly greater myocardial oxygen consumption; but again, the impact on total efficiency would be slight. The actual mechanism for the decrease in efficiency during pregnancy, if, in fact, efficiency decreases, is not fully understood and further research is needed.

Exercise Protocol

Another area of confusion within the field of exercise assessment relates to the standardization of testing modality and protocol. The modalities that have been used to assess fitness include step tests, bicycle ergometers, treadmills, swimming flumes, laddermills, and several others. Even within the literature related to pregnancy, several different testing devices have been employed (Table 12.4).

The most commonly used device is the bicycle ergometer. However, it is obvious that the protocols used vary greatly. Pollock (64) compared four major treadmill protocols and found that, for the most part, the protocols yielded similar results (Fig. 12.3) (65). The use of the treadmill protocol during pregnancy is questionable. In determining $\dot{V}_{O_2max}$ in pregnant subjects, Artal et al. (62) used a modified Balke treadmill protocol in which the speed was held constant at 2.5 mph while the elevation was increased by 2% each minute until the subject reached his or her maximum capacity. As in any weight bearing exercise, the metabolic cost is dependent upon the weight of the subject. During pregnancy, due to the increase in weight, the metabolic response to a similar increase in elevation or speed cannot be compared. For this reason, we recommend the use of a bicycle ergometer whenever attempting to evaluate the cardiovascular, respiratory, or metabolic response to submaximal exercise during pregnancy. If the purpose of study is to evaluate the effects of pregnancy on maximal aerobic power ($\dot{V}_{O_2max}$) during weight bearing exercise, the treadmill is the device of choice.

ACUTE METABOLIC RESPONSE TO EXERCISE

When an individual starts to exercise there is a brief lag in the increase in oxygen uptake. After a short period, depending on the intensity of the exercise and the fitness of the individual, the $\dot{V}_{O_2}$ reaches a plateau or steady-state. Many believe that in a dynamic system, such as the body during exercise, there are always homeostatic changes occurring. To suggest that a steady-state has been reached assumes some kind of static equilibrium within the system that, most likely, does not occur. The term steady-state exercise implies a more general adaption to a constant work load and does not attempt to imply a fixed physiological response.

For definitional purposes, any exercise intensity that results in a steady-level response in $\dot{V}_{O_2}$ is called submaximal exercise. If the work intensity is so great that $\dot{V}_{O_2}$ does not "level off" but continues to increase without changes in work load, the exercise will not result in steady-state $\dot{V}_{O_2}$ and maximal oxy-

Table 12.4. Different Protocols Used in Evaluating the Effect of Exercise on Pregnant Women

Widlund (50)	Step test	22, 40, 52 step frequency
Bader et al. (54)	Recumbent bicycle	10-min duration
Genzell et al. (55)	Bicycle ergometer	33, 66, 99 watts 6-min duration
Ueland et al. (56)	Bicycle ergometer	100, 200 kpm
Guzman and Caplan (57)	Bicycle ergometer	150, 250, 350 kgm; 4 m/10 m rest
Knuttgen and Emerson (48)	Treadmill and bike	4% grade 4.5 km·hr^{-1}; 60 watts
Pomerance et al. (58)	Bicycle ergometer	450 kpm (n = 49) 600 (4), 300 (1)
Pernoll et al. (59)	Bicycle ergometer	Submaximal test 6 min
Erkkola and Makela (60)	Bicycle ergometer	3-stage 150, 300, 450 kpm/min each lasting 4 min on the day after a voluntarily maximal test
Edwards et al. (52)	Bicycle ergometer	10 min @ 50 W
Collings et al. (61)	Bicycle ergometer	150 kpm @ 85 rpm or 4 min followed by 2-min rest; increments until subject reached HR = 150-160
Artal et al. (62)	Treadmill	2.5 mph, increased 2%/min until exhaustion
South-Paul et al. (63)	Bicycle ergometer	5 W @ 2 min, increased by 25 W to tolerance
Dibblee and Graham (37)	Step test	3 min step (Canadian Home Fitness) age and sex specific rhythm

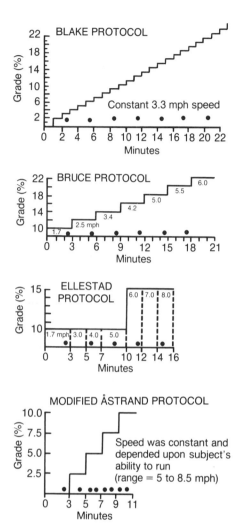

Figure 12.3. Commonly used exercise test protocols. ● = $\dot{V}_{O_2}$ determination. (From Pollock ML. A comparative analysis of 4 protocols for maximal exercise testing. Am Heart J 1976;93:39.)

gen consumption will be achieved. Any work load can lead to fatigue if performed long enough, but generally speaking, the test of $\dot{V}_{O_2max}$ is of reasonably short duration (8–14 min) and is of sufficient intensity to involve recruitment of the greater tension-producing glycolytic, fast-twitch muscle fibers.

Oxygen Deficit/Debt

During the initial phase of exercise, the cardiorespiratory system is not capable of providing O_2 rapidly enough to meet the metabolic demand. As a result, the muscle uses high-energy phosphates (ATP,CP) and

cellular oxygen to meet this transitional need. This leads to the so-called "oxygen deficit" (Fig. 12.4). At the end of exercise, during recovery, excess oxygen (above resting levels) is required to restore the muscles' energy pool back to equilibrium. This has been called the "oxygen debt." The rate of repayment or recovery is dependent on the work intensity and the fitness of the individual. The excess oxygen is used not just to replenish tissue O_2 stores and the high-energy phosphates, but must also be used to supply the energy for lactate removal and glycogen and glucose resynthesis. As well, the metabolic rate is elevated in recovery due, in part, to the increased body temperature (Q_{10} effect), and the very slow removal rate of several of the hormones that were released during the exercise.

Ready et al. (66) reported a decrease in maximal O_2 debt of 19.8% as a result of physical training for 6 weeks in young women. Pernoll et al. (59) reported a significant increase in exercise $\dot{V}_{O_2}$ in late pregnancy when compared to postpartum values. The oxygen debt incurred by standard nonweight bearing exercise was greater in late pregnancy than early in pregnancy or 14 weeks postpartum. This may indicate a reduced tolerance for exercise or, perhaps, a change in fuel utilization patterns during exercise and/or recovery. Widlund (50) and Seitchik (51) also reported increased oxygen debt during pregnancy.

Oxygen Pulse

Oxygen pulse, or the quotient of oxygen consumed divided by heart rate over the same period, is affected by and is an indirect measure of all of the aforementioned circulatory adjustments during exercise, a relationship that can be described by substitution as:

$$O_2 \text{ pulse} = \frac{\text{A-V } O_2 \text{ difference} \times \text{cardiac output}}{\text{heart rate}}$$

Therefore, any circulatory adjustment that improves A-V O_2 difference (e.g., redistribution of blood flow to the active muscle) or increases cardiac output (e.g., increased stroke volume due to greater venous return) will

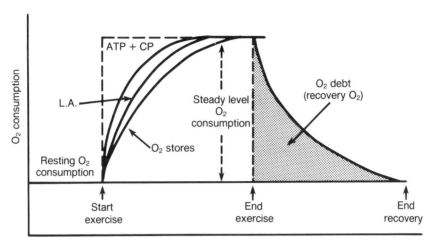

Figure 12.4. Oxygen deficit and debt. L.A. = lactic acid. (From DeVries HA. Physiology of exercise for physical education and athletics, ed. 2. Dubuque, IA: William C. Brown Co., 1974.)

effect an improvement in oxygen pulse. Hence, oxygen pulse becomes elevated in muscular exercise due to increased stroke volume as well as increased oxygen extraction in the working muscle. The increase in oxygen pulse with work load (relative work load in % of $\dot{V}_{O_2max}$) is linear above 50% relative work loads (60). While no information is available in the literature with regard to oxygen pulse in pregnancy, several studies have reported higher heart rates during submaximal exercise, thus implying a lower oxygen pulse during pregnancy. The work of Wiswell et al. (67) indicates a lowering of maximal heart rate during exercise but the $\dot{V}_{O_2max}$ was also reduced suggesting that maximal O_2 pulse may not change.

Ventilatory Equivalent for Oxygen (VE/$\dot{V}_{O_2}$)

Ventilatory equivalent, or the quotient obtained by dividing ventilation by $\dot{V}_{O_2}$, is often used as a measure of respiratory efficiency. During the initial few moments of exercise, the VE/$\dot{V}_{O_2}$ ratio rises rapidly, after which it gradually drops until reaching a lower stable value (Fig. 12.5). This is due to a rapid ventilatory acceleration (neural control) at the onset of exercise without a similar rise in $\dot{V}_{O_2}$. During steady-level submaximal exercise, the VE/$\dot{V}_{O_2}$ ratio reaches and maintains a plateau until certain anaerobic factors again begin to drive the ventilation up exponen-

tially. It is assumed that the lower the plateau value, the more efficient the respiratory system is in delivering O_2 to the working muscles. In this case, it is efficient to have a

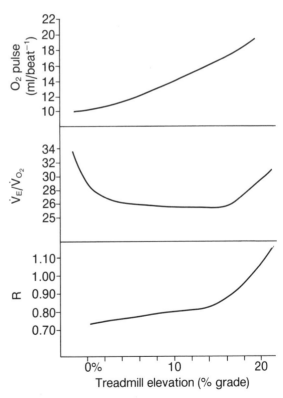

Figure 12.5. Time course of select metabolic parameters in pregnant women during maximal exercise. (From Wiswell et al. Hormonal and metabolic response to maximal exercise in pregnancy. Med Sci Sport Exerc 1985;17:206.)

higher $\dot{V}_{O_2}$ with a lower VE. Knuttgen and Emerson (48) reported an elevation in resting and submaximal exercise VE/$\dot{V}_{O_2}$ in prepartum versus postpartum subjects. The resting level decreased from 33.2 to 28.3, while the exercise value decreased from 33.7 to 29.3 after delivery. Submaximal VE/$\dot{V}_{O_2}$ has been used as a good predictor of $\dot{V}_{O_2max}$. However, due to the extremely high ventilation obtained by trained subjects, the maximal VE/$\dot{V}_{O_2}$ may not be a discriminator of fitness.

Respiratory Exchange Ratio (R)

The respiratory exchange ratio has been used to give an index of type of fuel being metabolized. The R equals the $\dot{V}_{CO_2}$ divided by the $\dot{V}_{O_2}$. By observing R during exercise one can obtain a rough idea of the foodstuff or substrate that is being utilized. Unfortunately, studies that have provided information about R and fuel metabolism do not always account for transient shifts in ventilation and the problems of interpreting the influence of protein metabolism on R (Table 12.5). This becomes relevant in the study of pregnancy due to the fact that there is a changing endocrine function, and some women become CHO intolerant during late pregnancy. The relationship between R and fuel metabolism in pregnancy is not well established. However, Knuttgen and Emerson (48) have reported a decrease in R from .83 to .77 in prepartum versus postpartum women. They postulated that the elevated R of pregnancy is due, in part, to the increased expired CO_2 caused by the abnormally high ventilation at rest and during submaximal exercise. Blackburn and Calloway (68, 69) reported a reduced R when comparing prepartum to postpartum values on both bicycle ergometer and treadmill.

Rating of Perceived Exertion (RPE)

When comparing individuals during exercise one would like to have an idea of the relative intensity of exercise. In most settings, information about the maximal oxygen consumption is not available. As a result, an indirect method for determining the relative intensity of a task to the individual has been developed. The rating of perceived exertion (RPE) is a means of obtaining such information by asking the subject to identify a relative level of fatigue experienced at a given work load. Table 12.6 provides the two methods of assessing RPE.

The use of the RPE scale in studies of exercise in pregnancy has been quite rare. In two studies (71, 72), RPE has been shown to decrease during exercise after physical conditioning. The application of the RPE in assessing maximal work capacity has not been reported but may provide supportive information as to the effect of pregnancy on maximal exercise capacity in the future.

EXERCISE PRESCRIPTION

With the increased interest in exercise, particularly endurance-type exercise, came methods to prescribe exercise for individuals. Prescription was based upon the individual's age, gender, physical fitness, and/or health status. To obtain an exercise prescription, the individual underwent a series of medical and physiological tests to ensure that he or she was physically competent to perform exhaustive exercise. Next, the clinician, physiologist, nurse, or technician would interpret the test results and devise a plan directed toward preventive health care and improvement of physical fitness. These prescriptions usually included information about what type of ex-

Table 12.5.   Using R in Determining Type of Fuel Used (Nonprotein R)[a]

Fuel	Respiratory Exchange Ratio		Example
Fats (Palmitic Acid)	R = .707	4.686 kcal/liter O_2	$C_{16}H_{32}O_2 + 23\ O_2 \rightarrow 16\ CO_2 + 16\ H_2O$ 16 CO_2/ 23 O_2 = .707
CHO (Glucose)	R = 1.0	5.047 kcal/liter O_2	$C_6H_{12}O_6 + 6\ O_2 \rightarrow 6\ CO_2 + 6\ H_2O$ 6 CO_2/6 O_2 = 1.0

[a]Adapted from Fox EL, Mathews DK. The physiological basis of physical education and athletics. Philadelphia: WB Saunders, 1981.

Table 12.6. Rating of Perceived Exertion[a]

Original RPE (6-20)		Modified RPE (0-10)		
6		0	Nothing at all	
7	Very, very light	0.5	Very, very weak	(just noticeable)
8		1	Very weak	
9	Very light	2	Weak	(light)
10		3	Moderate	
11	Fairly light	4	Somewhat strong	
12		5	Strong	(strong)
13	Somewhat hard	6		
14		7	Very Strong	
15	Hard	8		
16		9		
17	Very hard	10	Very, very strong	(almost max)
18				
19	Very, very hard			
20		*	Maximal	

[a]From Borg GA. Psychophysical bases of perceived exertion. Med Sci Sports Exerc 1982; 14:377-387.

ercise modality should be employed, as well as the duration, frequency, and intensity of the activity. Table 12.7 shows an example of guidelines that have been used in developing an exercise plan.

The American College of Sports Medicine (27) recommends exercise that uses large muscle groups, is rhythmical and aerobic in nature, and can be maintained continuously. They recommend that the intensity of training should be between 60–90% of maximum heart rate or 50–85% of $\dot{V}_{O_2max}$. The use of target heart rate has been a popular method of prescribing exercise. The target heart rate is determined by subtracting the individual's resting heart rate from his or her maximal heart rate. The difference is then multiplied by the desired exercise intensity (60–90%, depending on age and fitness of the subject) and added to the resting heart rate to produce the exercise heart rate range.

Unfortunately, there are major drawbacks in using heart rate as a means of prescribing exercise in pregnancy. Recent research in our laboratory causes us to question the usefulness of the above equation in determining the exercise heart rate during pregnancy. We have reported that maximal heart rate in pregnant females is considerably lower than that which has been estimated (67). This finding must be substantiated in a more controlled study before we eliminate the use of heart rate for exercise prescription, however. Further, it has been reported in an earlier chapter that there is a high frequency of mitral valve prolapse during pregnancy. This problem seems to be aggravated at heart rates above 140 bpm. It should also be noted that the physiological response to exercise is certainly related to the stage of pregnancy. Many of the precautions suggested only become relevant in the late second and third trimester.

Table 12.7. Guidelines for Estimating Frequency, Intensity, Duration, and Distance of Aerobic and Anaerobic Training Programs of Running[a]

Training Aspect	Endurance (Aerobic) Training	Sprint (Anaerobic) Training
Frequency	4–5 days/wk	3 days/wk
Intensity	Heart rate = 85–95% of maximal heart rate	Heart rate = 180 beats or greater
Sessions/day	One	One
Duration	12–16 wk or longer	8–10 wk
Distance/workout	3–5 miles	1.5–2 miles

[a]From Fox E. Sports physiology. Philadelphia: WB Saunders, 1984.

REFERENCES

1. Brown CH, Harrower JR, Deeter MF. The effects of cross-country running on pre-adolescent girls. Med Sci Sports 1972; 4:1–5.

2. Brown CH, Wilmore JH. The effects of maximal resistance training on the strength and body composition of women athletes. Med Sci Sports 1974; 6:174–177.

3. Drinkwater BL. Physiological responses of women to exercise. Exer Sport Sci Rev 1973; 1:125–153.

4. Drinkwater BL, Horvath SM, Wells CL. Aerobic power of females, ages 10–68. J Gerontol 1975; 30:385–394.

5. Plowman S. Physiological characteristics of female athletes. Res Quart 1974; 45:349–362.

6. Sinning DW. Body composition, cardiorespiratory function, and rule changes in women's basketball. Res Quart 1973; 44:313–321.

7. Spence DW, Disch JG, Fred HL, Coleman AE. Descriptive profiles of highly skilled women volleyball players. Med Sci Sports Exer 1980; 12:299–302.

8. Wilmore JH, Brown CH. Physiological profiles of women distance runners. Med Sci Sports 1974; 6:178–181.

9. Girandola RN, Wiswell RA, Frisch F, Wood K. VO_{2max} and anaerobic threshold in pre- and post-pubescent girls. In Borms J, Hebbelinck M, Venerando A, eds. Women and sport: an historical, biological, physiological and sportsmedical approach. Basel: S. Karger, vol 14, 1981; p 155–161.

10. Vaccaro P, Clarke DH. Cardiorespiratory alterations in 9- to 11-year-old children following a season of competitive swimming. Med Sci Sports 1978; 10:204–207.

11. Erdelyi GJ. Gynecological survey of female athletes. J Sports Med Phys Fitness 1962; 2:174–179.

12. Astrand PO, Engstrom L, Eriksson BO. Girl swimmers: gynaecological aspects. Acta Paediatr Scand 1963; 147:33–38.

13. Rebar RW, Cumming DC. Reproductive function in women athletes. JAMA 1981; 246:1950.

14. Feicht CB, Johnson TS, Martin BJ. Secondary amenorrhea in athletes. Lancet 1978; 2:1145–1146.

15. Dale E, Gerlach DH, Wilhite AL. Menstrual dysfunction in distance runners. Obstet Gynecol 1979; 54:47–53.

16. Speroff L, Redwine DB. Exercise and menstrual function. Phys Sports Med 1980; 8:42–52.

17. Fox E. Sports physiology. Philadelphia: WB Saunders, 1984.

18. Brooks GA, Fahey TD. Exercise physiology: human bioenergetics and its applications. New York: John Wiley & Sons, 1984.

19. Lamb DR. Physiology of exercise: responses and adaptations. New York: MacMillan, 1978.

20. Smith ML, Mitchell JH. Cardiorespiratory adaptation to training. In Blair SN, Painter P, Pate RR, Smith LK, Taylor CB, eds. ACSM resource manual for guidelines for exercise testing and prescription. Philadelphia: Lea & Febiger, 1988; p 48–54.

21. Holly RG. Measurement of the maximal rate of oxygen uptake. In Blair SN, Painter P, Pate RR, Smith LK, Taylor CB, eds. ACSM resource manual for guidelines for exercise testing and prescription. Philadelphia: Lea & Febiger, 1988; p 171–177.

22. Noble BJ. Physiology of exercise and sport. Chapter 5, St. Louis: Mosby, 1986.

23. Astrand PO, Rodahl K. Textbook of work physiology: physiological bases of exercise. New York: McGraw-Hill, 1977.

24. Pritchard J, MacDonald PC, Gant N. Williams obstretrics, ed 17. Norwalk, CN: Appleton-Century-Crofts, 1985.

25. Consolazio CF, Johnson RE, Pecora LJ. Physiological measurements of metabolic functions in man. New York: McGraw-Hill, 1963.

26. Wyndham CH. Submaximal tests for estimating maximum oxygen intake. Can Med Assoc J 1967; 96:736–745.

27. American College of Sports Medicine. Guidelines for graded exercise testing and exercise prescription. Philadelphia: Lea & Febiger, 1980.

28. Katch FI, McArdle WD. Nutrition, weight control and exercise. Philadelphia: Lea & Febiger, 1983.

29. Pernoll ML, Metcalfe J, Sclhlenker TL, Welch JE, Matsumoto JA. Oxygen consumption at rest and during exercise in pregnancy. Respir Physiol 1975; 25:285–293.

30. Drinkwater B. Training of female athletes In Dirix A, Knuttgen HG, Tittel K. The olympic book of sports medicine: Vol 1, The encyclopaedia of sports medicine. Blackwell Scientific, 1988; p 309–327.

31. Wyndham CH. Submaximal tests for estimating maximum oxygen intake. Can Med Assoc J 1977; 96:736–745.

32. Astrand PO, Rhyming I. A nomogram for calculation of aerobic capacity (physical fitness) from pulse rate during submaximal work. J Appl Physiol 1954; 7(2):218–221.

33. Wyndham CH, Strydom NB, Maritz JS, Morrison JF, Peter J, Potgieter ZU. Maximum oxygen intake and maximum heart rate during strenuous work. J Appl Physiol 1959; 14(6):927–936.

34. Issekutz B, Birkhead NC, Rodahl K. Use of respiratory quotients in assessment of aerobic work capacity. J Appl Physiol 1962; 17(1):47–50.

35. Mastropaolo JA. Prediction of maximal O_2 consumption in middle-aged men by multiple regression. Med Sci Sports 1970; 2(3):124–127.

36. Hermiston RT, Faulkner JA. Prediction of maximal oxygen uptake by a stepwise regression technique. J Appl Physiol 1971; 30(6):833–837.

37. Dibblee L, Graham TE. A longitudinal study of changes in aerobic fitness, body composition and energy intake in primi graud patients. Am J Obstet Gynecol 1983; 147:908–914.

38. Erkkola R, Rauramo L. Correlation of maternal physical fitness during pregnancy with maternal and fetal pH and lactic acid at delivery. Acta Obstet Gynecol Scand 1976; 55:441–446.

39. Morton JJ, Paul MS, Campos GR, Hart MV, Metcalf J. Exercise dynamics in late gestation: effects of physical training. Am J Obstet Gynecol 1985; 152:91–97.

40. Clausen JP. Circulatory adjustments to dynamic exercise and effects of physical training in normal subjects and in patients with coronary artery disease. Prog Cardiovasc Dis 1976; 18:459–495.

41. Lewis SF, Taylor WF, Graham RM, Pettinger WA, Schutte JE, Blomqvist CG. Cardiovascular responses to exercise as functions of absolute and relative work load. J Appl Physiol: Respirat Environ Exercise Physiol 1983; 54(5):1314–1323.

42. Passmore R, Durnin JVGA. Human energy expenditure. Physiol Rev 1955; 35:801.

43. Fox EL, Mathews DK. The physiological basis of physical education and athletics. Philadelphia: WB Saunders, 1981.

44. Donovan CB, Brooks GA. Muscular efficiency during steady rate exercise. J Appl Physiol 1977; 43:431–439.

45. Gaesser GA, Brooks GA. Muscular efficiency during steady-rate exercise: effects of speed and work rate. J Appl Physiol. 1975; 38(6):1132–1139.

46. Pendergast DR, diPrampero PE, Craig AB, Wilson DR, Rennie DW. Quantitative analysis of the front crawl in men and women. J Appl Physiol 1977; 43(3):475–479.

47. Howley ET, Glover ME. The caloric costs of running and walking one mile for men and women. Med Sci Sports 1974; 6:235–237.

48. Knuttgen HG, Emerson K Jr. Physiological response to pregnancy at rest and during exercise J Appl Physiol 1974; 36:549–553.

49. Teruoka G. Labour physiological studies on pregnant women. Arbeitsphysiol 1933; 7:259–279.

50. Widlund G. The cardio-pulmonary function during pregnancy. Acta Obstet Gynecol Scand 1945; 25(suppl 1):1–125.

51. Seitchik J. Body composition and energy expenditure during rest and work in pregnancy. Am J Obstet Gynecol 1967; 97:701–713.

52. Edwards MJ, Metcalfe J, Dunham MJ, Paul MS. Accelerated respiratory response to moderate exercise in late pregnancy. Respir Physiol 1981; 45:229–241.

53. Ueland KM, Novy J, Metcalfe J. Cardiorespiratory responses to pregnancy and exercise in normal women and patients with heart disease. Am J Obstet Gynecol 1973; 115:4–10.

54. Bader RA, Bader ME, Rose DJ, Braunwald E. Hemodynamics at rest and during exercise in normal pregnancy as studied by cardiac catherization. J Clin Invest 1955; 34:1524–1536.

55. Genzell D, Robbe H, Stron G. Total amount of hemoglobin and physical working capacity in normal pregnancy and puerperium (with iron medication). Acta Obstet Gynecol Scand 1957; 36:93–136.

56. Ueland KM, Novy MJ, Peterson EN. Maternal cardiovascular dynamics IV. The influence of gestational age on the maternal cardiovascular response to posture and exercise. Am J Obstet Gynecol 1969; 104:856.

57. Guzman CA, Caplan R. Cardiorespiratory response to exercise during pregnancy Am J Obstet Gynecol 1970; 108:600–605.

58. Pomerance JJ, Gluck L, Lynch VA. Physical fitness in pregnancy: Its effect on pregnancy outcome. Am J Obstet Gynecol 1974; 119:867–876.

59. Pernoll M, Metcalfe J, Kovach PA, Wachtel R, Dunham MJ. Ventilation during rest and exercise in pregnancy and postpartum. Respir Physiol 1975; 25:295–310.

60. Erkkola R, Makela M. Heart volumes and physical fitness of parturients. Ann Clin Res 1976; 8(1):15–21.

61. Collings CA, Curet LB, Mullin JP. Maternal and fetal responses to a maternal aerobic exercise program. Am J Obstet Gynecol 1983; 145:702–707.

62. Artal R, Wiswell RA, Romem Y. Hormonal response to exercise in diabetic and nondiabetic pregnant patients. Diabetes 1985; 34(2):78–80.

63. South-Paul JE, Rajagopak KR, Tenholder MF. The effect of participation in regular exercise program upon aerobic capacity during pregnancy. Obstet Gynecol 1988; 71:175–179.

64. Pollock ML. A comparative analysis of 4 protocols for maximal exercise testing. Am Heart J 1976; 93:39.

65. Ellestad MH. Stress testing: principles and practice. Philadelphia: FA Davis, 1980.

66. Ready AE, Eynon RB, Cunningham DA. Effect of interval training and detraining on anaerobic fitness in women. Can J Appl Sport Sci 1981; 6(3):114–118.

67. Wiswell RA, Artal R, Romen Y, Kammula R. Hormonal and metabolic response to maximal exercise in pregnancy. Med Sci Sports Exerc 1985; 17:206.

68. Blackburn M, Calloway D. Basal metabolic rate and work energy expenditure of mature pregnant women. J Am Dietet Assoc 1973; 69:24–28.

69. Blackburn M, Calloway D. Energy expenditure and consumption of mature pregnant and lactating women. J Am Dietet Assoc 1973; 69:29–37.

70. Borg GA. Psychophysical bases of perceived exertion. Med Sci Sports Exerc 1982; 14:377–387.

71. Ohtake PJ, Wolfe LA, Hall P, McGrath MJ. Physical conditioning effects on exercise heart rate and perception of exertion in pregnancy. Can J Sport Sci 1988; 13(3):71–73.

72. Wolfe LA, Lowe-Wylde SJ, Tranmer JE, McGrath MJ. Fetal heart rate during maternal static exercise. Can J Sport Med 1988; 13(3):95–96.

13

Exercise in Pregnancy in the Experimental Animal

Frederik K. Lotgering, Raymond D. Gilbert, and Lawrence D. Longo

During pregnancy, the fetus and placenta constitute a growing mass of tissue and, consequently, energy requirements gradually increase. During exercise, the energy demands of working muscles increase drastically. When the energy requirements of exercising muscles are superimposed upon those of pregnancy, they place additional demands on compensatory physiological mechanisms. If such compensatory mechanisms were inadequate to meet the combined demands of pregnancy and exercise either one, or both, functions could be curtailed.

In this review we will explore what is known about physiologic adjustments when exercise stress is imposed upon that of pregnancy. Among the issues which we will consider are: (*a*) differences in metabolic, endocrine, respiratory, and circulatory responses between pregnant and nonpregnant animals; (*b*) temperature changes; (*c*) uteroplacental blood flow and the placental transport of respiratory gases and substrates; and (*d*) metabolic, respiratory, and circulatory adjustments in the fetus. Because fetal physiologic functions are difficult to determine in humans, laboratory animals are commonly utilized for such studies. A more extensive review has been published elsewhere (1).

MATERNAL RESPONSES

A fundamental question concerns the extent to which responses to exercises during pregnancy differ from those in the nonpregnant state. This problem can be investigated only in carefully controlled studies against a background of knowledge of the physiological changes of both pregnancy and exercise. However, few well-controlled studies on the subject of exercise in pregnancy can be found in the literature. Unfortunately, it is therefore impossible in many instances to determine the exact extent to which exercise responses are different during pregnancy.

Oxygen Consumption

At rest, all energy is generated by oxidative metabolism of nutrients (2). Resting O_2 consumption ($\dot{V}_{O_2}$) is influenced by several factors, including species, body size and composition, sex, age, posture, and environmental factors (e.g., temperature) (2), and during pregnancy growth, metabolism, and muscular activity of the fetus. Strictly speaking, one cannot measure O_2 consumption or basal metabolic rate of the mother alone.

During pregnancy, O_2 consumption measured at rest increases with advancing gestational age to a maximum near term. In humans, this value is 16–32% above that of nonpregnant controls (3–5), while in near-term pygmy goats, it is increased 21% (6). The higher resting $\dot{V}_{O_2}$ during pregnancy results largely from the increased uterine, fetal, and placental tissue mass (7), with little change in metabolic rate per gram of maternal tissue or work for vital functions.

Maximal O_2 consumption during pregnancy has not been studied in great detail. In pregnant ewes, Lotgering and co-workers (8) observed a 5.6-fold increase in O_2 consumption to 32 ml·min^{-1}·kg^{-1} during maximal exercise, but it is unknown whether or not this is higher than in nonpregnant sheep. Although one might speculate that pregnancy weight increase could have some training effect, no change in $\dot{V}_{O_2max}$ has been demonstrated in two recent longitudinal studies in humans (9,10).

A study of physical training in rats has demonstrated 8% higher values for $\dot{V}_{O_2max}$ in those animals trained during pregnancy, as compared to sedentary pregnant animals

(11). Training only before pregnancy resulted in 13% higher values of $\dot{V}_{O_2max}$, whereas training both before and during pregnancy produced 23% higher values (11). Although this suggests that training is most effective if started before and continued during pregnancy, one might speculate that responses will be different in other species in which gestation is longer and weight gain more pronounced, as in humans.

Metabolism

Whereas plasma concentrations merely reflect the balance between production and utilization of different fuels, turnover rates are important from a quantitative standpoint (12). The maternal glucose concentration falls linearly with advancing gestational age in humans (13) and guinea pigs (14) but not significantly in sheep (15) and horses (16). The variations among these species may reflect their differences in blood volume increase with gestation. However, as pregnancy does not significantly affect the balance of carbohydrates and fats used for combustion, the turnover rates of the different substrates must increase linearly with O_2 consumption. The observation that the glucose turnover rate increases in absolute terms, but remains constant when normalized for body weight in humans (17) and horses (16) supports this suggestion.

Above about 50% $\dot{V}_{O_2max}$, the blood lactate concentration increases with the level of exercise. In pregnant sheep, lactate concentrations increase with both the level (8, 18) and the duration of exercise (8), and recovery is incomplete at 20 min following prolonged exercise at 70% $\dot{V}_{O_2max}$ (8).

Berg et al. (19) observed a slight decrease in the free fatty acid concentration during exercise in both pregnant and nonpregnant women. In sheep, in which acetate metabolism accounts for up to 30% (20) of the total energy expenditure at rest, the free fatty acid concentration during exercise is increased (21), while acetate metabolism is unaffected (22). In dogs, the contribution of free fatty acids to the energy expenditure increases with exercise duration until at very high levels the free fatty acid turnover rate is reduced (23).

It is unknown, however, whether the turnover rates during exercise in pregnancy are different from those in the nonpregnant state.

Body Temperature

During pregnancy, body temperature increases until about midgestation and declines thereafter to normal levels (23). These changes have been attributed to the opposing effects of progesterone and estrogen concentrations (24).

During exercise, 75–80% of energy is transformed into heat and total heat production may increase 20-fold. Most of the heat is lost to the environment, but some is stored, primarily in the exercising muscles. Physical training increases blood volume and enhances sweat production in humans. This permits greater cutaneous perfusion at a given thermal load and results in increased capability to dissipate heat.

Figure 13.1 depicts maternal body temperature during exercise in near-term pregnant ewes (8). Compared with that of humans, basal body temperature in sheep is approximately 2°C higher and heat loss across the

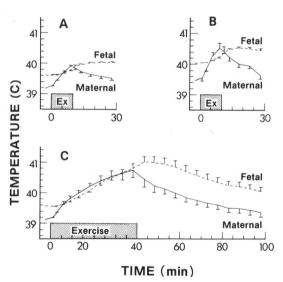

TIME (min)

Figure 13.1. Maternal and fetal temperature changes in response to three different exercise regimens. (From Lotgering et al. Exercise responses in pregnant sheep: blood gases, temperatures and fetal cardiovascular system. J Appl Physiol 1983;55:842–850.) *A,* Ten-minute exercise at 70% $\dot{V}_{O_2max}$. *B,* Ten-minute exercise at 100% $\dot{V}_{O_2max}$. *C,* Forty-minute exercise at 70% $\dot{V}_{O_2max}$.

skin is much lower as they pant rather than sweat. Within the first minutes of exercise, maternal body temperature increases rapidly, the rate of increase varying with the exercise level (Fig 13.1). After the initial rapid rise it continues to increase further, and a plateau was not observed during even relatively prolonged (40 min) exercise at 70% $\dot{V}_{O_2max}$. At exhaustion, reached either by short-term maximal exercise or by prolonged exercise at 70% $\dot{V}_{O_2max}$, the ewe's body temperature averaged 40.7°C (Fig. 13.1). After exercise, maternal temperature initially declined sharply, then gradually returned to normal. The recovery time varied with exercise intensity and duration.

Respiration and Blood Gases

The changes in resting respiratory function associated with pregnancy have been the subject of several reviews (25, 26).

Maternal blood gas values were not markedly affected by moderate short-term exercise in pregnant and nonpregnant pygmy goats (6). However, prolonged moderate exercise in sheep was found to be associated with an increase in pH (18, 27, 28) and either a decrease or only slight increase in O_2 tension (18, 28). However, in none of these studies were the blood gas values corrected for the exercise-induced temperature increase. Blood obtained anaerobically and analyzed for respiratory gases at a temperature below that of the body provides falsely low O_2 and CO_2 tensions and a falsely high pH (29). Therefore, consideration of exercise-induced temperature changes is essential for a correct assessment of the blood gases in vivo. Corrected for the temperature in vivo, no significant changes occurred during short-term (10 min) exercise at 70 and 100% $\dot{V}_{O_2max}$ in sheep, whereas during prolonged (40 min) exercise at 70% $\dot{V}_{O_2max}$, the ewe's arterial O_2 tension increased 13% (to 117 torr) and O_2 content 25% (to 13.3 ml·dl^{-1}), while CO_2 tension decreased 28% (to 28 torr) and H^+ concentration decreased 22% (with a pH increase to 7.56). Recovery was virtually complete within 20 min. The increase in arterial O_2 content resulted largely from hemoconcentration (8).

Hyperventilation during pregnancy results in a decrease in CO_2 tension and buffering capacity not only at rest but also during and after exercise. These changes are more pronounced in ungulates, in which hyperventilation has a more important role in heat dissipation than it does in humans. In other aspects, respiration during exercise in pregnancy does not seem to differ from that in the nonpregnant state.

Circulation

In human pregnancy, cardiac output is increased above nonpregnant levels by 12 weeks' gestation and Burwell et al. (30) reported a maximum increase of about 50% at about 30 weeks'. However, opinions differ as to the subsequent changes. Cardiac output may (31, 32) or may not (33, 34) increase further later in gestation. Lees et al. (34) suggested that the fall as observed in earlier studies during the third trimester may be attributed to decreased venous return in the supine position. Nonetheless, other investigators (32, 33) have observed a decrease in cardiac output during the third trimester also in the lateral and sitting positions. In sheep (35) and goats (6, 36), resting cardiac outputs during the third trimester remain markedly elevated above nonpregnant or postpartum control values. The cardiac output response to exercise in pregnancy has been studied in humans (4, 37–39), sheep (40, 41) and pygmy goats (6, 36). The increase in cardiac output during exercise is virtually unaffected by pregnancy and is mediated through a marked increase in heart rate and a less marked increase in stroke volume (36, 40, 41). Autonomic blockade reduces heart rate and cardiac output at rest and during exercise without affecting stroke volume, a response unaffected by pregnancy (36).

Early in human pregnancy, diastolic blood pressure decreases about 10% below nonpregnant vales, while systolic pressure decreases only slightly. During the third trimester both pressures return toward nonpregnant values (24). Sheep (35) and goats (6) do not show a clear gestational age trend and have slightly lower mean arterial pressures near term than postpartum. Total peripheral resistance in midpregnancy decreases as much as 30% in humans (37), sheep (35), and goats (6).

Upon the initiation of exercise, total peripheral resistance decreases immediately. The lowered resistance in the exercising muscles results from local vasodilatation and is inversely related to O_2 consumption (42). The systolic and mean arterial pressures increase with work intensity, while the diastolic pressure remains virtually constant. The arterial blood pressure response to exercise in pregnancy has been studied in humans (19, 37, 43–46); sheep (27, 28, 40, 41) and goats (6, 36). The mean arterial pressure and the systolic pressure increase proportionately with the level of exercise at moderate work loads (19, 44–46). However, in sheep, mean arterial pressure does not significantly increase any further when the exercise level is increased from 70 to 100% $\dot{V}_{O_2max}$, or when the duration of exercise is extended from 10 to 40 min (41). An increased pressure response has been reported in pregnant women in response to treadmill (38) and bicycle exercise (19, 46). Because both the cardiac output and the arterial pressure response to submaximal exercise are only slightly altered by pregnancy, the exercise-induced decrease in total peripheral resistance during pregnancy must be of a magnitude similar to that in the nonpregnant state. The more marked decrease in total peripheral resistance during exercise in pregnancy as reported in pygmy goats (6) probably reflects a higher work load as a result of pregnancy weight increase.

With advancing gestation, whole blood volume in humans increases gradually up to 50% near term, due to a 30–60% increase in plasma volume and a 20–30% increase in erythrocyte mass, but the increases are less pronounced in some other species such as sheep (47). During exercise, plasma volume decreases rapidly as a function of exercise intensity, reaching a maximal reduction of 14% at about 60% $\dot{V}_{O_2max}$ in man (48). Some workers (48) consider increased blood pressure the major force driving plasma filtrate across the capillary membrane in exercising muscles, while others (49) suggest a more important role for muscle tissue osmolality

changes. The hematocrit increases during exercise in pregnant sheep (18, 41), probably as the result of a decrease in plasma volume without a change in red cell mass (41) (Fig. 13.2). The 20% decrease in plasma volume observed in exercising pregnant sheep (Fig. 13.2) (41) was slightly larger than the maximum change observed in nonpregnant humans (48, 49) and was associated with a smaller increase in plasma protein concentration. However, if labeled red cells were released from the spleen and other reservoirs at the onset of exercise, the calculated whole blood and plasma volume decrease in sheep would be overestimated (41).

Cardiac Output Distribution

The most striking change in blood flow distribution during pregnancy is the increase in uterine blood flow with advancing gestational age. At present, uterine blood flow cannot be measured accurately under chronic unstressed conditions in women. In chronically catheterized sheep, uterine blood flow near-term is approximately 1300 ml·min^{-1}, or 240 ml·min^{-1}·kg^{-1} a 50 to 60-fold increase above nonpregnant values (50). Blood flow to placental cotyledons increases with fetal weight, whereas that to the myometrium and endometrium remains relatively constant (51), so that near-term cotyledonary flow is approximately 85% of total uterine blood flow (52, 53). Some factors affecting uterine blood flow have been reviewed (54–57). The large decrease in uterine vascular resistance during pregnancy probably results from vasodilation associated with increasing concentrations of estrogens produced by the fetoplacental unit and prostaglandins (PGE_2 and PGI_2) produced by the vessel wall. The uterine vasculature during pregnancy is less sensitive to the effects of vasoactive agents. This is true especially for cotyledonary flow, whereas the response of myoendometrial flow to catecholamines is similar in the pregnant and nonpregnant states (58).

The effects of exercise on uterine blood flow during pregnancy has been studied in humans (59), sheep (18, 27, 40, 41, 60, 61), and pygmy goats (62). Using the disappearance of ^{24}Na injected into the myometrium,

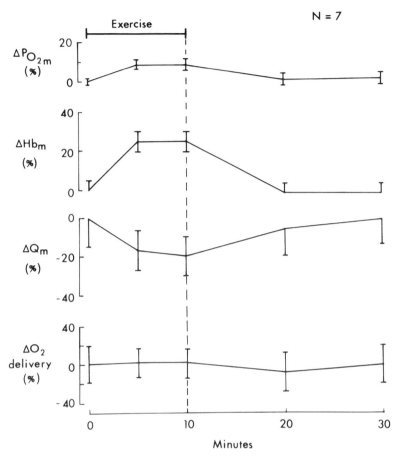

Figure 13.2. Changes in whole blood, plasma, and red cell volumes during exercise in pregnant sheep. (From Lotgering et al. Exercise responses in pregnant sheep: blood gases, temperatures and fetal cardiovascular system. J Appl Physiol 1983;55:842–850; and Lotgering et al. Exercise responses in pregnant sheep: oxygen consumption, uterine blood flow, and blood volume. J Appl Physiol 1983;53:834–841.)

Morris et al. (59) suggested a 25% decrease in perfusion of the human pregnant uterus during mild short-term bicycle exercise in the supine position. This probably represents an overestimate. In the supine position, the pregnant uterus may reduce venous return, cardiac output, and uterine blood flow. Furthermore, myometrial flow does not represent total uterine blood flow. Animal studies have shown that flow within the uterus is redistributed in response to exercise, favoring the cotyledons at the cost of the myometrium (40, 62).

Initial animal studies showed a variable change in uterine blood flow. In sheep, Orr et al. (61), using a Doppler flow probe around a distal branch of the uterine artery, and

Curet et al. (40), using microspheres, concluded that uterine blood flow remains constant during treadmill exercise. However, their measurements were made shortly after, rather than during, the exercise, and uterine flow returns rapidly to control levels when exercise is discontinued (41). Clapp reported no change in total uterine blood flow during mild exercise in sheep, and flow decreased 28% near the point of exhaustion during prolonged exercise. Chandler and Bell, however, reported a mean decrease of 36% (range 17–47%) in blood flow to the pregnant horn during prolonged, moderately strenuous exercise in sheep (18) and a decrease of 18–28% with the use of the antipyrine diffusion method (60). The exercise stress in these studies was expressed in work load rather than in physiological terms, which may explain some of the observed variability. Hohimer and co-workers (62) reported a mean decrease in uterine blood flow of 32% during short-term exercise in five pygmy goats in which maternal heart rate increased from 129–195 beats/min, whereas flow decreased only 18% in four other pygmy goats in which the mean heart rate increased to 210 beats/min.

Lotgering and co-workers (41) studied total uterine blood flow response to different levels (% $\dot{V}_{O_2max}$) and durations of exercise in sheep accustomed to the treadmill. The results are shown in Figure 13.3. Uterine blood flow decreased immediately at the onset of exercise, was significantly below control values throughout the exercise period, and returned to control values within 10 min of recovery. Mean uterine blood flow decreased significantly by 13% during a 10-min exercise period at 70% $\dot{V}_{O_2max}$, 17% during 10 min at 100% $\dot{V}_{O_2max}$, and 24% near the end of a 40-min period at 70% $\dot{V}_{O_2max}$ (Fig. 13.3). Thus, uterine blood flow decreases with both the level and the duration of exercise. In addition, uterine blood flow varies inversely with heart rate (41, 62) (Fig. 13.4).

The exercise-induced increase in uterine vascular resistance probably results from active vasoconstriction caused by increased

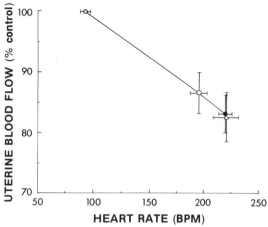

Figure 13.4.   Relation between heart rate and total uterine blood flow in near-term pregnant sheep. (From Lotgering et al. Exercise responses in pregnant sheep: oxygen consumption, uterine blood flow, and blood volume. J Appl Physiol 1983;55:834–841.) ○ = rest; □ = 10-min exercise at 70% $\dot{V}_{O_2max}$; ● = 10-min exercise at 100% $\dot{V}_{O_2max}$; △ = 40-min exercise at 70% $\dot{V}_{O_2max}$.

sympathetic activity. If it is true that the effects of increased sympathetic activity during exercise may be modified by local metabolic factors, one would expect myometrial flow to behave like the flow to the splanchnic bed, whereas cotyledonary flow would decrease only to such an extent that the fetoplacental O_2 demands can still be met. There

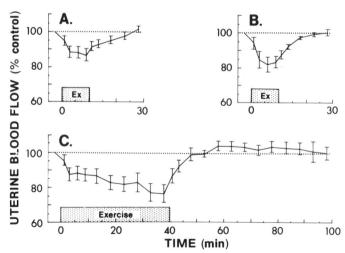

Figure 13.3.   Uterine blood flow response to three different exercise regimens in pregnant sheep. (From Lotgering et al. Exercise responses in pregnant sheep: oxygen consumption, uterine blood flow, and blood volume. J Appl Physiol 1983;55:834–841.) *A,* Ten-minute exercise at 70% $\dot{V}_{O_2max}$. *B,* Ten-minute exercise at 100% $\dot{V}_{O_2max}$. *C,* Forty-minute exercise at 70% $\dot{V}_{O_2max}$.

is some evidence that this is the case. Blood flow within the uterus is redistributed to the cotyledons at the expense of the myometrium, both during catecholamine infusion (63), as well as during (62) and after (40) exercise. Hohimer and colleagues (62) reported only an 8% decrease in cotyledonary flow when total uterine blood flow decreased 18%, while myometrial flow decreased 52%.

With the exception of uterine flow, there is little evidence that regional blood flow distribution during exercise is altered by pregnancy. Although Orr et al. (61) reported significant increases in carotid and iliac artery flow in pregnant ewes, they observed similar changes in nonpregnant sheep. Curet et al. (40) found no change in renal flow after exercise in pregnant sheep, but they made no comparison with nonpregnant ewes. Bell et al. (64) observed no major effect of additional heart stress on uterine or regional blood flow in pregnant sheep.

Physical training was found to have no effect on postexercise uterine and renal blood flows in a small number of sheep (40). However, training results in a lower physiological level of exercise (% $\dot{V}_{O_2max}$) of each work load and, consequently, trained individuals respond to a given work load with reduced sympathetic activity (65). Therefore, one would expect a given work load in a trained individual to result in a smaller reduction in uterine blood flow during exercise.

Uterine Oxygen Consumption

Uterine O_2 consumption increases during pregnancy in response to the increasing demands of the growing conceptus, as demonstrated in humans (66) and sheep (50, 67). With advancing gestational age, the uterine arteriovenous O_2 difference rises 3- (67) to 10-fold (50). Thus, uterine O_2 consumption increases much more than would be expected on the basis of the blood flow increase alone. Studies in chronically catheterized sheep showed a decreasing uterine blood flow per kg uterine contents, but constant (67) or increasing (50) O_2 consumption per kg tissue. About 45% of the O_2 used by the uterus is consumed by the placenta plus myoendometrium, so that the weight-specific O_2 consumption of this compartment is about three times that of the fetus (68).

Uterine O_2 consumption during exercise has not been studied in pregnant women, but it does not change significantly during prolonged submaximal treadmill exercise in sheep (8, 18, 27, 60). Although total uterine blood flow reported by Lotgering and co-workers was markedly reduced, O_2 consumption was maintained as the result of hemoconcentration and increased O_2 extraction (8) (Fig. 13.2). Uterine, umbilical and, by subtraction, uteroplacental O_2 consumption are unaffected by mild exercise (60). Because during maternal exercise myoendometrial flow decreases more markedly than cotyledonary flow (40, 62), it seems likely that the myoendometrium increases its O_2 extraction to a greater extent than do the cotyledons.

Table 13.1 summarizes some of the maternal responses to pregnancy and exercise.

FETAL RESPONSES

The fetus requires a continuous and increasing supply of oxygen and nutrients for its metabolism and growth. A prolonged severe reduction in this supply of substrates will result in fetal demise, but less severe reductions do not cause apparent damage. Our present understanding of the fetal adjustments and tolerance limits is limited for several reasons.

First, there is the absence of accurate and sensitive criteria for tolerance limits. Permanent structural or functional damage proves that tolerance was exceeded, but this criterion is relatively insensitive because small changes may be undetectable. Growth retardation demonstrates chronic adaptations within such limits, but this criterion lacks sensitivity because of the large normal variation. Physiological variables such as heart rate, O_2 consumption, and oxygen, substrate, or hormone concentrations are more sensitive to changes, but they represent temporary adjustments rather than provide information as to the fetal tolerance.

Second, it is difficult to obtain information about fundamental physiological variables in the fetus. Only heart rate can be determined in the human fetus with relative ease. Most

Table 13.1. Maximal Responses of Selected Maternal Physiological Variables to Pregnancy, Exercise, and Training

	Near Term Pregnancy[a]	Exercise[a]	Exercise during Pregnancy[b]	Training[b]	Training and Pregnancy[c]
O_2 consumption	↑ or ↑↑°	↑↑↑	↑	↑↑	↑ ?
Respiratory minute volume	↑ or ↑↑°	↑↑↑	↑ ?	↑	—
Tidal volume	↑	↑↑↑	↑ ?	— ?	— ?
Respiratory frequency	—	↑↑↑	— ?	↑	—
Cardiac output	↑ or ↑↑°	↑↑↑	↑ ?	↑ or ↑↑°	↑ ?
Stroke volume	↑	↑↑↑	↑ ?	↑ or ↑↑°	↑ ?
Heart rate	↑	↑↑↑	— ?	—	— ?
Mean arterial pressure	— or ↓°	↑	— ?	—	— ?
Plasma volume	↑ or ↑↑↑°	↓	— ?	—	— ?
Uterine blood flow	↑↑↑	↓↓↓ ?	↑ ?	— ?	— ?

[a]Change from nonpregnant, nontrained, resting values. ° = Marked species difference, ? = doubtful or unknown, — = change <5%, ↑ or ↓ increase or decrease of 6–20%, ↑↑ or ↓↓ 21–40%, ↑↑↑ or ↓↓↓ >40%.
[b]Change from nonpregnant, nontrained, exercise values.
[c]Change from pregnant, nontrained, exercise values.

other functions require invasive techniques. In certain experimental animals, chronic catheterization of the fetus can be used to study adaptive changes to a variety of stresses without the disadvantages of anesthesia or acute surgical stress.

Fetal Oxygen Consumption

Fetal oxygen consumption can be calculated from umbilical blood flow and umbilical arteriovenous O_2 content difference; in the lamb during the third trimester, it equals about 8.0 ml·min^{-1}·kg^{-1} fetus, (69, 70). O_2 consumption by the uterus as a whole is constant during maternal exercise in sheep (8, 18, 27, 60). This suggests the absence of major changes in fetal O_2 uptake and has been confirmed by observations of a constant umbilical uptake of oxygen during exercise (18, 60). During exhaustive exercise a 13% increase in uterine O_2 extraction was observed to compensate for a 10% decrease in umbilical blood flow (27).

According to the van't Hoff-Arrhenius law, the O_2 consumption of both total uterine contents and fetus should rise during exercise-induced hyperthermia. Assuming a Q_{10} of 2–3, Lotgering and co-workers (8) calculated that, with prolonged exercise, O_2 consumption of the fetus should increase 9–16% and that of the placental and uterine wall, 11–18%. However, they observed only a 6% increase in O_2 consumption of the total uter-

ine contents. Although this may suggest relative hypoxia, it is impossible to assess accurately whether or not the fetal and placental O_2 requirements are met during maternal exercise.

Fetal Metabolism and Endocrinology

In the fetus, substrates are used not only for "basal" metabolism and heat production, but also for growth and muscular activities. Furthermore, it is conceivable that under certain conditions the fetus relies on anaerobic metabolism for short time periods (71).

According to Battaglia and Meschia (69), about 65% of the caloric expenditure in the sheep fetus is used for oxidative metabolism and 35% for growth. The fetal respiratory quotient is 0.94 (72). This suggests the predominant metabolism of carbohydrates and amino acids. Glucose crosses the placenta by facilitated diffusion; thus, the rate is dependent upon the concentration in maternal blood. During prolonged exercise in sheep, uterine glucose uptake increases when uterine glucose extraction increases, probably because of the increased maternal to fetal glucose gradient (from about 2.0 to 3.1 mmol·l^{-1}) (18, 60, 73), whereas umbilical glucose uptake is virtually unaffected (60) and fetal blood glucose concentrations increase up to 75% with less pronounced changes occurring during short-term or mild exercise (Fig. 13.2) (8, 18, 60). Despite the hyperglycemia during exercise, fetal plasma insulin does not change significantly until after exercise (73). This may indicate that fetal glucose utilization does not increase until the recovery phase. However, unconfirmed observations in a small number of pregnant rats (n = 6) suggest that fetal glucose uptake after exercise is 40% lower than in control animals (74). It is conceivable that, during the recovery period, the fetus predominantly utilizes the readily available lactate instead of glucose for its metabolic needs. In addition, the fetal plasma concentrations of pancreatic glucagon, enteroglucagon, and growth hormone are not affected significantly by maternal exercise, whereas fetal corticosteroid concentrations increase gradually during and after exercise (73). The latter increase may have resulted, in part, from the increased maternal concentrations, as cortisol crosses the sheep placenta at a slow rate (75).

Although fetal lactate concentration is about twice that of the maternal, under normal conditions this does not result from anaerobic metabolism (76). The placenta produces large quantities of lactate, and lactate metabolism may constitute 25% of fetal O_2 consumption (69). Although fetal lactate concentrations increase up to 50–70% during prolonged moderate exercise (8, 18, 27, 73), they do not change significantly during short-term or mild exercise (8, 27). During exercise in sheep the normal placental release of lactate into the maternal circulation is reversed, with lactate being taken up by the pregnant uterus (18, 60). While Clapp (27) reported continued lactate uptake by the umbilical circulation during prolonged exercise, Chandler et al. noted a significant decrease in umbilical net uptake of lactate during exercise and suggested that the higher fetal lactate concentration during exercise resulted from increased fetal glycolysis (60). However, studies in rats suggest that fetal glycogenolysis does not occur as a result of maternal exercise (77). Further studies will have to resolve the question if the increased fetal levels result from anaerobic metabolism or from the high maternal lactate levels and reduced lactate transfer from the placenta to the mother during exercise.

Amino acids are actively transported across the placenta; about 60% is used as fuel and 40% for growth in fetal sheep (69). Free fatty acids represent a negligible fraction of the total caloric intake in the sheep fetus, in which fat accounts for 2% of the body weight at term, but may be more important in other species, such as man, in which it constitutes 16% of birth weight. Another substrate, acetate, has been studied during maternal exercise in sheep, and its uterine uptake does not change significantly (18). It is unknown to what extent maternal exercise affects the relative contribution of the different substrates to fetal metabolism.

The effects of exercise training during pregnancy on maternal metabolism has not been studied in great detail. In one study in rats, it was found that training increased the insulin responsiveness of adipocytes (78). This training effect was less pronounced in pregnant animals than in controls, but this may have resulted from the more strenuous training protocol in the control animals.

Body Temperature

Under normal resting conditions, the fetal temperature in the human (79), baboon (80), and sheep (81, 82) is about 0.5°C higher than the maternal. When the maternal temperature rises, the fetal temperature increases more slowly and the normal fetal-maternal temperature gradient diminishes (83) or reverses (79). Fetal and maternal placental blood flow also affect fetal temperature. The fetal-maternal temperature gradient increases with partial occlusion of the umbilical cord, the maternal aorta, or the inferior vena cava, as well as with uterine contractions (80).

Lotgering et al. (8) demonstrated that, during maternal exercise, the fetal temperature changes in sheep (Fig. 13.1) are comparable to those observed during maternal heating (79), lagging behind the relatively rapidly changing maternal temperature at the onset and cessation of exercise. This results in a smaller or reversed temperature gradient during the onset and a larger gradient immediately after exercise (Fig. 13.1). With heavier exercise (100 vs. 70% $\dot{V}_{O_2max}$) the maternal temperature increases more rapidly, resulting in a larger reversal of the temperature gradient (Fig. 13.1). After prolonged

(40 min) exhaustive exercise at 70% $\dot{V}_{O_2max}$, return of the fetal temperature to normal required over 1 hour.

Heat is stored in the body core during exercise at rates proportional to exercise intensity. Because dissipation of fetal heat is by convection and flow-limited diffusion, the fetal temperature will increase with that of the mother. A mathematical model of placental heat transfer developed by Schröder et al. had accurately predicted fetal temperature changes from changes in maternal temperature and uterine blood flow during exercise, when variables such as fetal metabolism were assumed constant (8). Further calculations (Schröder and Gilbert, unpublished data) suggest that maternal temperature is the major determinant, while changes in metabolism or uterine blood flow of up to 50% will change fetal temperature by less than 0.3°C.

Temperature changes will affect placental and fetal respiratory gas transfer, as a temperature increase shifts the oxyhemoglobin saturation curve to the right. This will tend to increase oxygen unloading in the fetal tissues. A mathematical model of placental O_2 transport (84) suggests that during maternal heating as in exercise, the larger shift in maternal than in fetal P_{50} will result in only a small increase in placental O_2 exchange and fetal O_2 tension. During exercise, this effect is opposed by other factors, as fetal O_2 tension decreases. One such factor is uterine blood flow, which is reduced not only by the sympathetic stimulation of exercise, but also by the temperature increase (84). The possible teratogenic effects of exercise hyperthermia are discussed in Chapter 24.

Respiration and Blood Gases

The fetus exchanges oxygen and carbon dioxide with the mother by passive diffusion across the placenta, a process affected by several factors, including maternal and fetal placental blood flows, arterial O_2 and CO_2 tensions, and hemoglobin concentrations (84). Several studies in exercising sheep (18, 27, 28) have reported significant decreases in fetal arterial O_2 tension and content of as much as 25%. However, in none of these reports were the respiratory blood gas values cor-

rected for the fetal temperature changes in vivo, resulting in underestimates of fetal O_2 and CO_2 tensions and overestimates of pH values. As noted previously, blood obtained anaerobically and analyzed at a temperature below that of the body shows a rise in pH and a fall in O_2 and CO_2 tensions (29). The failure to correct for a 1°C increase results in about a 1.9 and 2.7 torr underestimate for fetal O_2 and CO_2 tensions, respectively, while pH will be 0.015 unit too high (8). Failure to make temperature corrections largely explains the difference in blood gases between these studies and those of Lotgering et al. (8). In this latter study, fetal arterial O_2 and CO_2 tensions and O_2 content decreased with the level and the duration of exercise, but the values differed significantly from control only when the ewes were run to exhaustion. Near the end of prolonged (40 min) exercise at 70% $\dot{V}_{O_2max}$, ascending aortic O_2 tension decreased 3.0 torr, to 23.2 from 26.2 torr at rest. CO_2 tension decreased 4.5 torr from 54.1 torr at rest, and O_2 content decreased 1.5 ml·d1^{-1} from 5.8 ml·dl^{-1} at rest, while pH increased 0.02 unit. Figure 13.5 shows the percentage of changes in fetal blood gases under these circumstances. With the exception of O_2 content, all blood gases returned to control values within 20 min of termination of exercise. The cause of the decrease in fetal

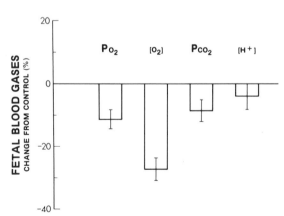

Figure 13.5. Percent changes in fetal sheep respiratory blood gases and hydrogen ion concentrations during prolonged (40 min) exercise at 70% $\dot{V}_{O_2max}$. (From Lotgering et al. Exercise responses in pregnant sheep: blood gases, temperatures and fetal cardiovascular system. J Appl Physiol 1983;55:842–850.)

O_2 tension and content during prolonged maternal exercise is not entirely clear. Theoretical calculations suggest that 30% of the decrease in O_2 saturation can be accounted for by the temperature and Bohr shifts of the oxyhemoglobin saturation curve (8). The remaining 70% of the decrease in O_2 saturation and the 3-torr decrease in O_2 tension probably result largely from the decrease in placental blood flow.

Circulation

Normally, the fetal heart operates near the plateau of its Starling function curve with cardiac output near its maximum (85). Consequently, decreases in fetal heart rate directly affect cardiac output, whereas large increases do not increase it further (86). Fetal cardiac output is a function of body weight, being about 500 $ml·min^{-1}·kg^{-1}$ in sheep (87, 88). Neither catecholamines (89) nor moderate degrees of hypoxia (90) appear to affect it. The increase in cardiac output with advancing gestation is associated with increases in whole blood and plasma volumes, which in sheep are about 110 and 77 $ml·(kg·fetus)^{-1}$ (91), respectively. During short-term maternal exercise in sheep fetal cardiac output is unaffected (87). In addition, fetal blood and plasma volumes are unaffected by prolonged, exhaustive treadmill exercise in the ewe (8). This confirms the absence of a change in hematocrit (18) and is indirect evidence of the absence of hypoxia.

About 40% of fetal cardiac output (or about 200 $ml·min^{-1}·kg^{-1}$), the largest proportion to a single organ, is directed to the placenta in sheep (88, 90). Umbilical flow in sheep is unaffected by hypoxia but changes in blood flow distribution to other organs (brain, heart, lungs, and adrenals) have been reported in response to hypoxia and norepinephrine infusion (89, 90, 92). Umbilical blood flow in sheep is also unaffected by short-term exercise at 70 and 100% $\dot{V}O_2max$ (8) and by prolonged but mild maternal exercise (27). In response to prolonged exhaustive exercise it has been reported to fall 10% (27), but this needs to be confirmed because the resting umbilical flow in these studies was 354

$ml·min^{-1}·kg^{-1}$, about 50% greater than accepted normal values. Lotgering et al. (8) found no change in cardiac output distribution to other organs during short-term maternal exercise, but this was not studied during prolonged exercise.

Fetal blood pressure gradually increases with advancing gestational age, reaching a value of about 40 mm Hg in near-term sheep when corrected for amniotic fluid pressure (93). Mean arterial pressure increases in response to norepinephrine infusion (89), whereas hypoxia may increase it (90). Fetal arterial blood pressure was unaffected by short-term (8) as well as prolonged exercise in sheep (8, 27, 28, 94) suggesting no great release of catecholamines. Although one study (94) reported a moderate increase in fetal norepinephrine levels during prolonged moderate exercise in sheep not accustomed to treadmill exercise, only insignificant increases in fetal catecholamine concentrations have been noted in fetal sheep in response to both strenuous short-term and moderate prolonged exercise in sheep accustomed to such exercise (8).

Table 13.2 summarizes some of the fetal variables in relation to prolonged and strenuous exercise. Most of the results as shown in the table are derived from studies in sheep. Although the studies of fetal cardiovascular responses during maternal exercise are limited, the available evidence suggests the absence of hypoxia or other "stress."

Table 13.2. Maximal Response of Selected Fetal Physiological Variables to Maternal Exercise

Variable	Response[a]
O_2 consumption	—
Cardiac output	—
Heart rate	— or ↑
Mean arterial pressure	—
Plasma volume	—
Umbilical blood flow	↓
Arterial O_2 tension	↓
Arterial O_2 content	↓ ↓
Arterial CO_2 tension	↓
Arterial H^+ concentration	—
Arterial catecholamine concentration	— ?

[a] ? = doubtful, — = change >5%, ↑ or ↓ = increase or decrease of 6–20%, ↓ ↓ = 21–40%.

PLACENTAL RESPONSES

The placenta has a multitude of functions that are only partially understood. Barron (95) has recently reviewed the discovery of its respiratory function. As early as 1796, Erasmus Darwin inferred from the color difference of the umbilical vessels that the placenta is a respiratory organ for the fetus, and Zweifel established definitive proof in 1876 [for references, see Barron (95)]. Placental physiology is difficult to study independently of the mother and fetus, because their functions are so interwoven.

The placenta uses several mechanisms to transport various substances: diffusion, facilitated diffusion, and active transport. Oxygen exchanges across the placenta by passive diffusion and may be considered flow limited. The placental diffusing capacity for O_2 cannot be quantified practically, but the diffusing capacity for carbon monoxide ($D_{P_{CO}}$), a diffusion-limited gas, provides a method to measure steady-state gas exchange. In sheep acute exercise does not affect $D_{P_{CO}}$ (8). However, this does not exclude the possibility that the amount of O_2 crossing the placenta per minute is reduced during exercise, as this is affected by the increased maternal hemoglobin concentration, P_{50}, and temperature, as well as by reductions in uterine and umbilical blood flows (84).

In guinea pigs which were exercised throughout gestation, $D_{P_{CO}}$ values were found to be up to 34% lower than in controls, the decrease being a function of the amount of daily exercise (85, 103). In other chronically exercised guinea pigs, a linear relation between placental diffusing capacity and maternal and fetal surface area per unit volume of placenta was observed (96). The reason for the smaller placental exchange areas in chronically exercised guinea pigs is unknown. Although theoretically O_2 transfer is affected by the decrease in surface area, it remains unclear whether O_2 transfer limitation caused the reduced birth weight observed in these fetuses.

Glucose diffuses across the placenta by facilitated diffusion, and the carrier system has been studied in detail (97–99). Glucose uptake increases rapidly with increasing maternal blood concentrations until the concentration is reached where the "carriers" are saturated and above which the rate of transport is slower. In chronically catheterized sheep at rest, glucose uptake by the fetus and the uteroplacental mass equals 28% and 72%, respectively, of the total uterine glucose uptake (100). Theoretical analysis (100) suggests that the net glucose transfer to the fetus is relatively insensitive to changes in uterine or umbilical blood flows. Despite a significant reduction in uterine flow, glucose uptake actually increased during prolonged exercise in sheep as the result of an increased transplacental glucose gradient and increased extraction during exercise (18, 73) (Fig. 13.2). Chandler et al. (60) showed that the increased uterine uptake of glucose during mild to moderate exercise in sheep resulted largely (80%) from increased glucose uptake by the placenta plus myoendometrium.

Lactate is the second most important substrate for fetal metabolism (69). It also diffuses across the placenta by a facilitated process (101). However, rather than being transferred from maternal blood, most of the lactate metabolized by the fetus is produced by the placenta. In chronically catheterized near-term sheep uteroplacental lactate production was 154 $\mu mol \cdot min^{-1}$, virtually all of which was taken up by the fetus (60). During prolonged exercise in sheep, Chandler and Bell (18, 60) observed increased uterine and uteroplacental uptake of lactate. It seems likely that this resulted from the increased maternal blood concentration and the resulting decreased placental-maternal lactate gradient. It is unknown to what extent placental lactate production itself is affected by exercise.

Of the other substrates, acetate is an important fuel for the resting ewe. Its role in fetal-placental metabolism is largely unknown, but uterine uptake of acetate (18) and 3-hydroxybutyrate (60) are unaffected by exercise in sheep. Amino acids are also important for combustion by both the placenta and the fetus. They are actively transported by the placenta (69), but it is unknown whether this energy-requiring transport mechanism is affected by exercise. The role of the placenta as a heat exchanger and its role in exercise has been discussed.

In conclusion, the effects of acute and chronic exercise on metabolic and transport functions of the placenta have been investigated only to a limited extent. The effect of exercise on placental endocrine function is unknown.

Fetal Outcome

Adverse effects on fetal outcome have been reported in pregnant animals forced to exercise strenuously in a laboratory during pregnancy. Intrauterine growth retardation with 8% weight reduction was reported in mice (102) and guinea pigs (103). Studies in mice (102) and rats (104) have reported an increased incidence of resorbed and macerated fetuses, but the numbers are too small to draw any definitive conclusions. In rats forced to swim (105) fetal weights were decreased 6% but in rats that were forced to run (104, 106) growth was not significantly retarded. Dhindsa et al. (6) reported fetal growth retardation with 20% weight reduction in exercising pygmy goats with multiple pregnancies, but a 12% increase in goats with singleton pregnancy; however, it is not clear whether the study included proper controls. In swine, moderate daily exercise did not reduce fetal weight (107). In some of these studies the "stress" of fear and handling in a laboratory rather than the exercise per se may have contributed to the growth retardation.

Several studies have reported the organ weights and functional development in neonates born from exercised mothers. Nelson et al. (103) observed brain "sparing" in the growth-retarded newborns of strenuously exercised guinea pigs. In contrast, body and organ weights and composition were not different from controls in neonatal rats born from exercised mothers (11, 104, 106, 108–110). Wilson and Gisolfi (11) reported that $\dot{V}_{O_2max}$, heart rate, blood pressure, myocardial blood flow, myocardial capillary density, and fiber-to-capillary ratio were not different from controls in male offspring of exercised rat mothers, although they did observe a lower fiber density in the right ventricle. These observations are in contrast with those of Parizková (109, 111), who reported increased capillary density and fiber-to-capillary ratio, and a decreased diffusion distance in hearts from neonatal rats born from exercised mothers. Bonner et al. (112) observed that cultured myocardial cells from offspring of exercised rat mothers were larger in size, showed an increased percentage of contracting cells, and beat at a slower rate than cells from controls. Butler et al. (113, 114) reported that such cultured cells have a higher calcium content, which protects against ethanol toxicity, and behave different from control cells when treated with Ca-antagonists, β-blockers, or ;β-agonists. Other studies have reported altered lipid metabolism (110), decreased glucose and higher insulin concentrations (105), delayed ossification (102), poorer motor performance (108), and unchanged skeletal muscle myosin ATPase, succinate dehydrogenase and phosphofructokinase in offspring of mothers exercised repeatedly (115). However, the available evidence is insufficient to conclude that exercise of the mother affects the functional development of the neonate.

In conclusion, there is some evidence that strenuous, repetitive maternal physical activity is associated with a small reduction in birth weight in some species. However, further well-controlled prospective studies are needed to confirm this. The mechanisms that might account for these effects are presently unresolved, but possibilities include decreases in uterine blood flow, substrate availability, or placental exchange area. Presently, there is neither sufficient evidence nor a physiological basis to suggest other adverse effects of maternal exercise on fetal and neonatal outcome.

SUMMARY

Exercise has numerous effects upon the pregnant mother, the developing fetus, and the placenta. In turn, pregnancy affects the ability to perform physical activity. Pregnancy affects maternal metabolism and the cardiovascular and respiratory systems. The increase in O_2 consumption of about 30% at rest results almost exclusively from the increased tissue mass. During pregnancy, a higher cardiorespiratory effort is required to perform a given amount of weight bearing exercise. However, a training effect of pregnancy weight gain has not been demonstrated. The sedentary life-style commonly adopted in late pregnancy in most western societies may reflect a cultural rather than a physiological phenomenon.

In contrast to the physiological alterations in the mother, and despite reductions in uterine blood flow during maternal exercise, such changes in the fetus are small. During prolonged exhaustive exercise, relatively minor changes occur in the blood concentrations of oxygen and substrates. In addition, despite a temperature increase of 1–2°C there is little evidence for significant alteration in fetal metabolism, cardiovascular hemodynamics, or blood catecholamine concentrations. This suggests that acute exercise normally does not represent a major stress for the fetus. Of course, most of the information concerning the fetus is derived from studies in experimental animals, particularly sheep. Conceivably, in humans, the upright position, increased uterine contractility, and increased susceptibility to venous pooling may affect the fetal responses differently.

Virtually nothing is known about the physiological effects of exercise training on the fetus. The most likely effect may be a relatively small reduction in birth weight, at least in some species; however, this needs to be further investigated. The data presently available do not allow any conclusions as to other possible fetal effects of physical training. Further studies are needed for a more complete understanding of the dynamics involved in the remarkably effective mechanisms that account for the relative homeostasis of the fetus during maternal exercise.

Acknowledgements—The authors wish to thank Mrs. J. Schot and Mrs. Y. de Roon for preparing the manuscript.

REFERENCES

1. Lotgering FK, Gilbert RD, Longo LD. Maternal and fetal responses to exercise during pregnancy. Physiol Rev 1985 65:1–36.
2. Astrand PO, Rodahl K. Textbook of work physiology. New York: McGraw-Hill, 1977.
3. Pernoll ML, Metcalfe J, Schlenker TL, Welch JE, Matsumoto JA. Oxygen consumption at rest and during exercise in pregnancy. Respir Physiol 1975; 25:285–293.
4. Ueland K, Novy MJ, Metcalfe J. Cardiorespiratory responses to pregnancy and exercise in normal women and patients with heart disease. Am J Obstet Gynecol 1973; 115:4–10.
5. Widlund G. The cardio-pulmonal function during pregnancy. A clinical-experimental study with particular respect to ventilation and oxygen consumption among normal cases in rest and after work tests. Acta Obstet Gynecol Scand 1945; 25 (Suppl 1):1–125.
6. Dhindsa DS, Metcalfe J, Hummels DH. Responses to exercise in the pregnant pygmy goat. Respir Physiol 1978; 32:299–311.
7. Clapp III JF. Cardiac output and uterine blood flow in the pregnant ewe. Am J Obstet Gynecol 1978; 130:419–423.
8. Lotgering FK, Gilbert RD, Longo LD. Exercise responses in pregnant sheep; blood gases, temperatures and fetal cardiovascular system. J Appl Physiol 1983; 55:842–850.
9. Sady SP, Carpenter MW, Thompson PD, Sady MA, Haydon B, Coustan DR. Cardiovascular response to cycle exercise during and after pregnancy. J Appl Physiol 1989; 66:336–341.
10. Lotgering FK, Van Doorn MB, Struyk PC, Wallenburg HCS. Maximal exercise in pregnant women: a longitudinal study. In Society for Gynecologic Investigation, Abstracts of the 35th Annual Meeting, Baltimore, March 17–20, 1988, p 62.
11. Wilson NC, Gisolfi CV. Effects of exercising rats during pregnancy. J Appl Physiol 1980; 48:34–40.
12. Issekutz Jr B, Miller HI, Rodahl K. Lipid and carbohydrate emtabolism during exercise. Fed Proc 1966; 25:1415–1420.
13. Knopp RH: Fuel metabolism in pregnancy. Contemp OB/GYN 1978; 12:83–90.
14. Sparks JW, Pegorier J-P, Girard J, Battaglia FC. Substrate concentration changes during pregnancy in the guinea pig studied under unstressed steady state conditions. Pediatr Res 1981; 15:1340–1344.
15. Steel JW, Leng RA. Effect of plane of nutrition and pregnancy on glucose entry rates in sheep. Proc Aust Soc Anim Prod 1968; 7:242.
16. Evans JW. Effect of fasting, gestation, lactation and exercise on glucose turnover in horses. J Anim Sci 1971; 33:1001–1004.
17. Kalhan SC, D'Angelo LJ, Savin SM, Adam PAJ. Glucose production in pregnant women at term gestation. Sources of glucose for human fetus. J Clin Invest 1979; 63:388–394.
18. Chandler KD, Bell AW. Effects of maternal exercise on fetal and maternal respiration and nutrient metabolism in the pregnant ewe. J Dev Physiol 1981; 3:161–176.
19. Berg A, Mross F, Hillemans HG, Keul J. Die Belastbarkeit der Frau in der Schwangerschaft. Med Welt 1977; 28:1267–1269.
20. Pethick DW, Lindsay DB, Barker PJ, Northrop AJ. Acetate supply and utilization by the tissues of sheep in vivo. Br J Nutr 1981; 46:96–110.
21. Bird AR, Chandler KD, Bell AW. Effects of exercise and plane of nutrition on nutrition utilization by the hind limb of the sheep. Austral J Biol Sci 1981; 34:541–550.
22. Judson GJ, Filsell OH, Jarrett IG. Glucose and acetate metabolism in sheep at rest and during exercise. Austral J Biol Sci 1976; 29:215–222.
23. Issekutz Jr B, Miller HI, Paul P, Rodahl K. Aerobic

work capacity and plasma FFA turnover. J Appl Physiol 1965; 20:293–296.

24. Hytten FE, Leitch I. The physiology of human pregnancy. Oxford: Blackwell, 1964.

25. Bonica JJ. Maternal respiratory changes during pregnancy and parturition. In Marx GF, ed. Clinical anesthesia, parturition & perinatology. Philadelphia: FA Davis, 1973, vol 10/2.

26. Weinberger SE, Weiss ST, Cohen WR, Weiss JW, Johnson TS. Pregnancy and the lung. Am Rev Respir Dis 1980; 121:559–581.

27. Clapp III JF. Acute exercise stress in the pregnant ewe. Am J Obstet Gynecol 1980; 136:489–494.

28. Emmanouilides GC, Hobel CJ, Yashiro K, Klyman G. Fetal responses to maternal exercise in the sheep. Am J Obstet Gynecol 1972; 112:130–137.

29. Severinghaus JW. Blood gas calculator. J Appl Physiol 1966; 21:1108–1116.

30. Burwell CS, Strayhorn WD, Flickinger D, Corlette MD, Bowerman EP, Kennedy JA. Circulation during pregnancy. Arch Intern Med 1938; 62:979–1003.

31. Hamilton HFH. The cardiac output in normal pregnancy as determined by the Cournand right heart catheterization technique. J Obstet Gynaecol Br Emp 1949; 56:548–552.

32. Ueland K, Novy MJ, Peterson EN, Metcalfe J. Maternal cardiovascular dynamics; IV. The influence of gestational age on the maternal cardiovascular response to posture and exercise. Am J Obstet Gynecol 1969; 104:856–864.

33. Atkins AFJ, Watt JM, Milan P, Davies P, Selwyn Crawford J. A longitudinal study of cardiovascular dynamic changes throughout pregnancy. Eur J Obstet Gynecol Reprod Biol 1981; 12:215–224.

34. Lees MM, Taylor SH, Scott DB, Kerr MG. A study of cardiac output. Am J Psychol 1980; 239:R115–R122.

35. Metcalfe J, Parer JT. Cardiovascular changes during pregnancy in ewes. Am J Physiol 1966; 210:821–825.

36. Hosenpud JD, Hart MV, Rowles JR, Morton MJ. Maternal heart rate and stroke volume in the pygmy goat: effect of exercise and cardiac autonomic blockade. Quart J Exp Physiol 1986; 71:59–65.

37. Bader RA, Bader ME, Rose DJ, Braunwald E. Hemodynamics at rest and during exercise in normal pregnancy as studied by cardiac catheterization. J Clin Invest 1955; 34:1524–1536.

38. Knuttgen HG, Emerson Jr K. Physiological response to pregnancy at rest and during exercise. J Appl Physiol 1974; 36:549–553.

39. Krukenberg H. Arbeitsphysiologische Studien an graviden Frauen. I. Mitteilung: Über den Einfluss der körperlichen Arbeit auf den Muskelstoffwechsel. Arch Gynaekol 1932; 149:250–277.

40. Curet LB, Orr JA, Rankin JHG, Ungerer T. Effect of exercise on cardiac output and distribution of uterine blood flow in pregnant ewes. J Appl Physiol 1976; 40:725–728.

41. Lotgering FK, Gilbert RD, Longo LD. Exercise responses in pregnant sheep: oxygen consumption, uterine blood flow, and blood volume. J Appl Physiol 1983; 55:834–841.

42. Rowell LB. Human cardiovascular adjustments to exercise and thermal stress. Physiol Rev 1974; 54:75–159.

43. Artal R, Platt LD, Sperling M, Kammula RK, Jilek J, Nakamura R. Exercise in pregnancy; I. Maternal cardiovascular and metabolic responses in normal pregnancy. Am J Obstet Gynecol 1981; 140:123–127.

44. Lehmann V, Regnat K. Untersuchung zur körperlichen Belastungsfähigkeit schwangeren Frauen. Der Einfluss standardisierter Arbeit auf Herzkreislaufsystem, Ventilation, Gasaustausch, Kohlenhydratstoffwechsel und Säure-Basen-Haushalt. Z Geburtshilfe Perinatol 1976; 180:279–289.

45. Lehmann V. Die köperliche Leistungsfähigkeit während der Schwangerschaft. Med Klin 1977; 72:1313–1319.

46. Soiva K, Salmi A, Grönroos M, Peltonen T. Physical working capacity during pregnancy and effect of physical work tests on fetal heart rate. Ann Chir Gynaecol 1963; 53:187–196.

47. Longo LD, Ching KS. Placental diffusing capacity for carbon monoxide and oxygen in unanesthetized sheep. J Appl Physiol 1977; 43:885–893.

48. Greenleaf JE, Convertino VA, Stremel RW, Bernauer EM, Adams WC, Vignau SR, Brock PJ. Plasma (Na$^+$), (Ca^{2+}), and volume shifts and thermoregulation during exercise in man. J Appl Physiol 1977; 43:1026–1032.

49. Lundvall J, Mellander S, Westling H, White T. Fluid transfer between blood and tissues during exercise. Acta Physiol Scand 1972; 85:258–269.

50. Huckabee WE, Crenshaw MC, Curet LB, Barron DH. Uterine blood flow and oxygen consumption in the unrestrained pregnant ewe. Q J Exp Physiol 1972; 57:12–23.

51. Makowski EL, Meschia G, Droegemueller W, Battaglia FC. Distribution of uterine blood flow in the pregnant sheep. Am J Obstet Gynecol 1968; 101:409–412.

52. Power GG, Longo LD, Wagner Jr HN, Kuhl DE, Forster RE. Uneven distribution of maternal and fetal placental blood flow, as demonstrated using macroaggregates, and its response to hypoxia. J Clin Invest 1967; 46:2053–2063.

53. Rosenfeld CR, Morriss FH Jr, Makowski EL, Meschia G, Battaglia FC. Circulatory changes in the reproductive tissues of ewes during pregnancy. Gynecol Invest 1974; 5:252–268.

54. Bell C. Control of uterine blood flow in pregnancy. Med Biol 1974; 52:119–228.

55. Bruce NW, Abdul-Karim RW. Mechanisms controlling maternal placental circulation. Clin Obstet Gynecol 1974; 17:135–151.

56. Rankin JHG, McLaughlin MK. The regulation of the placental blood flows. J Dev Physiol 1979; 1:3–30.

57. Wallenburg HCS. Modulation and regulation of uteroplacental blood flow. Placenta 1981; 2 (suppl 1):45–64.

58. Greiss Jr FC. Differential reactivity of the myoendometrial and placental vasculatures: adrenergic responses. Am J Obstet Gynecol 1972; 112:20–30.

59. Morris N, Osborne SB, Wright HP, Hart A. Effective uterine blood-flow during exercise in normal and pre-eclamptic pregnancies. Lancet 1956; 2:481–484.

60. Chandler KD, Leury BJ, Bird AR, Bell AW. Effects of undernutrition and exercise during late pregnancy on uterine, fetal and uteroplacental metabolism in the ewe. Br J Nutr 1985; 53:625–635.

61. Orr J, Ungerer T, Will J, Wernicke K, Curet LB. Effect of exercise stress on carotid, uterine, and iliac blood flow in pregnant and nonpregnant ewes. Am J Obstet Gynecol 1972; 114:213–217.

62. Hohimer AR, Bissonnette JM, Metcalfe J, McKean TA. Effect of exercise on uterine blood flow in the pregnant pygmy goat. Am J Physiol 1984; 246:H207–H212.

63. Rosenfeld CR, West J. Circulatory response to systemic infusion of norepinephrine in the pregnant ewe. Am J Obstet Gynecol 1977; 127:376–383.

64. Bell AW, Hales JRS, Fawcett AA, King RB. Effects of exercise and heat stress on regional blood flow in pregnant sheep. J Appl Physiol 1986; 60:1759–1764.

65. Clausen JP. Effect of physical training on cardiovascular adjustments to exercise in man. Physiol Rev 1977; 57:779–815.

66. Assali NS, Douglass RA Jr, Baird WW, Nicholson DB, Suyemoto R. Measurement of uterine blood flow and uterine metabolism; IV. Results in normal pregnancy. Am J Obstet Gynecol 1953; 66:248–253.

67. Morriss Jr FH, Rosenfeld CR, Resnik R, Meschia G, Makowski EL, Battaglia FC. Growth of uterine oxygen and glucose uptakes during pregnancy in sheep. Gynecol Invest 1974; 5:230–241.

68. Meschia G, Battaglia FC, Hay WW, Sparks JW. Utilization of substrates by the ovine placenta in vivo. Fed Proc 1980; 39:245–249.

69. Battaglia FC, Meschia G. Principal substrates of fetal metabolism. Physiol Rev 1978; 58:499–527.

70. Lorijn RHW, Longo LD. Clinical and physiological implications of increased fetal oxygen consumption. Am J Obstet Gynecol 1980; 136:451–457.

71. Parer JT. Fetal oxygen uptake and umbilical circulation during maternal hypoxia in the chronically catheterized sheep. In Longo LS, Reneau RR, eds. Fetal and newborn cardiovascular physiology. New York: Garland, 1978, vol 2, pp. 231–247.

72. James EJ, Raye JR, Gresham EL, Makowski EL, Meschia G, Battaglia FC. Fetal oxygen consumption, carbon dioxide production, and glucose uptake in a chronic preparation. Pediatrics 1972; 50:361–371.

73. Bell AW, Bassett JM, Chandler KD, Boston RC. Fetal and maternal endocrine responses to exercise in the pregnant ewe. J Dev Physiol 1983; 5:129–141.

74. Treadway JL, Young JC. Decreased glucose uptake in the fetus after maternal exercise. Med Sci Sports Exerc 1989; 21:140–145.

75. Beitins IZ, Kowarski A, Shermeta DW, De Lemos RA, Migeon CJ. Fetal and maternal secretion rate of cortisol in sheep: diffusion resistance of the placenta. Pediatr Res 1970; 4:129–134.

76. Burd LI, Jones MD Jr, Simmons MA, Makowski EL, Meschia G, Battaglia FC. Placental production and foetal utilisation of lactate and pyruvate. Nature 1975; 254:710–711.

77. Carlson KI, Yang HT, Bradshaw WS, Conlee RK, Winder WW. Effect of maternal exercise on fetal liver glycogen late in gestation in the rat. J Appl Physiol 1986; 60:1254–1258.

78. Craig BW, Treadway J. Glucose uptake and oxidation in fat cells of trained and sedentary pregnant rats. J Appl Physiol 1986; 60:1704–1709.

79. Adamsons K Jr. The role of thermal factors in fetal and neonatal life. Pedriatr Clin North Am 1966; 13:599–619.

80. Morishima HO, Yeh M, Niemann WH, James LS. Temperature gradient between fetus and mother as an index for assessing intrauterine fetal condition. Am J Obstet Gynecol 1977; 129:443–448.

81. Abrams R, Caton D, Clapp J, Barron DH. Thermal and metabolic features of life in utero. Clin Obstet Gynecol 1970; 13:549–564.

82. Power GG, Schröder H, Gilbert RD. Measurement of fetal heat production using differential calorimetry. J Appl Physiol 1984; 57:917–922.

83. Cefalo RC, Hellegers AE. The effect of maternal hyperthermia on maternal and fetal cardiovascular and respiratory function. Am J Obstet Gynecol 1978; 131:687–694.

84. Longo LG, Hill EP, Power GG. Theoretical analysis of factors affecting placental O_2 transfer. Am J Physiol 1972; 222:730–739.

85. Gilbert RD, Cummings LA, Juchau MR, Longo LD. Placental diffusing capacity and fetal development in exercising or hypoxic guinea pigs. J Appl Physiol 1979; 46:828–834.

86. Rudolph AM, Heymann MA. Cardiac output in the fetal lamb: the effects of spontaneous and induced changes of heart rate on right and left ventricular output. Am J Obstet Gynecol 1976; 124:183–192.

87. Gilbert RD. Effects of afterload and baroreceptors on cardiac function in fetal sheep. J Dev Physiol 1982; 4:299–309.

88. Rudolph AM, Heymann MA. Circulatory changes during growth in the fetal lamb. Circ Res 1970; 26:289–299.

89. Lorijn RHW, Longo LD. Norepinephrine elevation in the fetal lamb: oxygen consumption and cardiac output. Am J Physiol 1980; 239:R115–R122.

90. Longo LD, Wyatt JF, Hewitt CW, Gilbert RD. A comparison of circulatory responses to hypoxic and carbon monoxide hypoxia in fetal blood flow and oxygenation. In Longo LD, Reneau DD, eds. Fetal and newborn cardiovascular physiology. New York: Garland, 1978, vol 2, pp. 259–287.

91. Brace RA. Blood volume and its measurement in the chronically catheterized sheep fetus. Am J Physiol 1983; 244:H487–H494.

92. Peeters LLH, Sheldon RE, Jones Jr MD, Makowski EL, Meschia G. Blood flow to fetal organs as a function of arterial oxygen content. Am J Obstet Gynecol 1979; 135:637–646.

93. Faber JJ, Green TJ. Foetal placental blood flow in the lamb. J Physiol (Lond) 1972; 223:375–393.

94. Palmer SA, Oakes GK, Champion JA, Fisher DA, Hobel CK. Catecholamine physiology in the ovine fetus. III. Maternal and fetal response to acute maternal exercise. Am J Obstet Gynecol 1984; 149:426–434.

95. Barron DH. A history of fetal respiration: from Harvey's question (1651) to Zweifels answer (1876). In Longo LD, Reneau DD, eds. Fetal and newborn physiology. New York: Garland, 1978, vol I, Developmental Aspects, pp. 1–32.

96. Smith AD, Gilbert RD, Lammers RJ, Longo LD. Placental exchange area in guinea pigs following long-term maternal exercise: a stereological analysis. J Dev Physiol 1983; 5:11–21.

97. Bissonnette JM, Black JA, Wickham WK, Acott KM. Glucose uptake into plasma membrane vesicles from the maternal surface of human placenta. J Membr Biol 1981; 58:75–80.

98. Bissonnette JM, Hohimer AR, Cronan JZ, Black JA. Glucose transfer across the intact guinea-pig placenta. J Dev Physiol 1979; 1:415–426.

99. Yudilevich DL, Eaton BM, Short AH, Leichtweiss H-P. Glucose carriers at maternal and fetal sides of

the trophoblast in guinea pig placenta. Am J Physiol 1979; 237:C205–C212.

100. Simmons MA, Battaglia FC, Meschia G. Placental transfer of glucose. J Dev Physiol 1979; 1:227–243.

101. Moll W. Girard H, Gros G. Facilitated diffusion of lactic acid in the guinea-pig placenta. Pflugers Arch 1980; 385:229–238.

102. Terada M. Effect of physical activity before pregnancy on fetuses of mice exercised forcibly during pregnancy. Teratology 1974; 10:141–144.

103. Nelson PS, Gilbert RD, Longo LD. Fetal growth and placental diffusing capacity in guinea pigs following long-term maternal exercise. J Dev Physiol 1983; 5:1–10.

104. Treadway J, Dover EV, Morse W, Newcomer L, Craig BW. Influence of exercise training on maternal and fetal morphological characteristics in the rat. J Appl Physiol 1986; 60:1700–1703.

105. Levitsky LL, Kimber A, Marchichow JA, Uehara J. Metabolic response to fasting in experimental intrauterine growth retardation induced by surgical and nonsurgical maternal stress. Biol Neonate 1977; 31:311–315.

106. Blake CA, Hazelwood RL. Effect of pregnancy and exercise on actomyosin, nucleic acid, and glycogen content of the rat heart. Proc Soc Exp Biol Med 1971; 136:632–636.

107. Hale CM, Booram CV, McCormick WC. Effects of forced exercise during gestation on farrowing and weaning performance of swine. J Anim Sci 1981; 52:1240–1243.

108. Jenkins RR, Ciconne C. Exercise effect during pregnancy on brain nucleic acids of offspring in rats. Arch Phys Med Rehabil 1980; 61:124–127.

109. Parizková J. Cardiac microstructure in female and male offspring of exercised rat mothers. Acta Anat 1979; 104:382–387.

110. Parizková J, Petrasek R. The impact of daily work load during pregnancy on lipid metabolism in the liver of the offspring. Bibl Nutr Dieta 1979; 27:57–64.

111. Parizková J. Impact of daily work-load during pregnancy on the microstructure of the rat heart in male offspring. Eur J Appl Physiol 1975; 34:323–326.

112. Bonner HW, Buffington CK, Newman JJ, Farrar RP, Acosta D. Contractile activity of neonatal heart cells in culture derived from offspring of exercised pregnant rats. Eur J Appl Physiol 1978; 39:1–6.

113. Butler AW, Farrar RP, Acosta D. Effects of cardioactive drugs on the beating activity of myocardial cell cultures isolated from offspring of trained and untrained pregnant rats. In vitro 1984; 20:629–634.

114. Butler AAW, Smith MA, Farrar RP, Acosta D. The effects of ethanol on cellular calcium content in primary myocardial cell cultures from offspring of sedentary and swim-trained pregnant rats. Bioch Biophys Res Comm 1987; 142:496–500.

115. Corbett K, Brassard L, Taylar AW. Skeletal muscle metabolism in the offspring of trained rats. Med Sci Sports Exerc 1979; 11:107.

14

Hormonal Responses to Exercise in Pregnancy

Raul Artal Mittelmark

Very few studies are available on the hormonal adaptation to exercise in pregnancy. Ample literature is available on the endocrine changes in pregnancy and the related pertinent literature has been reviewed in Chapter 2. To assess the effects of physical activity on the endocrine system properly, a distinction has to be made between responses to acute exercise and physical training. The endocrine responses to exercise in pregnancy have to be examined against a background of various endocrine adaptations to pregnancy superimposed by acute oxygen and fuel requirements of exertion.

One of the major physiological requirements of pregnancy is the constant need for an adequate supply of nutrients to the fetus. Pregnancy is characterized by a state of reduced peripheral insulin sensitivity and hyperinsulinemia that leads to an increase in peripheral glucose utilization, a decrease in plasma glucose levels, increased tissue storage of glycogen, and decreased hepatic glucose production. Late in pregnancy there is a sparing of maternal glucose utilization resulting in decreased maternal levels of glucose and amino acids and ketones, pancreatic islet hypertrophy, and increased insulin response to glucose. As such, pregnancy has been described as a diabetogenic state during which various degrees of carbohydrate intolerance are observed (1–3). For additional details, see Chapters 3 and 4.

To maintain even the lightest type of exercise, there is a continuous uptake of glucose from the blood (4). Exercise favors the release of glucose from the liver (glycogenolysis and gluconeogenesis) and the release of fatty acids from adipose tissue (lipolysis). To maintain such a steady glucose production, there is a delicate interplay between an increased sympathoadrenal and neurohumoral activity, which results in a decline in plasma insulin and increased concentration of norepinephrine, epinephrine, cortisol, glucagon, and growth hormone. Figure 14.1 illustrates glucose, glucagon, and insulin levels before and after mild exercise; Figure 14.2 illustrates

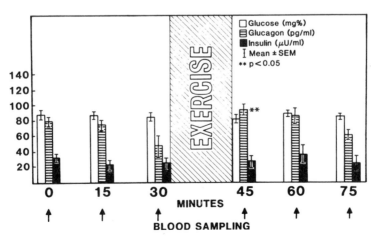

Figure 14.1. Effect of exercise on maternal glucose, glucagon, and insulin concentrations. The *asterisks* indicate a significant difference for that value when compared to the preexercise value. (From Artal R, et al. Exercise in pregnancy. Maternal cardiovascular and metabolic response in normal pregnancy. *Am J Obstet Gynecol* 1981; 140:123.)

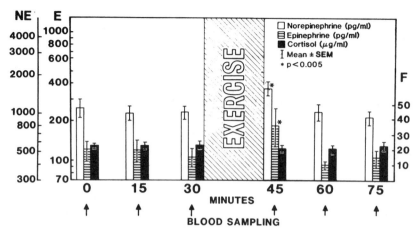

Figure 14.2.   Comparison of preexercise and postexercise concentrations of norepinephrine, epinephrine, and cortisol. The data for norepinephrine *(NE)* and epinephrine *(E)* are illustrated on a logarithmic scale to the *left* of the figure and those for cortisol *(F)* are on a separate scale to the *right* of the figure. The *asterisks* indicate a significant statistical difference for that value when compared to the preexercise value. (From Artal R, et al. *Am J Obstet Gynecol* 1981; 140:123.

the sympathoadrenal responses (norepinephrine, epinephrine, cortisol) (5).

The extent of the hormonal alterations is increased as the intensity of the exercise increases, this process favors lipolysis. With mild exercise, the mobilized energy stores come predominantly from fat, the reduction in insulin coupled with elevation in catecholamines results in mobilization of free fatty acids. As the level of exercise increases, there is a greater contribution from carbohydrates. One method to assess substrate use is indirect calorimetry through determinations of respiratory exchange ratio (R) (6). R is a respiratory variable that reflects the ratio between carbon dioxide output ($\dot{V}_{CO_2}$) and oxygen uptake ($\dot{V}_{O_2}$) and provides information on the proportion of substrate derived from various foodstuffs. If carbohydrates are completely oxidized to CO_2 and water (H_2O), one volume of CO_2 is produced for each volume of O_2 consumed. An R value of 1.0 would indicate that only carbohydrates are being used (Fig. 14.3). An R value of 0.7 would indicate that fats are being burned. Comparative measurements by indirect calorimetry in pregnancy indicate preferential carbohydrate use during nonweight bearing exercise. (7) (Fig 14.4). Studies confirm that with light exercise, plasma glucose concentrations are

maintained at a remarkably constant level in pregnancy: this is facilitated by a fall in insulin and a rise in glucagon concentrations (8,9). The decrease in plasma insulin level is proportionate to the duration and intensity of exercise. With mild exercise we have not observed a change in insulin concentrations, but we did observe a very small rise in glu-

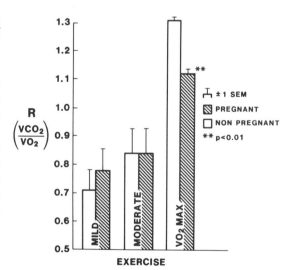

Figure 14.3.   Comparison of R in pregnant and nonpregnant subjects during mild, moderate, and strenuous exercise.

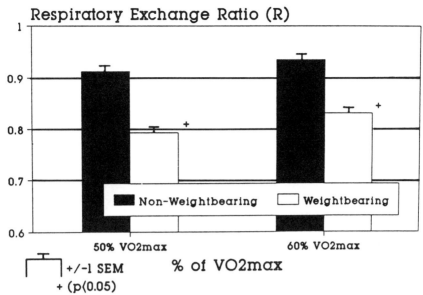

Figure 14.4.   Respiratory exchange ratio during nonweight bearing (bicycle ergometry) and weight bearing (treadmill) exercise at incremental work loads. From Artal R, et al. Am J Obstet Gynecol 1989; 161:1464–1469.

cagon (Fig. 14.1). The interactions between glucose, glucagon, free fatty acids (FFA), epinephrine, and norepinephrine in diabetic and nondiabetic pregnant patients after a light exercise routine are illustrated in Figure 14.5 (10).

With more intense exercise, glucagon levels increase significantly. Glucagon increases glycogenolysis and gluconeogenesis in the liver and has an important role in the physiological adaptation to exercise. During recovery from exercise glucagon concentrations remain elevated for as long as 30 min, a reflection of the increased hepatic uptake of gluconeogenic precursors.

Acute changes in hormones are very sensitive to the type, intensity, and duration of exercise. The physical fitness and the basic condition of the individual, for example, fasting or postprandial, are crucial in determining hormonal responses. It is important, however, to point out that the change in the hormone plasma concentrations may be a result of the shift of fluids that occurs during exercise and, thus, is a reflection of the reduction in plasma volume. Furthermore, we have to recognize the pulsatile nature of some of these hormonal responses with unknown rates of delivery. Figure 14.6 illustrates a comparison of the percentage change in the plasma glucose level at the ends of mild, moderate, and strenuous exercise in pregnant and nonpregnant subjects. It appears that glucose levels are maintained at more stable levels during mild and moderate exercise in pregnancy (11,12). During short-term exercise, insulin, glucagon, and the catecholamines modulate glucose homeostasis. During prolonged exercise, other hormones, i.e., cortisol and growth hormone participate in the metabolic homeostasis of exercise. For prolonged exercise, continuous production of adenosine triphosphate (ATP) is essential.

During mild to moderate exercise, blood glucose regulation is balanced between liver output and peripheral uptake so that plasma glucose remains constant (13). In pregnancy, this function appears to be strictly guarded (10). In the nonpregnant woman, when exercise of mild to moderate intensity (30–60% $\dot{V}_{O_2max}$) continues for an hour, plasma glucose varies very little (13). Nevertheless, if the exercise intensity is lower and longer, plasma glucose will decrease and, at times, hypoglycemia may develop (14). In pregnancy, prolonged continuous stationary bicycle exercise of 1 hour at 50–60% $\dot{V}_{O_2max}$

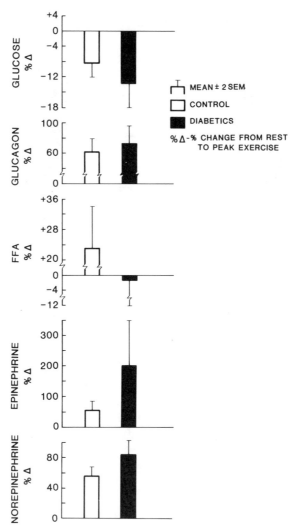

Figure 14.5.   Hormonal responses to mild exercise in pregnant, healthy, and diabetic patients.

lowered blood glucose from 5.17 ± 0.2 mmol/liter to 3.66 ± 0.17 mmol/liter (16) (Fig. 14.7).

Exercise has been often prescribed to achieve normoglycemia in the nonpregnant woman (see Chapters 4 and 28). Presently, research is being conducted to establish exercise programs for the type II pregnant diabetic patients (10). It appears that under strict medical supervision, pregnant diabetic patients can benefit from prescription exercise. Studies indicate that, in such patients, the response to mild exercise is similar to the one observed in the healthy pregnant subject. As illustrated in Figure 14.5, plasma glucose fell similarly with exercise in pregnant diabetic women and controls who underwent a 15-min walk on a motorized treadmill at a speed of 2 mph.

The significant increase in glucose utilization during exercise is accompanied by simultaneous increases in glucose production, but hypoglycemia remains the major clinical problem in diabetic patients during and after exercise. Such occurrences are highly undesirable in pregnancy because of their adverse effects on the outcome. At this time, it is not known if pregnancy could be a contributing factor to exercise-related hypoglycemia, but it appears that prolonged strenuous exercise may induce hypoglycemia more rapidly in pregnancy (15, 16, 27).

Mild exercise levels are of sufficient inten-

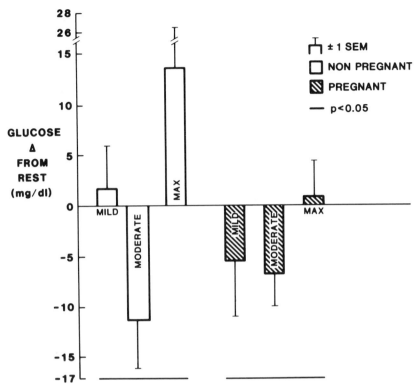

Figure 14.6. Comparison of plasma glucose change with mild, moderate, and strenuous exercise in pregnant and nonpregnant healthy subjects.

sity to induce a training effect, sensitize insulin receptors, and increase glucose utilization in type II pregnant diabetics. (10, 15). We consider this level of activity if repeated three to four times weekly to be of benefit to these patients (17); recognizing that a single bout of exercise may have a 48-hour effect on insulin sensitivity (18).

Plasma insulin concentrations decrease significantly during prolonged exercise in normal pregnancy (16) (Fig. 14.8).

The catecholamines are known to promote both liver glycogenolysis and adipose tissue lipolysis. Epinephrine modulates both the release of glucagon and FFA. FFA provide an important energy substrate during prolonged exercise. Studies of acute exercise, revealed limited change in FFA during mild and moderate exercise but during continuous prolonged stationary bicycle exercise of 1 hour, FFA increased significantly in pregnancy (16).

The level of the sympathoadrenal activity correlates with the severity of the work performed (19). Increases in circulating norepinephrine appear even at mild work loads as illustrated in Figures 14.2 and 14.9. The increments for absolute concentrations appear to be higher during $\dot{V}_{O_2max}$ exercise in pregnant as compared to nonpregnant controls; however, the relative percentage of increase from the resting state to the end of exercise is significantly blunted in pregnancy.

As stated many times in this text, the major hemodynamic response to exercise is the selective redistribution of blood flow to the working muscles, with a reduction in blood flow to the splanchnic organs and potentially to the pregnant uterus as well as to the fetus. The mechanism for blood flow redistribution is catecholamine mediated.

Studies have observed a predominant rise in norepinephrine in comparison to epinephrine, confirming that exercise activates sympathetic nerves to a greater extent than it

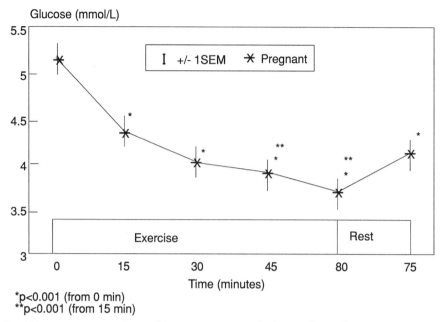

*p<0.001 (from 0 min)
**p<0.001 (from 15 min)

Figure 14.7.   Glucose concentrations of pregnant women during prolonged exercise. (From Soultanakis HN, et al. Dissertation Graduate School, USC)

does the adrenal medulla, in both pregnant and nonpregnant subjects alike. It is important to recognize that norepinephrine can act as a stimulant to the uterus and induce uterine activity (20).

During mild and moderate exercise, the changes in circulating epinephrine are minimal; however during heavy strenuous exercise, epinephrine increases to a greater degree in the nonpregnant subject (19), (10; Fig. 14.10). The smaller increment in epinephrine would facilitate glucose uptake and maintain

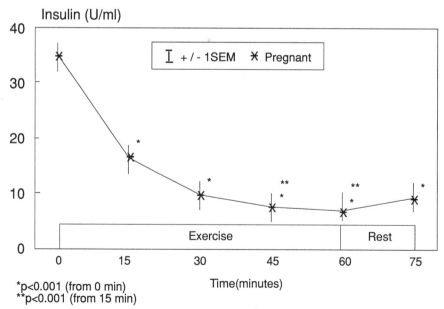

*p<0.001 (from 0 min)
**p<0.001 (from 15 min)

Figure 14.8.   Insulin concentrations of pregnant women during prolonged exercise. (From Soultanakis HN, et al. Dissertation Graduate School, USC.)

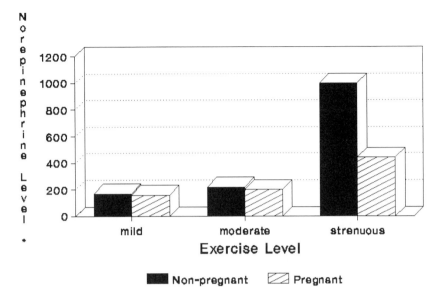

* Expressed as a percent of baseline

Figure 14.9.   Comparison of plasma norepinephrine *(NE)* change with mild, moderate, and strenuous exercise in pregnant and nonpregnant healthy subjects. Data expressed as percentage of increase from the resting state to the peak exercise.

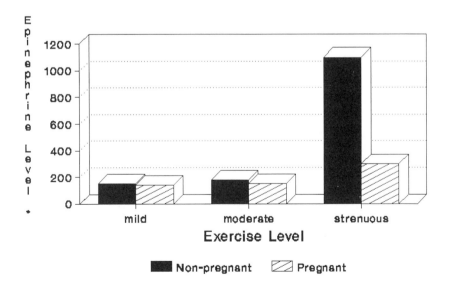

* Expressed as a percent of baseline

Figure 14.10.   Comparison of plasma epinephrine *(E)* change with mild, moderate, and strenuous exercise in pregnant and nonpregnant healthy subjects. Data expressed as percentage of increase from the resting state to the peak exercise.

stable glucose levels. This steady-state is desirable in pregnancy and is essential to the well-being of the fetus. A further surge in epinephrine would inhibit glucose uptake and create a glut of circulating glucose. The hormonal changes observed during mild and moderate exercise are transient and return to control values within 15 min; with strenuous exercise, the changes could last as long as 30 min and beyond (11).

The hormonal changes at any absolute work load can be significantly diminished with training. Typical is a diminished catecholamine response in individuals after training (21). As a result, such training also blunts both the glucagon increase and the insulin decrease (22).

The role of glucocorticoids during exercise has yet to be determined. Under normal conditions, glucocorticoids are known to increase and enhance liver gluconeogenesis, and induce lypolysis. It appears that short-term administration of glucocorticoids can improve exercise performance; this has been demonstrated under laboratory conditions (23). The mechanism behind the enhanced performance seems to be related to the in-

creased ability to induce gluconeogenesis and provide further supply of glucose during exercise. In addition, anti-inflammatory properties have been attributed to them as well.

The ability to release glucocorticoids during exercise appears to be related to the work load itself, and to increase significantly during strenuous exercise (24). As with catecholamines, plasma glucocorticoids tend to increase less with exercise in trained subjects.

Plasma concentrations of cortisol increase with the advancement of gestation and primarily through an increase in the specific cortisol-binding protein, transcortin (25). Theoretically, along with increased levels of cortisol in pregnancy we should observe enhanced exercise performance and endurance; but there is no evidence for such effects. Mild exercise produces only a limited adrenal response; along with minimal changes in epinephrine levels, there are limited changes in circulating cortisol (Fig. 14.2) (5). Insignificant changes in circulating cortisol are also observed after submaximal exercise (Fig. 14.11) (26). Thus, it appears that cortisol plays only a limited role during mild activity in the pregnant and nonpregnant woman.

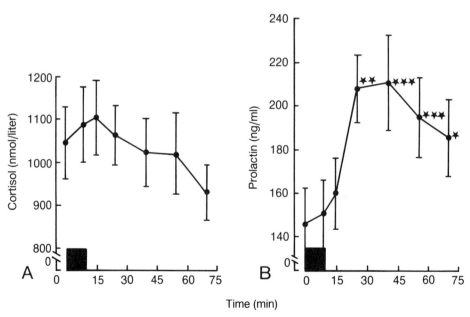

Figure 14.11. Serum cortisol *(A)* and prolactin *(B)* concentrations (means ± SEM). ■ = Submaximal exercise. Significance of differences: *$P > 0.02$; **$P > 0.01$; ***$P > 0.005$. (From Rauramo I, et al. Stress hormones and placental steroids in physical exercise during pregnancy. *B Obstet Gynaecol* 1982; 89:921.)

Prolactin is a peptide hormone with similarities to growth hormone. Prolactin has been reported to have a multitude of actions and because of its role in water electrolyte balance it has certain physiological significance in response to exercise (27). Submaximal exercise in pregnancy significantly elevates serum prolactin concentrations for at least 1 hour (Fig. 14.11) (26).

The ovarian hormones, estradiol and progesterone, increase during exercise, with a most prominent response during strenuous exercise (28). It is unclear if the circulating hormones or their administration cause improved exercise performance. During normal human pregnancy, there is a hyperestrogenic state with a disproportionate increase in estriol. The close involvement of the fetus in the biosynthesis of estriol has been utilized in the past to monitor fetal status. Low values of estriol have been interpreted to reflect fetal distress. During submaximal exercise in pregnancy, there is a significant transient rise in serum estriol concentrations, as illustrated in Figure 14.12 (26). This temporary rise may be interpreted in different ways, it could reflect fetal well-being and be considered a normal response to a state of increased sympathetic

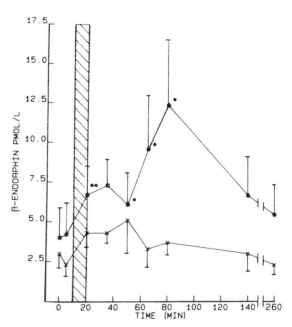

Figure 14.13. Mean concentrations (+ SE) of β-endorphin in plasma in relation to exercise test in nonpregnant (*lower curve*) and in pregnant women (*upper curve*). Shaded column indicates the 10-min period of the exercise. ^{x}p < 0.02, ^{xx}p < 0.01, paired comparison with value at start of exercise. (From Rauramo I, et al. Acta Obstet Gynecol Scand 1986; 65:610.)

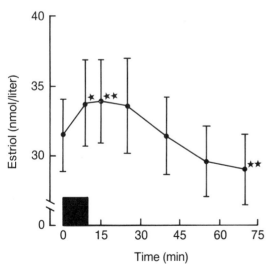

Figure 14.12. Serum estriol concentration (means ± SEM). ■ = Submaximal exercise. Significance of differences: *P > 0.05; **P > 0.02. (From Rauramo I, et al. Stress hormones and placental steroids in physical exercise during pregnancy. *Obstet Gynaecol* 1982; 89:921.

activity, or it could be explained by an increased flow of estriol-rich uteroplacental blood into the maternal circulation immediately after the exercise.

Physical activity stimulates the secretion of the endogenous opioids, β-endorphin and β-lipotropin. During submaximal exercise, the plasma concentrations are virtually doubled and tripled (29) (Fig. 14.13). Exercise training during pregnancy persistently elevated opioids in these women, which might have benefited them during labor and delivery by decreasing pain perception (29).

The endocrine responses to exercise in pregnancy are presently being investigated. The limited information that is available indicates that, in the healthy pregnant woman, the changes are transitory and reversible with no deleterious lasting effects. The complete complex interactions between mother and fetus during maternal activity have yet to be described.

REFERENCES

1. Kalkhoff RK, Schalch DS, Walker JL, et al. Diabetogenic factors associated with pregnancy. Trans Assoc Am Physicians 1964;77:270.
2. Spellacy WN, Goetz FC. Plasma insulin in normal late pregnancy. N Engl J Med 1963; 268:988.
3. Kuhl C. Serum preinsulin in normal and gestational diabetic pregnancy. Diabetologia 1976; 12:295.
4. Wahren J, Ahlborg G, Felig P, Jorfeldt L. Glucose metabolism during exercise in man. In: Pernoe B, Saltin B, eds. Muscle metabolism during exercise. New York: Plenum, 1971; p. 189.
5. Artal R, Platt LD, Sperling M, Kammula KR, Jilek J, Nakamura P. Exercise in pregnancy. Maternal cardiovascular and metabolic responses in normal pregnancy. Am J Obstet Gynecol 1981; 140:123.
6. Artal R, Wiswell R, Romem Y. Pulmonary responses to exercise in pregnancy. Am J Obstet Gynecol 1986; 154:378–383.
7. Artal R, Masaki DI, Khodigman N, Romem Y, Rutherford SE, Wiswell RA. Exercise prescription in pregnancy: weight-bearing versus non-weight-bearing exercise. Am J Obstet Gynecol 1989; 161:1464–1469.
8. Pruett EDR: Plasma insulin concentrations during prolonged work at near maximal oxygen intake. J Appl Physiol 1970; 29:155.
9. Bottiger I, Schlein FM, Faloona GR, et al. The effect of exercise on glucagon secretion. J Clin Endocrinol Metab 1972; 35:117.
10. Artal R, Wiswell R, Romem Y. Hormonal responses to exercise in diabetic and nondiabetic pregnant patients. Diabetes 1985; 34(2):78–80.
11. Artal R, Farmer R, Wiswell R, Romem Y, Kammula R. Hormonal changes during exercise in pregnancy (unpublished observations).
12. McMurray RG, Katz VL, Berry J, Cefalo RC. The effect of pregnancy on metaolic responses during rest. Am J Obstet Gynecol 1988; 158:481–486.
13. Chisholm DJ, Jenkins AB, James DE, Kraegen EW. The effect of hyperinsulinemia on glucose homeostasis during moderate exercise in man. Diabetes 1982; 31:603–608.
14. Felig PA, Cherif A, Minagawa A, Wahren J. Hypoglycemia during prolonged exercise in normal man. N Engl J Med 1982; 306:895–900.
15. Artal R: Exercise and diabetes mellitus in pregnancy: A brief review. Sports Med 1990; 9(5):261–265.
16. Soultanakis H. Glucose homeastasis during pregnancy in response to prolonged exercise. Dissertation, Graduate School, USC.
17. Mikines KJ, Sonne B, Farrell PA, Golbo H: Insulin sensitivity and responsiveness after acute exercise. Med Sci Sports Exec 1985; 17:242.
18. Hartley LH, Mason JW, Hogan RP, Jones LG, Kotchen TA, Mongey EH, Wherry FE, Pennington LL, Ricketts PT. Multiple hormonal responses to graded exercise in relation to physical training. J Appl Physiol 1972; 33:602.
19. Zuspan FP, Cibls LA, Pose Sy. Myometrial and cardiovascular responses to alterations in plasmus epinephrine and norepinephrine. Am J Obstet Gynecol 1962; 84:841.
20. Scheuer J, Tipton CM: Cardiovascular adaptations to physical training. Annu Rev Physiol 1977; 39:221.
21. Gyntelberg F, Rennie MJ, Hickson RC, Holloszy JO. Effect of training on the response of plasma glucagen to exercise. J Appl Physiol 1977; 43:302.
22. Isekutz B, Allen M. Effect of methylprednisolone on carbohydrate metabolism of exercising dogs. J Appl Physiol 1977; 31:813.
23. Dessypris A, Kuoppasalmi K, Adlercrentz H. Plasma cortisol, testosterone, androstenedione and luteinizing hormone in a noncompetitive marathon run. J Steroid Biochem 1976; 7:33.
24. Rosenthal HE, Slaunwhite WR Jr, Sandberg AA. Transcortin: a corticosteroid-binding protein of plasma. Cortisol and progesterone interplay and unbound levels of these steroids in pregnancy. J Clin Endocrinol Metab 1969; 29:352.
25. Rauramo I, Andersson B, Laatikainen T. Stress hormones and placental steroids in physical exercise during pregnancy. Br J Obstet Gynaecol 1982; 89:921.
26. Yen SSC. Physiology of human prolactin. In: Yen SSC, Jaffe RB, eds. Reproductive endocrinology. Philadelphia: WB Saunders, 1978; p. 150.
27. Jurkowski JE, Jones NL, Walker WC, Younglai EV, Sutton JR. Ovarian hormonal responses to exercise. J Appl Physiol 1978; 44:109.
28. Rauramo I, Salminen K, Laatikainen T. Release of Beta-endorphin in response to physical exercise in non-pregnant and pregnant women. Acta Obstet Gynaecol Scand 1986; 65:609–612.
29. Varrassi G, Bazzano C, Edwards T. Effects of physical activity on maternal plasma beta-endorphin levels and perception of labor pain. Am J Obstet Gynecol 1989; 160:707–712.

15

Pulmonary Responses to Exercise in Pregnancy

Raul Artal Mittelmark, Jeffrey S. Greenspoon, Robert A. Wiswell, and Yitzhak Romem

The physiological requirements and normal changes of pregnancy include close interactions between cardiovascular and respiratory functions. The mechanism by which O_2 and CO_2 are transported between the atmosphere and the cells, mother, and fetus is quite complex and is described in detail in Chapter 12.

As pregnancy progresses, individuals who exercise may experience increasing intolerance to exercise, which is caused by the inability to transfer gas (O_2 and CO_2) between the atmosphere and cells. Such deficiencies are usually compensated in nonpregnant individuals by increased pulmonary diffusing capacity and increased alveolar ventilation. In addition, in pregnancy, hemoglobin, oxygen-carrying capacity, and cardiac output increase significantly and in excess of demands, leading to decreased arteriovenous oxygen difference.

The purpose of this chapter is to review the adaptive changes in the respiratory system during exercise in pregnancy.

As described in Chapter 2, pregnancy is characterized by various anatomical changes. The most significant are summarized below. The upper respiratory tract is often affected by changes in the mucosa of the nasopharynx such as hyperemia, edema, and excessive secretion, all causing obstructive symptoms. The rib cage undergoes changes in pregnancy that result in an expansion of the chest circumference due to the elevation of the diaphragm by the growing uterus (1–4). These changes are more prominent during the second half of pregnancy, and lead to an increase in inspiratory capacity of 300 ml (tidal volume + inspiratory volume) and a reduction in functional residual capacity (5, 6) to maintain intact total lung and vital capacity. Significantly, pregnancy is characterized by

a 10–20% increase in oxygen consumption. The combination of reduced functional residual capacity and increased oxygen consumption results in lower oxygen reserve. If not properly compensated, the oxygen reserve could be further lowered during heavy exercise and potentially could lead to hypoxia. The resting minute ventilation is increased by 40–50%, leading to a decrease of arterial P_{CO_2} to 30 torr and an arterial P_{O_2} of approximately 105 torr (7). Lung compliance increases approximately 36% and airway resistance decreases. These changes are attributed to effect of progesterone relaxing smooth muscle (8).

The respiratory alkalosis is due to the effect of estrogen and progesterone on the respiratory center of the brain (9). Acid-base status is maintained by a compensatory metabolic acidosis. This results in a decrease in serum bicarbonate of approximately 20 mEq/liter. The arterial pH is maintained in the normal range at approximately 7.44 as a result of the primary respiratory alkalosis and the compensatory metabolic acidosis. These physiological changes have appeared in large part by the 7th week of normal pregnancy, but are not observed in women who will experience spontaneous abortion (10). The primary purpose of the increased maternal ventilatory responses during pregnancy is to reduce arterial P_{CO_2}. The result is a mild maternal alkalosis that promotes placental gas exchange and prevents fetal acidosis (11).

Arterial P_{O_2} can be significantly reduced in pregnancy in the supine position due to ventilation-perfusion mismatch. Fetal hypoxia may occur directly as a result of maternal hypoxia or indirectly as a result of maternal hyperventilation leading to maternal alkalosis, which then causes fetal hypoxia. (See later in this chapter and Fig. 15.8.) Functionally, the

Table 15.1.   Comparison of Pulmonary Function of Pregnancy and Postpartum[a]

Author (Ref.)	No. of Patients	VC	IC	EC	MV	TV	RF	FRC	RV	TLC
Prowse and Gaensler (15)	9	—		↓				↓	↓	—
Gee et al. (8)	10	↓		↓				↓	↓	
Gazioglu et al. (5)	8	↑	↑	↓	↑	↑	—	↓	↓	
Lehmann and Fabel (16)	23	—	↑	↓	↑	↑	—	↓	↓	
Knuttgen and Emerson (6)	13	↑	↑			↑	↑	—	↓	—
Pernoll et al. (17)	12					↑	↑	↓		
Alaily and Carrol (14)	38	—	↑	↓	↑	↑	↑	↓	↓	

[a]VC = vital capacity; IC = inspiratory capacity; EC = expiratory capacity; MV = minute volume; TV = tidal volume; RF = respiratory frequency; FRC = functional residual capacity; RV = residual volume; TLC = total lung capacity; ↑ = increase; — = no difference; ↓ = decrease.

changes described are a result of the deeper breathing done by the pregnant woman. In other words, the pregnant woman has a greater tidal volume, while respiratory frequency is not substantially increased. In pregnancy, even individuals with moderate to severe lung disease do well in contrast to women with cardiac disease (12). In the non-pregnant state, subjects with lung disease, e.g., chronic obstructive lung disease, can exercise to a maximum breathing capacity of 80–100% while individuals with heart disease only to about 55% of their predicted maximum heart rate (13).

PULMONARY RESPONSES TO EXERCISE DURING PREGNANCY

As stated previously, pulmonary functions change in pregnancy. Several studies have reviewed this topic and the findings are summarized in Table 15.1, adapted from Alaily and Carrol (14).

Few of these studies have conducted the measurements in the same individuals in the pregnant and nonpregnant state. Furthermore, fewer have studied the same functions in humans during exercise. Several related studies have been completed in experimental animals and are described in detail in Chapter 13.

Exercise studies conducted or performed on pregnant women, by and large, lacked controls and standardization, ignored state of fitness, or extrapolated it from estimated $\dot{V}_{O_2max}$ data. Only a few studies carried their subjects to $\dot{V}_{O_2max}$. Very little attention has been paid to distinguishing between weight bearing and nonweight bearing exercise. The limitations and advantages of utilizing each such testing are detailed in Chapter 12.

Weight bearing exercises are performed less efficiently and are more energy-costly in pregnancy because they contain a component of body weight. Few studies have been published on pulmonary responses to exercise in pregnancy and postpartum (6, 15–20). Because the methods, intensity of exercise, and level of fitness in the different studies cannot be compared in absolute values, we have summarized the data published by their relative changes (Table 15.2).

From these studies, it appears that respiratory frequency tends to increase with either weight bearing or nonweight bearing exercises. Such an increase is quite similar to that occurring in nonpregnant controls. Most of the studies have found a significant increase in minute ventilation and tidal volume, not only at rest, but also during and after exercise. The changes were significantly higher for the degree of exercise than in nonpregnant controls. The disproportionate increase in minute ventilation as compared to oxygen consumption is reflected in a relatively high ventilatory equivalent for oxygen.

In our studies (19), we compared the pulmonary responses to mild, moderate, and $\dot{V}_{O_2max}$ exercise (Fig. 15.1). During mild exercise (approximately 210 kpm or 35 W, the respiratory frequency of pregnant women (43 subjects) was significantly higher than con-

Table 15.2. Comparison of Pulmonary Responses to Exercise in Pregnancy Versus Controls[a]

Author	No. of Patients	RF	$\dot{V}_E$	$\dot{V}_{O_2}$	VT	$\dot{V}_E/\dot{V}_{O_2}$	R	Exercise	Intensity[b]
Bader et al. (18)	46				↑			Ergometer	Steady rate
Guzman and Caplan (20)	8	↑—		↑	—	—		Ergometer	150 kpm
Ueland et al. (21)	22			↑				Ergometer	16.3 W (100 kpm)
Knuttgen and Emerson (6)	13	—	↑	↑	↑	↑	↑	Treadmill	62.3 W (380 kpm)
Knuttgen and Emerson (6)	13	—	↑	—	↑	↑	—	Ergometer	60 W (367 kpm)
Pernoll et al. (22)	12	↑—	↑	↑	↑	—		Ergometer	50.1 W (306 kpm)
Collings et al. (23)	20			↑				Ergometer	Submax
Artal and Wiswell (19)	58	↑	—↑	—	—	↑	—↑	Treadmill	34 W (210 kpm)
	34	↓	—	—	—	—↓	—	Treadmill 10% grade	57.2 W (~350 kpm)
	35	↓	↓	↓	↓	↑	↓	Treadmill	$\dot{V}_{O_2max}$ 106.2 W (~650 kpm)

[a] RF = respiratory frequency; $\dot{V}_E$ minute ventilation; $\dot{V}_{O_2}$ = oxygen uptake; VT = tidal volume; $\dot{V}_E/\dot{V}_{O_2}$ = ventilatory equivalent; R = respiratory exchange ratio; ↑ = increase; — = no difference; ↓ = decrease.
[b] 100 kpm = 16.35 watts.

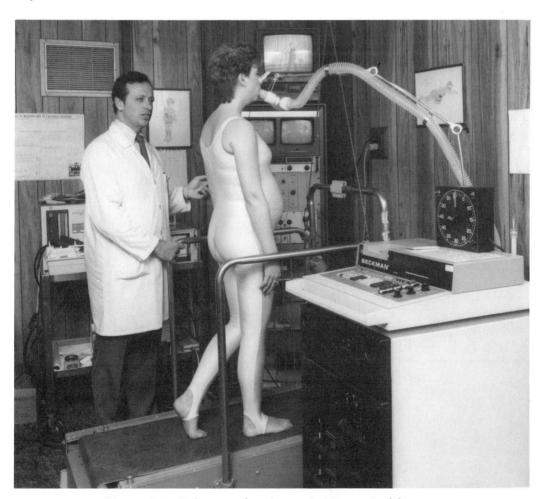

Figure 15.1. Pulmonary function testing in exercise laboratory.

trols (15 subjects), although there was no significant difference between pregnant and nonpregnant subjects at moderate (350 kpm or 60 W) and $\dot{V}_{O_2max}$ exercise (Fig. 15.2). Oxygen consumption, C_{O_2} production, and tidal volume at mild and moderate exercise levels were no different among pregnant and nonpregnant controls, but all were significantly decreased in pregnant subjects at $\dot{V}_{O_2max}$ exercise (Figs. 15.3–15.5) Pregnant women performed significantly less work at $\dot{V}_{O_2max}$ than control subjects. The ventilatory equivalent ($\dot{V}_E/\dot{V}_{O_2}$) was no different among pregnant and nonpregnant subjects at similar exercise levels (Fig. 15.6). However, there was a trend toward higher $\dot{V}_E/\dot{V}_{O_2}$ among pregnant women, as the level of work approached the maximal $\dot{V}_{O_2}$ (15.7).

Sady et al. (25) reported no difference in maximal heart rate at 25 weeks' gestation and at 8 and 24 weeks postpartum. They also measured $\dot{V}_{O_2max}$ at the three different times and reported 1.99 ± 0.42; and 1.89 ± 0.36; 2.03 ± 0.28 liters·min^{-1}, respectively. This suggests no effect of gestation on absolute $\dot{V}_{O_2max}$. We found a similar lack of difference in the absolute $\dot{V}_{O_2max}$ but a decrease in pregnancy when $\dot{V}_{O_2max}$ was expressed relative to body weight.

By and large, the pregnant subjects responded to exercise with increased ventilation during mild exercise. Most studies indicate that pregnant subjects respond with higher minute ventilation ($\dot{V}_E$) than nonpregnant subjects at the same level of work. Pregnant subjects have a similar ventilatory response to exercise when compared with nonpregnant controls as demonstrated by similar ventilatory equivalents at the same level of exercise ($\dot{V}_E/\dot{V}_{O_2}$) (see Fig. 15.6). It is important to appreciate that in pregnancy $\dot{V}_{O_2max}$ is achieved at lower exercise levels than that of nonpregnant subjects (see Fig. 15.7). The pregnant woman has a physiological limitation due to her increase in weight. When the $\dot{V}_{O_2}$ is indexed as liters per minute per kilogram, the $\dot{V}_{O_2}$ values are similar for pregnant and nonpregnant subjects performing mild and moderate work. The only group in which the $\dot{V}_{O_2max}$ could be properly evaluated is among world class athletes who cannot improve their $\dot{V}_{O_2max}$ through further training. This group could be studied before and throughout pregnancy while maintaining their optimal fitness to determine whether $\dot{V}_{O_2max}$ changes. In our own studies, two world class athletes showed only a minimal decline of $\dot{V}_{O_2max}$ during pregnancy, South-Paul

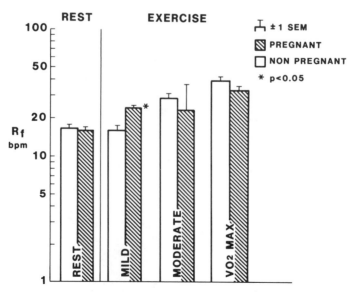

Figure 15.2. Respiratory frequency during mild, moderate, and $\dot{V}_{O_2max}$ exercise. (From Artal R, et al. Pulmonary responses to exercise in pregnancy. Am J Obstet Gynecol 1986; 154:378–383.)

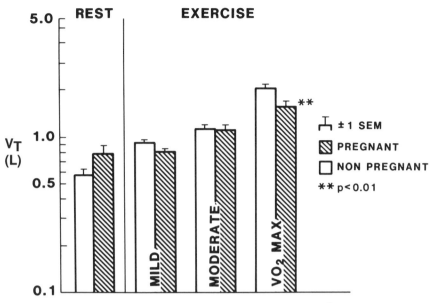

Figure 15.3.   Comparison of tidal volumes during mild, moderate and $\dot{V}_{O_2max}$ exercise. (From Artal R, et al. Pulmonary responses to exercise in pregnancy. Am J Obstetr Gynecol 1986; 154:378–383.)

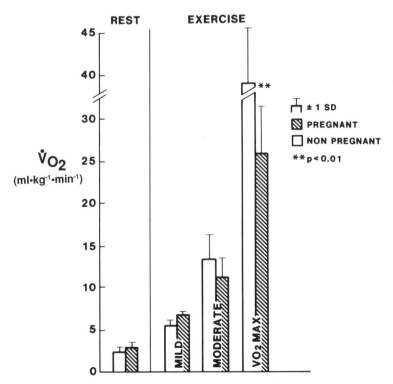

Figure 15.4.   Oxygen consumption during mild, moderate and $\dot{V}_{O_2max}$ exercise. (From Artal R, et al. Pulmonary responses to exercise in pregnancy. Am J Obstet Gynecol 1986; 1954:378–383.)

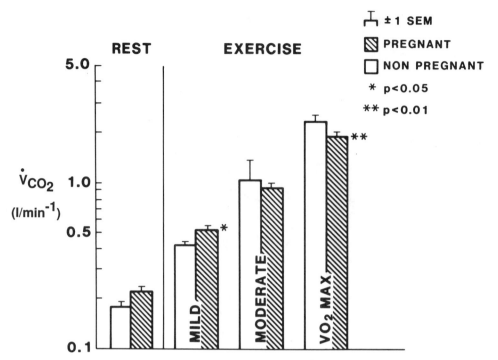

Figure 15.5. CO_2 production during mild, moderate, and $\dot{V}_{O_2max}$ exercise. (From Artal R, et al. Pulmonary responses to exercise in pregnancy. Am J Obstet Gynecol 1986; 154:378–383.)

et al. (26) studied pregnant women at 20 and 30 weeks' gestation using a cycle ergometer at 75 W and $\dot{V}_{O_2max}$. One group of pregnant women exercised regularly, the other group did not. There was no effect of training on respiratory frequency or $\dot{V}_{O_2max}$/ ml·kg^{-1}·min^{-1}. Tidal volumes at 75 W were similar, but a significant increase in V_T occurred at $\dot{V}_{O_2max}$ in the training group compared with the nonexercising group of pregnant women.

This state of hyperventilation that occurs

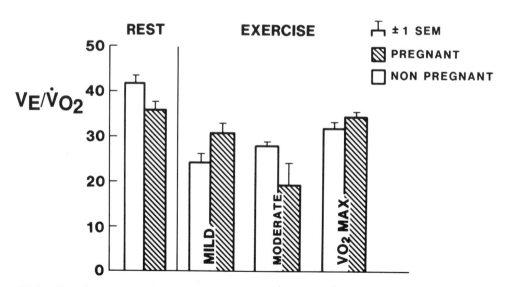

Figure 15.6.   Ventilatory equivalents during mild, moderate and $\dot{V}_{O_2max}$ exercise. (From Artal R, et al. Pulmonary responses to exercise in pregnancy. Am J Obstet Gynecol 1986; 154:378–383.)

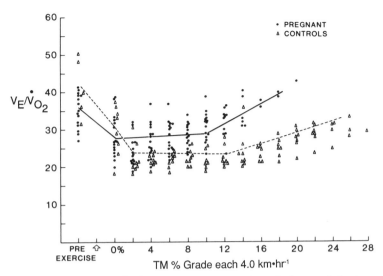

Figure 15.7.   Ventilatory equivalent ($\dot{V}_E/\dot{V}_{O_2}$) determinations done before and during symptom-limited maximal oxygen consumption exercise. The *solid line* illustrates the mean values for the pregnant subjects and the *broken line* the nonpregnant control subjects.

at rest in pregnancy persists and increases with exercise, resulting in lower CO_2 tension, lower bicarbonate concentrations, lower buffering capacity, a modest increase in pH, with negligible changes in O_2 tension.

It has been recognized for a long time that maternal hyperventilation, when producing respiratory alkalosis in the mother, may lead to fetal respiratory alkalosis (27). The fall in maternal and fetal P_{CO_2} is associated with a corresponding fall in fetal P_{O_2} (Fig. 15.8).

The issue of fuel utilization is important because of the possible effects of exercise-induced maternal hypoglycemia on the fetus. Higher R values were observed by Clapp et al. (28) suggesting that there is enhanced utilization of carbohydrate rather than fat. This is consistent with our observations. The higher R values (V_{CO_2}/V_{O_2}) calculated from our data indicate that, during intensive exercise, pregnant women utilize proportionately more carbohydrates as their fuel source and use less fat as an energy source (Fig. 15.9).

One important factor that may account for the different R values reported in various studies is the requirement that the subject be in a physiological steady-state during respiratory gas analysis.

The R value is also affected by the subject's diet or lactation (29). This may indicate an inability to exercise anaerobically, a protective mechanism from hypoxia, or reflect a protective mechanism to maintain steady levels of carbohydrates. However, caution must be exercised when trying to assess fuel substrate utilization pattern derived from R, in the presence of hyperventilation of pregnancy. We know of no studies that have evaluated substrate turnover during exercise in pregnancy and therefore, we submit the above as a possible hypothesis.

Berry et al. (30) studied pulmonary response during immersion. They concluded that, during pregnancy, exercise during immersion resulted in pulmonary functions that were altered but not compromised. The increase in minute ventilation V_E occurring with exercise during immersion was mediated by increases in both the tidal volume (V_T) and respiratory frequency. In comparison, the exercise-induced increase in V_E during ordinary (nonimmersed) exercise was mediated by increases in V_T, while respiratory frequency remains unchanged.

PULMONARY HEMODYNAMICS

Bader et al. (18) performed a unique study in which 46 normal pregnant women had right heart and pulmonary artery catheteriza-

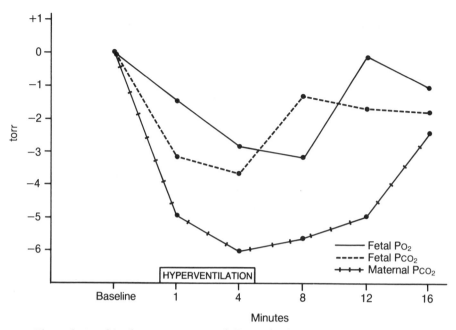

Figure 15.8. The relationship between maternal P_{CO_2}, fetal P_{CO_2}, and fetal P_{O_2} during maternal hyperventilation. (From Miller FC, et al. Am J Obstet Gynecol 1974; 120:489.)

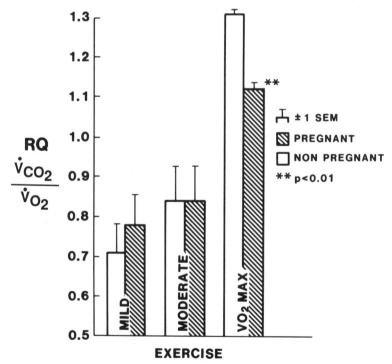

Figure 15.9. Comparison of respiratory exchange ratio *(R)* during mild, moderate, and $\dot{V}_{O_2max}$ exercise. (From Artal R, et al. Pulmonary responses to exercise in pregnancy. Am J Obstet Gynecol 1986; 154:378–383.)

tion at rest and during 10 minutes of exercise in a recumbent position. These authors found that resting oxygen consumption increased as gestational age advanced. However, oxygen consumption during exercise (which was not quantitated) was similar throughout pregnancy. The mean of oxygen consumption during exercise ranged from 230–250 $ml\cdot kg^{-1}\cdot min^{-1}$. Conversely, they found a decrease in cardiac index with exercise at and beyond 28 weeks' gestation. In retrospect, the decrease in cardiac index at rest and with exercise that was noted in the third trimester was probably due to the recumbent position impairing venous blood return to the heart. The phenomenon of supine caval occlusion decreasing cardiac output was described later (31).

The arteriovenous O_2 difference was significantly lower early in pregnancy when compared to late pregnancy. Pulmonary artery diastolic pressure was normal at rest, increased slightly with exercise, and exceeded 12 torr in five subjects. Mean pulmonary artery pressure was normal through pregnancy, rose with exercise by 15 torr in six subjects, and in two subjects, the increment was 20 torr. Pulmonary capillary pressure did not change either at rest or with exercise as pregnancy progressed.

An elevation in right ventricular and diastolic pressure at rest was noted in some patients, a finding consistent with a congested circulatory state. It also appears from this study that pregnant women respond to exercise with an increase in pulmonary diffusing capacity identical to nonpregnant subjects. Conversely, the pulmonary alterations associated with pregnancy and exacerbated by exercise (e.g., hyperventilation) are an important factor in regulating utilization of fuel and buffering the effect of lactate production that could limit exercise tolerance.

REFERENCES

1. Schofman MA. The nose and pregnancy. J Fla Med Assoc 1961; 48:160.
2. Thomson KJ, Cohen ME. Studies of the circulation in pregnancy: vital capacity observations in normal pregnant women. Surg Gynecol Obstet 1938; 66:591.
3. Marx GF, Orxin LR. Physiological changes during pregnancy: a review. Anesthesiology 1958; 19:258.
4. Leoutic EA. Respiratory disease in pregnancy. Med Clin North Am 1977; 61:111.
5. Gazioglu K, Kaltreider NL, Rosen M, Yu PN. Pulmonary function during pregnancy in normal women and in patients with cardiopulmonary disease. Thorax 1970; 25:445.
6. Knuttgen HG, Emerson K. Physiological response to pregnancy at rest and during exercise. J Appl Physiol 1974; 36:549.
7. Bonica JJ. Maternal respiratory changes during pregnancy and parturition. Clin Anesth 1974; 10:1–19.
8. Gee JGL, Packer BS, Millen JE, Robin ED. J Clin Invest 1967; 46:945–952.
9. Regensteiner JG, Woodard WD, Hagerman DD, Weil JV, Pickett CK, Bender PR, Moore LG. Combined effects of female hormones and metabolic rate on ventilatory drives in women. J Appl Physiol 1989; 66:808–813.
10. Clapp JF III, Seaward BL, Sleamaker RH, Hiser J. Maternal physiologic changes to early human pregnancy. Am J Obstet Gynecol 1988; 159:1456–1460.
11. Liboratore SM, Pistelli R, Patalano F, Moneta E, Incarzi RA, Ciappi G. Respiratory function during pregnancy. Respiration 1984; 46:145–150.
12. Bedell GN, Adams RW. Pulmonary diffusing capacity during rest and exercise. A study of normal persons and persons with atrial septal defect, pregnancy and pulmonary disease. J Clin Invest 1962; 41:1908.
13. Kanarek DJ, Hand RW. The response of cardiac and pulmonary disease to exercise testing. Clin Chest Med 1984; 5:181.
14. Alaily AB, Carrol KB. Pulmonary ventilation in pregnancy. Br J Obstet Gynaecol 1978; 85:518.
15. Prowse CM, Gaensler EA. Respiratory and acid-base changes during pregnancy. Anesthesiology 1965; 26:381.
16. Lehmann V, Fabel H. Lung enfunktion untersuchungen an schwangeren; Tell I: Lungenvolumina. Z Geburtshilfe Perinatol 1973; 177:387.
17. Pernoll ML, Metcalfe J, Schlenker TL, Welch JE, Matsumoto JA: Oxygen consumption at rest and during exercise in pregnancy. Respir Physiol 1975; 25:285.
18. Bader RA, Bader ME, Rose DJ, Braunwald E. Hemodynamics at rest and during exercise in normal pregnancy as studied by cardiac catheterization. J Clin Invest 1955; 34:1524.
19. Artal R, et al. Pulmonary responses to exercise in pregnancy. Am J Obstet Gynecol 1986; 154:378–383.
20. Guzman CA, Caplan R. Cardiorespiratory response to exercise during pregnancy. Am J Obstet Gynecol 1970; 108:600.
21. Ueland K, Navy JM, Metcalfe J. Cardiorespiratory responses to pregnancy and exercise in normal women and patients with heart disease. Am J Obstet Gynecol 1973; 115:4.
22. Pernoll ML, Metcalf J, Kovach PA, Wachtel R, Dunham MJ. Ventilation during rest and exercise in pregnancy and postpartum. Respir Physiol 1975; 25:295.
23. Collings CA, Curet LB, Mullin JP. Maternal and fetal responses to a maternal aerobic exercise program. Am J Obstet Gynecol 1983; 145:702.
24. Edwards MJ, Metcalfe J, Dunham MY, Raul MS. Accelerated respiratory response to moderate exercise in late pregnancy. Respir Physiol 1981; 45:229.

25. Sady M, Haydon D, Sady S, Carpenter M, Coustan D, Thompson P. Maximal exercise during pregnancy and postpartum [Abstract]. Med Science Sports Exer 1988; 20:511.

26. South-Paul JE, Rajagopal KR, Tenholder MF. The effect of participation in a regular exercise program upon aerobic capacity during pregnancy. Obstet Gynecol 1988; 71:175–179.

27. Miller FC, Petrie RH, Arce JJ, Paul RH, Hon EH. Hyperventilation during labor. Am J Obstet Gynecol 1974; 120:489.

28. Clapp JF, III, Wesley M, Sleamaker RH. Thermoregulatory and metabolic responses prior to and during pregnancy. Med Science Sports Exer 1987; 19:124–130.

29. Blackburn NW, Calloway DH. Energy expenditure and consumption of mature pregnant and lactating women. J Am Diet Assoc 1976; 69:29–37.

30. Berry MJ, McMurray RG, Katz VL. Pulmonary and ventilatory responses to pregnancy, immersion, and exercise. J Appl Physiol 1989; 66:857–862.

31. Lees MM, Taylor SH, Scott DB, Kerr MG. A study of cardiac output at rest throughout pregnancy. J Obstet Gynaecol Br Commonw 1967; 74:319–328.

16

Maternal Cardiovascular Response to Exercise During Pregnancy

Janet P. Wallace and Robert A. Wiswell

Important questions frequently arise regarding the influence of maternal exercise on pregnancy and its outcome. Because the metabolic demands of pregnancy effect many changes in maternal resting physiological status, it is of particular relevance that we recognize whether the additional stress of exercise induces adjustments that might exceed the threshold of safety for mother and/or child. In this chapter, we will review the information published on adaptations of the pregnant circulatory system to exercise stress, emphasizing the potential benefits attributable to physical conditioning.

In Chapter 5, Morton provides information related to the changes occurring with regard to maternal hemodynamics in pregnancy. Significant changes occur in the resting circulatory system, such as increases in blood volume, heart rate, and cardiac output and a decrease in resting arterial blood pressure. Table 16.1 summarizes the most significant changes and provides information about the possible effect of acute exertion on these variables. It is obvious that such changes could affect women's ability to perform exercise, particularly at higher exercise levels.

Most of these circulatory adaptations arise from the need to compensate for the continuing normal alterations of pregnancy. In addition to the specific changes presented in Table 16.1, a general adaptation toward blood redistribution occurs. Blood flow to the kidney may increase up to 400 ml/min at rest whereas to the uterus a 500 ml/min increase occurs. In general there is a greater distribution of blood to the splanchnic organs (1). The major shift in blood distribution to the various organs is part of the normal changes associated with pregnancy. The demands of exercise require a major redistribution of blood away from the splanchnic organs toward the working muscles. Figure 16.1 provides an example of the magnitude of these changes in blood flow based upon studies on nonpregnant subjects. The possible negative effect of shunting blood away from the reproductive organs, as reported in animals, is of major concern during exercise in pregnancy. Although several studies have been conducted investigating this problem, there is no conclusive evidence as to whether the human fetus actually is affected as a result of this apparent deprivation.

This review focuses on the cardiovascular effects of acute exercise on the mother and the possible effect of physical conditioning on maternal function.

CARDIOVASCULAR RESPONSE TO MATERNAL EXERCISE

The earliest investigations of maternal cardiovascular response to exercise were performed using a variety of different step tests (2). During the exercise bout (Table 16.1), attempts were made to measure several parameters noninvasively, such as heart rate, blood pressure, oxygen uptake, and respiratory capacity. These measurements gave the researchers some insights as to what to expect during exercise, but because maximal work capacity is difficult to attain using step testing procedures, the results were limited to inference about low level weight bearing submaximal exercise response. Further, due to the fact that testing is a weight-dependent exercise, interpretation of metabolic and circulatory response was very difficult. Although submaximal tests are of limited value in describing the possible circulatory responses at maximal exercise intensities, they do provide important information about oxygen cost of submaximal exercise. From steady-state submaximal data one can address the

Table 16.1. Cardiovascular Changes at Rest and During Various Work Intensities That Influence Exercise Capacity During Normal Pregnancy

Function	Nonpregnant	Pregnant	Percentage Difference
Blood volume (ml)	2500	3900	55
Heart volume (ml)			12
Heart rate (bpm)			
Rest	70	84	20
Submaximal exercise[a]	130	140	8
Maximal exercise	190	170–175	−7.5
Cardiac output (ml/min)			
Rest[b]	4500	6000	30
Submaximal exercise	10000	11400	−14
Stroke volume (ml/beat)			
Rest[c]	60–70	75–85	30
Submaximal exercise	85–95	85–95	0
A-V oxygen difference (ml/liter)			
Rest	45	40	−12
Submaximal exercise	100–110	80–90	−20
Maximal exercise	160–200		
Arterial pressure (systolic/diastolic mm/Hg)			
Rest	120/75	112/70	−5
Submaximal exercise	150/70	140/82	
Maximal exercise	180/80		
Systemic vascular resistance (dynes/sec/cm-5)	1700	1250	−30

[a]Submaximal exercise of approximately 3–4 METs.
[b]Greatest during midpregnancy.
[c]Greatest by the end of the second trimester.

issues of circulatory reserve and metabolic efficiency. Several investigators have reported metabolic data during submaximal bicycle ergometry with equivocal results. Widlund (2) found no significant differences in the metabolic cost or the oxygen debt incurred during low intensity exercise (step test) in his pregnant subjects. These results are surprising in view of the fact that the subjects were gaining weight. The possible implication is that pregnancy is associated with improved efficiency, at least during low intensity exercise. At the higher intensity, Widlund reported a 10% increase in oxygen cost and a 15% higher oxygen debt.

It is of relevance to analyze work efficiency in pregnancy in relation to the circulatory system. If the pregnant woman is more efficient in the use of oxygen, the circulatory demands associated with a given load may be lessened. As a result, many physiological changes that might lead us to interpret submaximal response to exercise as indicative of improved fitness may prove incorrect or at least misleading.

Using bicycle ergometers, a non-weight-dependent exercise, several investigators have reported an increase in oxygen cost of exercise in pregnancy and an increase in oxygen debt (3–5). As a result one must assume that the same amount of work in the pregnant woman represents a greater physiological stress than during nonpregnancy. Thus, we expect the circulatory system to adjust accordingly, that is, by increasing heart rate, blood pressure, and cardiac output for any given exercise task. However, the literature is not in universal agreement that this is the case.

Bader et al. (6) catheterized the right heart and pulmonary artery of 46 healthy pregnant women to observe hemodynamic changes during 10 min of supine exercise on a cycle ergometer. Intensity of exercise was not indicated, but the mean exercise heart rate (HR) of 108 beats/min (rest HR = 94) suggested a

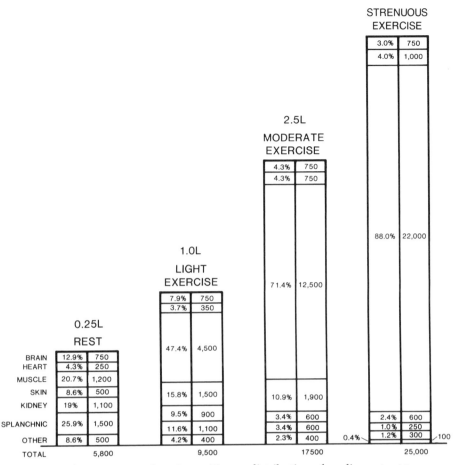

Figure 16.1.   Effects of exercise at various intensities on distribution of cardiac output to organ systems. (Adapted from Horvath SM. Diabetes 1979; 28 (Suppl):33–38.)

rather light exercise intensity. The authors concluded that the decrease in total peripheral resistance and the increase in cardiac output, arterial blood pressure, heart rate, and arteriovenous oxygen difference were all within normal limits for exercise of such intensity in nonpregnant women. The difficulty in interpreting these results relates to the lack of appropriate controls and the fact that the exercise intensity was at such a low level. Again, the failure to show a significant effect in cross-sectional research of this nature may relate to the fact that the general circulatory effects of pregnancy, that is, increased blood volume, reduced peripheral resistance and arterial blood pressure are effective at increasing the efficiency of the circulatory and metabolic response to exer-

cise during light activity. As the intensity increases the response may lead to an entirely different interpretation.

Rose et al. (7), employing the same subjects and exercise protocol as Bader et al. (6), calculated left ventricular work using cardiac output and mean brachial arterial pressure. Left ventricular work increased during exercise, but in subjects near term the increase was somewhat smaller. The authors concluded that because the increase in cardiac output was proportional to the increase in V_{O_2}, this relationship was normal; pregnancy effected no impairment of myocardial reserve during exercise. This was a cross-sectional study and did not attempt to extrapolate the observed effects to adaptations and requirements of pregnancy. Although our own studies suffer from some of the same design weaknesses, by using maximal exercise rather than low intensity exercise, our data suggest that pregnancy may impose a major detriment to maximal exercise tolerance.

More appropriate design strategies appeared in the late 1960s and employed longitudinal designs or, at least, compared pregnancy with a postpartum condition. In a longitudinal study throughout the duration of pregnancy, Dahlstrom and Irhman (8) measured the cardiorespiratory response and predicted maximal work capacity of pregnant and nonpregnant women performing cycle ergometry. Exercise heart rates at the lower intensity and heart rate recovery after all three exercise intensities increased as pregnancy progressed. Exercise heart rates at the higher intensities did not change and were similar to controls. As a result, the predicted maximal work capacity, which was the same for both groups, remained constant throughout the study. Maximal exercise capacity was not assessed.

Ueland et al. (9) measured cardiac output, heart rate, stroke volume, and arterial blood pressure of pregnant women at rest, during exercise, and after recovery by catheterization of the brachial artery and the antecubital vein. Exercise was performed on a cycle ergometer at light and moderate intensities. Heart rate ranges were 116–128 bpm (rest = 92) for light and 125–135 bpm (rest = 83) for moderate exercise intensities, increasing through pregnancy. The exercise-induced increase in cardiac output for moderate exercise decreased progressively throughout pregnancy. These investigators concluded that the increase in cardiac output was well within the normal limits for nonpregnant women, indicating no impairment in myocardial reserve during pregnancy; yet because of the smaller rise in cardiac output later in pregnancy, there may be a progressive decline in circulatory reserve most likely due to peripheral blood pooling. These findings suggest that submaximal exercise does in fact require a greater cardiac output for the pregnant woman and that the requirement for enhanced cardiac output to meet the demands of the exercise

may diminish in late pregnancy. This does not imply that the system responds better to stress in late pregnancy but that the process of homeostasis to adjust the maternal circulation to the needs of pregnancy has perhaps become more refined or permanent.

Morton and Metcalfe (10) provided further comment on the acute adjustment to exercise in pregnancy and presented some of their own results in the first edition of this text:

The enlarged heart of pregnancy might be ideally suited for exercise. Distance athletes also show significant cardiac enlargement (although with more hypertrophy) in response to training (22) [Ref. 11 this edition]. Bicycle exercise, when performed in the supine position during pregnancy, produces changes in cardiac output which parallel those observed at rest; the level of cardiac output achieved during standard exercise falls in the third trimester. Even with the active muscle pump and elevated legs, cardiac output during exercise achieves a value similar to that recorded in resting subjects early in the second trimester. This observation suggests two possible explanations; either the dilated heart of pregnancy is poorly suited to perform work at the higher arterial pressures characteristic of exercise, or venous return is so impeded in the supine position that the heart is continually "running dry," even during leg exercise.

Subsequent studies made during upright bicycle exercise suggests a better cardiac reserve. Guzman and Caplan (23) [Ref. 12 this edition] showed that maternal cardiac output at work loads of 150, 250, 350 kpm was increased throughout gestation. It is of interest that stroke volume at the highest work load was 77 ml near term compared with a nonpregnant value of 74 ml. Heart rate was higher throughout gestation at all work loads than corresponding control values. Ueland and colleagues (4) studied subjects at 100 and 200 kpm during upright bicycle exercise. At both work loads, cardiac output increased with exercise and was minimally increased or unchanged with respect to postpartum values: in agreement with Guzman and Caplan's findings, stroke volume fell progressively at both work loads as gestation advanced. Near-term values could not be distinguished from postpartum value; however, stroke volume fell progressively as gestation advanced, reaching values near term similar to those found postpartum.

We have recently begun to measure maternal cardiac output before, during and after exercise using impedance cardiography and echocardiography. Our preliminary data strongly suggest that impaired venous return restricts cardiac performance during upright bicycle exercise near term. The ability of the left ventricle to increase contractility during exercise appears to be normal in late gestation. Figure 16.2 shows cardiac output, heart rate, and stroke volume before, during and after 6 min of upright bicycle exercise at 50 watts (300 kpm)

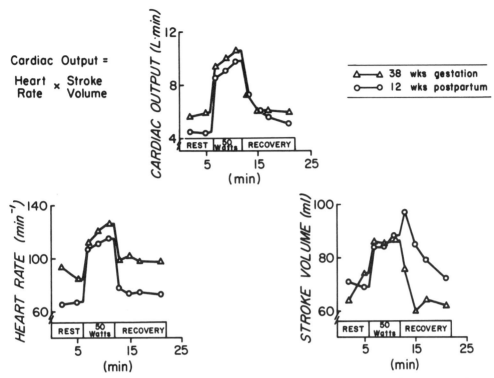

Figure 16.2.   Exercise hemodynamics at 38 weeks of gestation ($N = 9$). Cardiac output, heart rate, and stroke volume are shown in late gestation and postpartum during an upright bicycle exercise protocol. Stroke volume was determined by impedance cardiography.

intensity. Nine women were studied at 38 weeks of gestation and again 12 weeks postpartum. Steady-state values, both at rest and during exercise, are similar to those of Guzman and Caplan (23) [Ref. 12 this edition] and Ueland et al. (4). In late gestation, stroke volume during exercise is not significantly different from the postpartum value. The most striking finding is a precipitous drop in stroke volume when exercise stops in late gestation. We interpret this to mean that the leg muscle pump is crucial for maintenance of venous return during upright exercise in late gestation. Even with active pedaling, however, stroke volume in late gestation does not exceed postpartum levels. This is difficult to reconcile with the finding of a larger heart unless venous return in impeded, even during exercise. We do not believe that these findings can be attributed to a reduced contractile response to exercise. We are studying the problem with M-mode echocardiography (Fig. 16.3). Figure 16.4 shows left ventricular dimension and normalized dimension shortening (Delta D/D) obtained by echocardiography performed on one woman serially before and during pregnancy. A small increase in end-diastolic dimension is noted early in exercise except in the first trimester. The increase of fractional shortening in response to exercise remains stable throughout gestation. When exercise stops, end-diastolic dimension falls sharply, especially in the third trimester, these findings support

the concept that a restriction of venous return causes the reduction in stroke volume after exercise. The fact that the response of fractional shortening to exercise is normal throughout pregnancy is strong evidence that contractility is maintained during gestation (p. 117–120).

Summarizing the findings of Guzman and Caplan (12), one could conclude that, compared with postpartum values, oxygen uptake during non-weight bearing exercise remains essentially unchanged throughout pregnancy except for an increase at the lowest intensity. Stroke volume and cardiac output are also significantly higher throughout pregnancy but lower than postpartum levels. It was further concluded that the pregnant woman reaches her maximal exercise capacity at lower levels of exertion than in the nonpregnant state. One must be careful in accepting conclusions about maximal aerobic capacity in that there are no data published in the literature of responses to maximal exercise.

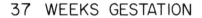

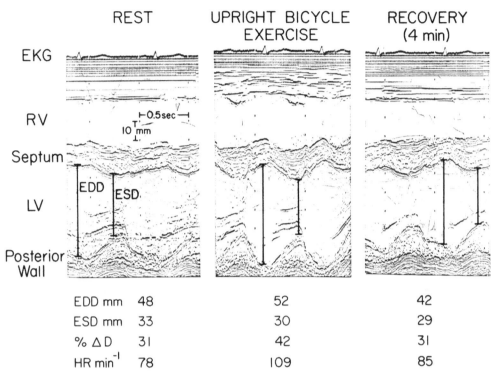

	REST	UPRIGHT BICYCLE EXERCISE	RECOVERY (4 min)
EDD mm	48	52	42
ESD mm	33	30	29
% ΔD	31	42	31
HR min^{-1}	78	109	85

Figure 16.3. M-mode echocardiograms of the left ventricle with the subject sitting on the ergometer at rest, during upright bicycle exercise, and during recovery. Measurements of end-diastolic *(EDD)* and end-systolic dimension *(ESD)* are indicated. Cardiac output is increased during exercise by increases in both EDD and percent shortening *(%ΔD)*. During recovery in this subject in late gestation, impaired venous return results in a marked reduction in EDD. This appears to be the mechanism for the reduced stroke volume after exercise that is shown in Figure 16.2.

CARDIOVASCULAR CONDITIONING IN PREGNANCY

There are two major statistical designs that have been employed in studying the effects of exercise training in pregnancy. The most common design found in the literature uses a cross-sectional comparison between either pregnant and nonpregnant subjects or between active pregnant versus inactive pregnant subjects. The obvious flaw in research of this nature relates to the ability to match subjects to eliminate the confounds of weight, activity level, or initial fitness status. A second design used in the literature is the longitudinal study. In research of this nature, a group of women are measured at sequential points during gestation and compared with either a prepregnancy or a postpregnancy level. It is obvious that the latter of these two statistical methodologies is preferable. Unfortunately, the longitudinal study is more time-consuming and requires a considerable commitment from the subject. As a result few well-controlled training studies employing a longitudinal design have reported.

The cross-sectional studies related to fitness that have been conducted using a comparison of pregnant with nonpregnant subjects (13–15) or fit (active) pregnant subjects compared with their sedentary pregnant counterparts (16–18) provide interesting information, yet inference from their results is difficult. In these studies the fit pregnant subjects have a similar response to acute exercise as fit nonpregnant subjects although the pregnant subjects are usually less fit than their nonpregnant control. Pregnant women

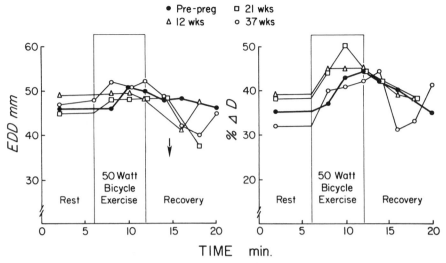

Figure 16.4.   Left ventricular end-diastolic dimension *(EDD)* and percent fractional shortening *(%ΔD)* are shown before and throughout gestation in one subject. The decrease in EDD that occurs after exercise during pregnancy is evident; so is the falling %ΔD that occurs after exercise in the 37th week of pregnancy.

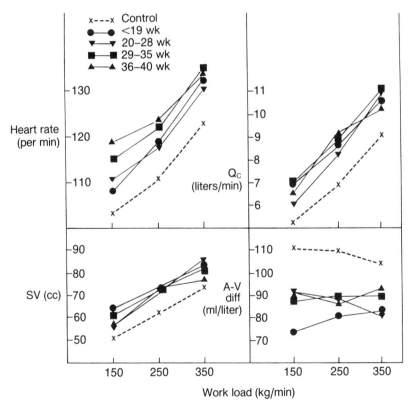

Figure 16.5.   Effects of pregnancy on heart rate, cardiac output *(Qc)*, stroke volume *(SV)* and A-V difference at 3 work loads. *Dotted lines* represent measurements in the nonpregnant state; *solid lines*, values during various stages of pregnancy. (From Guzman C, Caplan R. Am J Obstet Gynecol 108:600–605, 1970 (11).)

who demonstrate higher fitness also exhibited lower resting heart rates (16, 18), lower exercise heart rates at a submaximal intensity rate (16), higher predicted oxygen uptakes (16–18), greater stroke volume (18), and lower lactates at a submaximal intensity (17) than sedentary pregnant women. Resting and exercise blood pressures (16) and resting cardiac outputs (18) are not different.

Unfortunately, the results of these cross-sectional studies can be questioned. Two important assumptions required in interpreting exercise results have not been addressed, which leaves their results open to criticism. The first is the validity of the technique for measuring physical fitness or cardiovascular endurance. The second is the applicability of the measurement technique to a pregnant population.

The problem inherent in studies assessing physical fitness is the measurement of fitness itself (19). Maximal oxygen uptake ($\dot{V}_{O_2max}$) is the criterion measure of cardiovascular endurance (20). None of these studies actually measured this variable of fitness. The majority of studies predicted $\dot{V}_{O_2max}$ from submaximal tests (16, 17, 20, 21). Some estimated fitness by questionnaire (18, 22) or by interview (23). Even though Erkkola and Rauramo (17, 24) exercised subjects to maximal levels, they failed to collect gases and determine a valid measure of $\dot{V}_{O_2max}$ (25). Thus, these data are subject to criticism because the independent variable may not have been measured correctly.

Furthermore, the validity of a predicted $\dot{V}_{O_2max}$ for a pregnant population can be criticized. The basic assumption of these prediction methodologies is that maximal heart rates are predictable and unchanging during pregnancy. Some studies (26, 28) have demonstrated that maximal heart rates during pregnancy do not reach nonpregnant values and that the maximal heart rate during pregnancy cannot be predicted at this time. Thus, these studies further violate the basic assumption for the predicted $\dot{V}_{O_2max}$ that may not be a valid measurement for pregnant populations studies.

A question that has not been raised in the literature but must soon be addressed if we are to continue to study fitness variables relates to the validity of maximal exercise testing in the pregnant population. As stated in Chapter 12, several criteria must be met in order for a subject to have achieved $\dot{V}_{O_2max}$. There are only three studies in the literature that report $\dot{V}_{O_2max}$ data, and all can be criticized for not stating whether the criteria for $\dot{V}_{O_2max}$ was actually met. In one of these studies, maximal serum lactate levels have been reported to be very low. (27) This suggests that the 10-mmol concentration criteria for maximal exercise may not be possible in pregnancy, although, in about 35% of the subjects the maximal lactate levels exceeded the criterion value. Similarly, a plateauing in $\dot{V}_{O_2}$ was not reported in any of the three studies. It seems that the only true criterion that has been met by the subjects in these studies is that they reached volitional fatigue and could not continue with further exercise. These results, or lack of results, imply that maximal testing in pregnancy requires further validation. Until validity measures have been established to ensure that the maximal values reported are in fact maximal, the research community must interpret the result with caution. Furthermore, to our knowledge, there are no studies that have reported test-retest reliabilities in performing $\dot{V}_{O_2max}$ in pregnancy. The test-retest reliabilities of $\dot{V}_{O_2max}$ in pregnancy may be very low due to the physiological changes that occur with the passage of time, and they may give a misrepresentation of the true reliability coefficient.

Results of Physical Conditioning Programs

The studies utilizing a conditioning intervention (26–35) are more abundant than the population studies comparing physically fit women with sedentary women (16–18, 22–24, 36). In contrast to the latter studies, the focus of the conditioning studies is more on physical fitness than on pregnancy outcome (28, 30, 34, 37, 38). A summary of the exercise training studies during pregnancy are presented in Table 16.2.

The conditioning stimulus used in these studies was one that would have resulted in typical physiological changes in a nonpregnant population. However, the only changes

ble 16.2. Summary of the Cardiovascular Conditioning Studies During Pregnancy

| Investigators | Date | Subjects | | Mode | Frequency | Intensity | Duration | |
		Experimental	Control				Workout	Study
rman (31)	1960	26	46	Running, stride-strike- and star-jumping	2/wk[a]	HR 140/min	35 min	9 Weeks @ 20 to 30 wk of gestation
kola (29)	1976	31	31	Individual preference	3/wk	HR 140/min or onset of sweat	60 min	Last 28 wk of gestation
kola and Makela (30)	1976	23	21	Individual preference	3/wk	HR 140/min or onset of sweat	60 min	Last 28 wk of gestation
ollins et al. (28)	1983	12	8	Flexibility, cycle ergometry	3/wk	65–70% of capacity HR 152/min	25 min	7 to 19 wk
all and Kaufmann (37)	1987	82 low attendance 309 med 61 high	393	Weight training, cycle ergometry	3/wk	1 set 12 reps 300 kpm/min @ 85% max, <140 HR	45 min	Continuous
lpa et al. (38)	1987	38	47	Swimming, aerobics, jogging, walking, cross country skiing, racquetball	NS	75% of max HR	NS	Continuous
olfe et al. (35)	1987	16	8	Cycle ergometry	3/wk	70% of HR reserve	25 min	2nd and 3rd trimesters
ebb et al. (34)	1988	33	23	Cycle ergometry, muscle conditioning	3/wk	70% of HR reserve	25 min	2nd and 3rd trimesters
htake et al. 32, 33	1988	27	20	Cycle ergometry, muscle conditioning	3/wk	70% of HR reserve	25 min	2nd and 3rd trimesters
outh-Paul et al. (26)	1988	10	7	Conditioning, cycle ergometer	3/wk	60%–80% of max HR	60 min	20 wk to parturition

k, week; HR, heart rate; NS, not significant.

that were detected when comparing pregnant exercisers with pregnant control groups were a higher aerobic capacity (28, 30–32, 38), lower exercise heart rates (32, 35), lower exercise perceived exertion (32, 35), and greater heart volume (31) for pregnant women who exercise. These results were not consistent. Other investigators found no difference in exercise heart rates (26, 29, 31). The only investigator (26) who actually measured maximal oxygen uptake found no difference when compared with the control group, whereas the five other studies (28, 30–32, 38) that

predicted V_{O_2max} found changes. In addition, a second study found no change in heart volume for exercising women (30). All other variables measured demonstrated no differences between exercise and control groups of pregnant women.

The data from the cross-sectional studies differed from the longitudinal studies when similar variables were measured. Lower resting heart rates, which would be expected of more fit subjects, were reported in the population studies (16, 18) but not in the conditioning studies (26, 30–32, 35). Stroke volume was reported to increase in the study of Morton and associates (18), but not in the training study of Wolfe and associates (35). The most consistent finding from exercise intervention studies is an increase in the predicted aerobic capacity (16, 18, 28–32, 38); however, when maximal oxygen uptake was actually measured, it demonstrated no change (26). Table 16.3 summarizes the findings of the experimental trials on physical fitness variables.

SUMMARY AND CONCLUSIONS

It is difficult to draw conclusions from the present published literature because of study design and measurement problems. There needs to be good control over the exercise stimulus, supervision of the exercise sessions, adherence to the exercise program, and measurement of the confirmation of a change in exercise capacity. Population studies need to be larger in number of subjects. However, from the information provided, it can be concluded that as a result of physical conditioning in pregnancy, one could expect that:

1. Similar exercise intensities will be perceived as less strenuous in the conditioned subjects.
2. Exercise capacity, as estimated from submaximal performance, can increase as a result of training.
3. Submaximal exercise heart rates may be lower in trained pregnant subjects.
4. Low intensity training in pregnancy does not influence submaximal cardiac output or stroke volume.
5. There is no evidence that the low intensity training performed in these studies have any negative cardiovascular effects on the mother.

In summary, we have tried to provide a basic overview of the effects of acute exercise and/or the effect of conditioning during pregnancy on the cardiovascular system. The pregnant subject demonstrates a significant loss in cardiovascular reserve during gestation that seems to limit her ability to perform strenuous exercise. When training is imposed on the pregnant woman, she is able to improve cardiovascular function and to tolerate the exercise intervention. Exercise studies have employed very low intensity training regimens, and the value of these results may be minimal when trying to address the issue of high intensity training in pregnancy.

Table 16.3. Physiological Variables Measured in Response to Physical Conditioning in Pregnancy

No Difference	Changes with Conditioning
Skinfold thickness (32, 35)	
Maternal weight gain (32)	
	< RPE[a] at submax (32, 35)
Resting heart rate (31, 32, 35)	
Exercise heart rate (26, 29, 31)	< Exercise heart rates (32, 35)
Maximal heart rate (26)	
Cardiac output at submax (35)	
Stroke volume at submax (35)	
Resting blood pressure (29, 31)	
Orthostatic blood pressures (31)	
Exercise blood pressures (29)	
Hemoglobin (31)	
Total blood volume (31)	
Heart volume (30)	> Heart volume (31)
Resting metabolism (35)	
Oxygen uptake at submax (26, 35)	
Maximal oxygen uptake (26)	
	> Physical work capacity (28, 29, 31, 32, 38)
R.Q. at max and submax (26)	

[a]RPE, rating of perceived exertion, R.Q., respiratory quotient.

REFERENCES

1. deSweit M. The cardiovascular system. In: Hytten F, Chamberlain G, eds. Clinical physiology in obstetrics. Oxford: Blackwell Scientific Publications, 1980, p. 3–42.
2. Widlung G. Cardio-pulmonal function during pregnancy. Acta Obstet Gynecol Scand 25 (Suppl 1), 1945.
3. Seitchik J. Body composition and energy expenditure during rest and work in pregnancy. Am J Obstet Gynecol 1967; 97:701–713.

4. Pernoll M, J Metcalfe, T Schlenker, et al. Oxygen consumption at rest and during exercise in pregnancy. Respir Physiol 1975; 25:285–293.
5. Pernoll M, J Metcalfe, P Kovach, et al. Ventilation during rest and exercise in pregnancy and postpartum. Respir Physiol 1975; 25:295–310.
6. Bader R, M Bader, D. Rose, E Braunwald. Hemodynamics at rest and during exercise in normal pregnancy as studied by cardiac catheterization. J Clin Invest 1955; 34:1524–1536.
7. Rose D, M Bader, R Bader, et al. Catheterization studies of cardiac hemodynamics in normal pregnant women with reference to left ventricular work. Am J Obstet Gynecol 1956; 72:233–246.
8. Dahlstrom H, K Irhman. Clinical and physiological study of pregnancy in material from northern Sweden. V. The results of work tests during and after pregnancy. Acta Soc Med Upsal 1960; 65:305–314.
9. Ueland K, M Novy, E Peterson, et al. Maternal cardiovascular dynamics. VI. The influence of gestational age on maternal cardiovascular response to posture and exercise. Am J Obstet Gynecol 1969; 104:856–864.
10. Morton, MJ, J Metcalfe. Changes in maternal hemodynamics during pregnancy. In: Artal R, Wiswell RA, eds. Exercise in pregnancy. Baltimore: Williams & Wilkins, 1986, p. 113–126.
11. Morganroth, J, BJ Maron, WL Henry, SE Epstein. Comparative left ventricular dimensions in trained athletes. Ann Intern Med 1975; 82:521–524.
12. Guzman, CA, R Caplan. Cardiorespiratory response to exercise during pregnancy. Am J Obstet Gynecol 1970; 108:600–605.
13. Banerjee, B, KS Khew, N Saha. A comparative study of energy expenditure in some common daily activities on non-pregnant and pregnant Chinese, Malay and Indian women. J Obstet Gynecol Br Comm 1971; 78:113–116.
14. Erkkola, R. The physical fitness of Finnish primigravidae. Ann Chir Gynecol Fenniae 1975; 64:394–400.
15. Seitchik, J. Body composition and energy expenditure during rest and work in pregnancy. Am J Obstet Gynecol 1967; 97:701–713.
16. Dibblee L, Graham TE. A longitudinal study of changes in aerobic fitness, body composition and energy intake in primi graud patients. Am J Obstet Gynecol 1983; 147:908–914.
17. Erkkola R, Rauramo L. Correlation of maternal physical fitness during pregnancy with maternal and fetal pH and lactic acid at delivery. Acta Obstet Gynecol Scand 1976; 55:441–446.
18. Morton MJ, Paul MS, Campos GR, Hart MV, Metcalfe J. Exercise dynamics in late gestation: effects of physical training. Am J Obstet Gynecol 1985; 152:91–97.
19. LaPorte RE, Montoye HJ, Casperson CJ. Assessment of physical activity in epidemiologic research: problems and prospects. Pub Health Rep 100:131–146, 185.
20. Astrand PO, Rodahl K. Textbook of Work Physiology. Philadelphia: McGraw-Hill, 1985.
21. Wong SC, McKinzie DC. Cardiorespiratory fitness during pregnancy and its effect on outcome. Int J Sports Med 1987; 8:79–83.
22. Dale E, Mullinax KM, Bryan DH. Exercise during pregnancy: effects on the fetus. Can J Appl Spt Sci 1982; 7:98–103.
23. Clapp JF, Dickstein S. Endurance exercise and pregnancy outcome. Med Sci Sports Exer 1984; 16:556–562.
24. Erkkola R. The physical work capacity of the expectant mother and its effect on pregnancy, labor and the newborn. Int J Gynaecol Obstet 1976; 14:153–159.
25. Arstila M. Pulse-conducted triangular exercise-ECG test. Acta Med Scand (Suppl.) 1972; 529:29–39.
26. South-Paul JE, Rajagopal KR, Tenholder MF. The effect of participation in regular exercise program upon aerobic capacity during pregnancy. Obstet Gynecol 1988; 71:175–179.
27. Artal R, Khodiguian N, Rutherford S, Wiswell RA. Cardiopulmonary and metabolic responses to bicycle ergometry in pregnancy. Proc Soc Gyn Invest 1987.
28. Collings CA, Curet LB, Mullin JP. Maternal and fetal responses to a maternal aerobic exercise program. Am J Obstet Gynecol 1983; 145:702–707.
29. Erkkola R. The influence of physical training during pregnancy on physical work capacity and circulatory parameters. Scand J Clin Lab Invest 1976; 36:747–754.
30. Erkkola R, Makela M. Heart volumes and physical fitness of parturients. Ann Cin Res 1976; 8:15–21.
31. Ihrman K. A clinical and physiological study of pregnancy in a material form northern Sweden. VIII. The effects of physical training during pregnancy on the circulatory adjustment. Acta Soc Med Upsal, 1960; 65:335–347.
32. Ohtake PJ, Wolfe LA, Hall P, McGrath MJ. Physical conditioning effects on exercise heart rate and perception of exertion in pregnancy. Can J Spt Sci 1988; 13(3):71–73 P.
33. Ohtake PJ. Wolfe LA, Hall P, McGrath M. Ventilatory responses to physical conditioning during pregnancy. The physiologist 1988; 31:A158.
34. Webb KA, Wolfe CA, Tranmer JE, McGrath MJ. Pregnancy outcome following physical fitness training, Can J Spt Sci 1988; 13(3):98–94P.
35. Wolfe LA, Hall P, McGrath MJ, Burgffrat GW, Tranmer JE. Cardiovascular responses to physical conditioning during pregnancy. Can J Spt Sci 12:27P 2987.
36. Pomerance J, Lynch L, Lynch V. Physical fitness in pregnancy: its effect on pregnancy outcome. Am J Obstet Gynecol 1974; 119–867.
37. Hall DC, Kaufmann DA. Effects of aerobic and strength conditioning on pregnancy outcomes. Am J Obstet Gynecol, 1987; 157:1199–1203.
38. Kulpa PJ, White BM, Visscher R. Aerobic exercise in pregnancy. Am J Obstet Gynecol 1987; 156:1395–1403.

17

Maternal Exercise Performance and Early Pregnancy Outcome

James F. Clapp III

The goals of this chapter are first, to provide the reader with a working knowledge of some of the physiological adaptations to various types of exercise and to early pregnancy, and second, to use this information to assess the interaction between the two. The latter will include a theoretical and practical assessment of the effects of early pregnancy on maternal exercise performance as well as an assessment of the effects of exercise in early pregnancy on early pregnancy outcome.

PHYSIOLOGICAL ADAPTATIONS

As the physiological adaptations to both exercise and pregnancy are detailed elsewhere in this volume, only a few salient features will be discussed here. The exercise-induced perturbations of concern to the well-being of the conceptus in early pregnancy include: the redistribution of cardiac output; the rise in core temperature; the change in hormonal milieu; the type, intensity, and duration of the exercise; and the timing of the exercise in relation to the time course of the pregnancy. The pregnancy-associated perturbations that may have an impact on exercise performance include specific changes in metabolism; increased or hyperdynamic cardiorespiratory function; and, usually, a fairly marked change in an individual's sense of well-being.

Physiological Adaptations to Exercise

During exercise, there is a redistribution of cardiac output and regional blood flow away from visceral to muscular and cutaneous vascular beds. The magnitude of the flow redistribution increases linearly with an increase in the intensity of the exercise (1). As detailed elsewhere (2, 3), this may have a significant effect on the rate of utero-ovarian blood flow

with an estimated reduction of about 50% at usual training intensities. Theoretically, any embryonic effect of this reduction in oxygen and substrate delivery should be minimized by a balanced increase in tissue substrate extraction (4). However, some experimental data suggest that this may not be the case (3).

The increased energy expenditure associated with exercise results in an increase in core temperature the magnitude of which is again directly related to the intensity of exercise (5). Also, it is important to note that the slope of this relationship can be dramatically increased by environmental factors such as high ambient temperature and humidity (6). Thus, the core temperature increase of 1–1.5°C, routinely observed in female nonpregnant recreational runners under thermoneutral conditions (7), could easily exceed 2–2.5°C under environmental conditions that decrease the efficiency of heat dissipation. As a positive thermal gradient must exist between the conceptus and mother (8), an exercise-induced rise in maternal core temperature produces a similar rise in embryonic temperature that should exceed the absolute maternal temperature by 0.5–1.0°C during sustained physical activity.

The impact of exercise on the hormonal milieu is complex, and discussed in chapter 14. Suffice it to say that exercise induces an acute stress response in which catecholamines, prolactin, cortisol, endorphins, and glucagon increase while insulin and gonadotropins are decreased. Its effects on the sex steroid milieu are mixed due to its variable effects on clearance versus production and its more chronic effects on hypothalamic function. These changes are obviously further modified by a host of exercise variables. In any case, there is concern that these changes may alter the hormonal signaling responsible for successful implantation and the maintenance of uterine quiescence in early pregnancy.

The type, intensity, duration, and frequency of the exercise are important variables as they directly influence the magnitude and duration of the disruption in regional blood flow, thermal equilibrium, and hormonal milieu. The type of exercise is important because it determines the muscle mass involved and whether the activity is continuous or intermittent. The greater the muscle mass utilized, the greater the flow redistribution requirement, and continuous exercise requires unremitting adaptation without the opportunity for intermittent recovery (2). Thus, running and cross country skiing require well-defined and sustained physiological adaptation whereas the same is not true for most racquet and ball sports.

As stated earlier, under any defined set of conditions, the magnitude of the exercise-associated changes in regional flow and core temperature is directly dependent on exercise intensity, and the duration of the exercise obviously determines the overall duration of the change. The overall rhythm or frequency of an individual's exercise performance may also be an important exercise variable. For example, the organism may readily adapt to the chronic stimulus of a daily 45- to 60-min exercise routine whereas a biweekly or weekend regimen may, due to its intermittent nature and intensity, be a physiologically stressful experience.

The timing and frequency of the physiological adaptations to exercise in the timecourse of early pregnancy should theoretically influence any effects that they might have on early pregnancy outcome. For example, if they occurred in the preovulatory phase of the cycle of attempted conception, they could suppress ovulation or alternately induce a luteal phase defect followed by an early unrecognized loss. Conversely, if they occurred at a specific time point during organogenesis, they could induce a specific anatomical defect. Alternatively, the local effects of a diminution in blood flow and oxygen

availability might, like altitude, stimulate the process of placentation.

Physiological Adaptations to Early Pregnancy

Recent experimental data support the concept that early pregnancy is associated with extensive preparatory physiological changes that could influence both exercise performance and the physiological adaptations required by the exercise (9).

These serial studies demonstrate that fat deposition and significant weight gain occur early in the first trimester along with a striking increase in postprandial resting oxygen consumption and a fall in core temperature. These factors suggest that exercise efficiency should change early, requiring perhaps a greater exercise intensity for the same work load in early pregnancy. Interestingly, the opposite appears to be the case (10).

Hematocrit and the cardiovascular responses to both gravitational stress and exercise are altered in a fashion suggesting that relative hypovolemia is the norm in early pregnancy. In addition, minute ventilation at rest and during exercise is increased in very early pregnancy. Thus, the usual exercise-induced changes in heart rate and minute ventilation, used by most athletes to monitor exercise intensity, are radically altered at this time.

In early pregnancy, several symptoms often adversely affect an individual's sense of well-being. These include an overwhelming sense of fatigue and/or lassitude as well as semi-continuous feelings of nausea and/or gastrointestinal upset. These are said to be related to ill-defined changes in hormonal milieu and clearly may have an impact on exercise performance.

THE INTERACTION

Theoretical Considerations

As noted above, the physiological adaptations to exercise and early pregnancy interact in an additive fashion in at least three areas. These include a demand for regional redistribution of cardiac output, a demand for the dissipation of increased heat production, and an increased demand for oxygen and energy substrate.

REDISTRIBUTION OF BLOOD FLOW

In terms of flow redistribution, exercise induces redistribution away from the viscera to skin and skeletal muscle whereas early pregnancy is associated with maintenance of flow in all circulations with increases in renal, uterine, and perhaps splanchnic and skin blood flow (11). This difference, combined with the evidence of relative hypovolemia in early pregnancy, should magnify the inferred exercise-induced reduction in utero-ovarian blood flow. This flow limitation in substrate delivery to the conceptus could have adverse effects as, in animal models, flow reductions of this magnitude in early pregnancy have been associated with an adverse outcome (3). Likewise, if one accepts the unlikely assumption that the demands of the pregnancy override those of exercise, then a relative restriction in muscle blood flow could theoretically decrease exercise performance.

INCREASED HEAT PRODUCTION

Both early pregnancy and exercise increase metabolic rate and heat production. Thus, the combination of early pregnancy and exercise should generate more heat than the same exercise in the nonpregnant state. Theoretically, all else being equal, this should increase the absolute core and intrauterine temperature attained during exercise. As hyperthermia of 39.2°C or greater is believed to have possible teratogenic effects, this potential additive effect is of real concern in early pregnancy. As hyperthermia is also a limiting factor in peak exercise performance, this should be limited as well.

However, several pieces of information suggest that the thermal effect of exercise may actually be decreased in early pregnancy. First, the fact that both exercise and early pregnancy are associated with an increase in skin blood flow suggests that excessive flow redistribution to the skin may improve the ability to dissipate heat during exercise in early pregnancy. Second, the ob-

served early weight gain should increase thermal inertia by about 4%, which should buffer any rise in core temperature. Third, the observed fall in resting core temperature, along with the initial cooling effects from peripheral venous pooling, should also buffer the absolute temperature attained during exercise in early pregnancy (7, 9).

INCREASED NEED FOR SUBSTRATE

Both exercise and early pregnancy increase oxygen consumption and the need for energy substrate by different tissues. Thus, the combination of the two could limit the maximal availability of oxygen and other metabolic substrates for either purpose. However, given the limited mass of the products of conception in early pregnancy, it is unlikely that the availability of oxygen and nutrients in the intrauterine environment would be reduced to a critical level. Likewise, it is unlikely that the increased demands of the pregnancy at this stage would significantly affect oxygen and nutrient availability during a routine exercise regimen.

On the other hand, several lines of evidence suggest that the potential for nutrient compromise does exist. First, until the process of placental vascularization is complete, the conceptus is more subject to diffusional and gradient limitation of substrate availability than it is thereafter. Second, the combination of a sustained reduction in blood flow coupled with this diffusional limitation and the potential for a hypoglycemic response to exercise (7) could theoretically reduce substrate availability below a critical level. Third, experimental evidence in both the sheep and the guinea pig suggests that this may be the case (3).

CHANGE IN OVERALL ENERGY EXPENDITURE

An additional area where a potentially important interaction may occur is the opposite effects that exercise and pregnancy may have on an individual's sense of well-being and overall energy expenditure. On the one hand, a regular exercise program is said to improve a variety of biological functions and perceptions including productivity and overall activity as well as self-image and the sense of personal well-being. On the other, the fatigue and lassitude of early pregnancy coupled with gastrointestinal upset may alter the type, frequency, intensity, and duration of exercise performance as well as overall activity in order to maintain a sense of well-being. This potential combination theoretically could minimize any negative and emphasize any positive effects of exercise performance in early pregnancy.

Practical Observations

IMPACT OF EARLY PREGNANCY ON EXERCISE

Three earlier studies have assessed the impact of the physiological adaptation to early pregnancy on exercise performance (12–14). The initial study dealt exclusively with runners and was retrospective. It reported that all aspects of running performance measurable by recall were reduced in the first trimester. The second was prospective, dealt with runners, aerobic dancers, and cross country skiers, but used only two brief interviews (one at initial registration and one in the third trimester) to assess exercise performance. It reported that in approximately 60% of subjects, exercise performance was reduced in early pregnancy. The two principal reasons for this behavioral change were unanticipated fatigue and gastrointestinal upset. The third was prospective limited to runners, and exercise performance was carefully monitored in the 22 subjects. It reported that exercise performance in this small group of well-conditioned recreational runners decreased by only 10% in the first 4 postconceptional weeks of pregnancy. In the ensuing 4 weeks it fell somewhat further to 75% of preconceptional levels.

In a recent study (15), we have obtained prospective exercise performance data in 51 recreational runners, 17 aerobic dance instructors, and 28 aerobic dance participants before pregnancy and throughout the first trimester. Details of their preconceptional exercise regimens are given in Table 17.1. All of these women were physically fit, in excellent general health, and had engaged in a regular exercise program for a minimum of 2

Table 17.1.   Exercise Performance before Pregnancy[a]

Parameter	Runners	Parameter	Aerobic Dancers
Miles/wk	22	Classes/wk	4.4
	(12–55)		(3–11)
Intensity	68	Intensity	70
(% max)	(52–83)	(% max)	(55–88)
Time/wk	221	Time/wk	129
(min)	(93–397)	(min)	(90–330)
Pace	8:03		
(min/mi)	(6:30–9:50)		

[a]Data presented as the mean with the range given in parentheses. The data for aerobics includes only the high intensity portion of each session, which accounts for approximately 70% of the overall energy expenditure.

years before enrollment. To date, data regarding the impact of pregnancy on exercise performance are quite similar to those observed in the earlier limited study. The mean decrease in exercise performance in the first 4 weeks after conception averaged 14% in runners and 14% and 16% in the aerobic dance instructors and participants, respectively. In the second 4-week interval, it fell to 81% of preconceptional levels in the runners and to 85% of preconceptional levels in aerobic dance instructors and participants alike. It is of interest that individual performance over both time intervals was extremely variable and skewed to the left in both the recreational runners and the aerobic dance participants. In the runners, exercise performance ranged from 0 to 110% of preconceptional levels with seven women (15%) averaging less than 75%. In the aerobic dance group the range was from 0 to 104%, and 13 or 30% averaged less than 75% of preconceptional levels.

Again, the reasons for the reduction in overall exercise performance were primarily related to the symptoms of early pregnancy (fatigue and nausea). In three instances injury played a major role. In many instances, although overall performance was not reduced, individual concern over a rapid pulse rate and/or a feeling of breathlessness during exercise in early pregnancy caused a change in the quality of performance. Namely, it resulted in a voluntary decrease in exercise intensity coupled with an increase in exercise duration so that overall performance (intensity × duration) was either unchanged or slightly increased.

Thus, all available data support two tentative conclusions: first, that the physiological adaptation to early pregnancy has a defined impact on exercise performance in recreational runners, aerobic dancers, and cross country skiers; second, that there is an enormous degree of individual variation in the response ranging from a total cessation of exercise to a minimal increase in overall performance with a significant reduction in intensity and a marked prolongation of each exercise bout. Finally, it should be pointed out that these conclusions may not apply to numerous other types of physical activity and sport for which no data are currently available.

IMPACT OF EXERCISE ON EARLY PREGNANCY OUTCOME

Aside from data obtained in animal models, there are few objective data dealing with the effects of a variety of types of exercise on various aspects of early pregnancy outcome. Unfortunately, the potential bias produced by the stress of experimental circumstance itself, coupled with the known differences in cardiovascular and thermal regulation in these animal models, suggest that the animal data may not be relevant to the human condition (2). This concern, coupled with the suggestion that early wastage was increased in physically active women (11), leads us to begin the prospective study noted above (15). The study is specifically designed to examine the impact of various forms of significant (three times per week or more) recreational endurance exercise on four aspects of early pregnancy outcome. These include the inability to conceive, the incidence of abortion, the incidence of congenital malformations, and the occurrence of pregnancy events suggesting abnormalities of placentation.

To date, data available from the subjects noted above and a group of 35 controls matched for life-style and socioeconomic, morphometric, and obstetrical characteristics have not demonstrated any significant between-group differences in any of these outcome variables. The incidence of a failure of conception, defined as no documented conception in 6 months, is 5% in the exercise groups and 11% in the controls. Carefully documented (hCG done if menses 48 hours late followed by an ultrasound exam at 5.5 weeks conceptual age) early pregnancy loss has occurred in 17% of the conceptions of the recreational runners, in 19% of those of the aerobic dancers, and in 23% of those of the controls. In addition, no differences in the pattern of exercise performance have been observed between those who abort and those who carry to term during either the periconceptional period or early pregnancy. Details are presented in Table 17.2.

Only three congenital abnormalities have been seen at birth: a single case of hypospadias in the offspring of an aerobic dancer, webbing of the toes (present in three members of the family including the father) in the offspring of a runner, and a child with trisomy 21 born to a control subject. To date there have been no cases of ectopic pregnancy, placenta previa, placental abruption, or clinically diagnosed uteroplacental insufficiency in either the exercise or control groups. There have been two cases of clinically diagnosed mild pregnancy-induced hypertension without proteinuria. One occurred in an aerobic dancer, the other in a control subject. There have been five cases of preterm labor evenly distributed between the groups.

Thus, the data available do not support the hypothesis that the continuation of endurance types of antigravitational exercise in well-

Table 17.2.   Exercise Performance in the Cycle of Conception and Early Pregnancy by Exercise Type and Outcome[a]

Group	Follicular Phase	Weeks 1–4	Weeks 5–8
Runners			
Aborted (8)	88 ± 13	88 ± 16	83 ± 14
Term delivery (41)	94 ± 15	86 ± 20	80 ± 19
Dancers			
Aborted (8)	81 ± 20	80 ± 21	81 ± 22
Term delivery (35)	92 ± 27	87 ± 26	88 ± 25

[a]Data presented as the mean (±sd) percent of preconceptional exercise performance during the stated time interval. The numbers in parentheses indicate the number of subjects with a given pregnancy outcome.

conditioned women at levels at or near pre-conceptional levels have a significant impact on these four indices of early pregnancy outcome. Given the theoretical concerns discussed earlier, the interesting question, which is currently under investigation, is why. Finally, it must be pointed out that the data discussed above only apply to a highly select group of women and, as they all are volunteers, selection bias may be a confounding factor. Therefore, although this data is reassuring, the same may not be true for other types of physical activity or for a different group of women.

SUMMARY

In summary, the interaction between the physiological adaptations to exercise and early pregnancy are complex and suggest that they should have an impact on one another. Objective data to support this concern is sparse. The data currently available indicate that several types of commonly performed antigravitational exercise are not associated with evidence of an adverse early pregnancy outcome in a select populace and that early pregnancy appears to minimally modulate exercise performance.

REFERENCES

1. Rowell LB. Human cardiovascular adjustments to exercise and thermal stress. Physiol Rev 1974; 54:75–159.
2. Clapp JF. The effects of exercise on uterine blood flow. In: Rosenfeld CR, ed. The uterine circulation. Ithaca, Perinatology Press, 1989, p. 300–310.
3. Clapp JF. The effects of maternal exercise during pregnancy on uterine blood flow and pregnancy outcome. In: Moawad AH, Lindheimer MD, eds. Uterine and placental blood flow. New York, Masson Press, 1982, p. 177–184.
4. Clapp JF. The relationship between blood flow and oxygen consumption in the uterine and umbilical circulations. Am J Obstet Gynecol 1978; 132:410–413.
5. Saltin, B, Hermansen L. Esophageal, rectal and muscle temperature during exercise. J Appl Physiol 1966; 21:1757–1762.
6. Rowell LB. Cardiovascular aspects of human thermoregulation. Circ Res 1983; 52:367–379.
7. Clapp JF, Wesley M, Sleamaker RH. Thermoregulatory and metabolic responses to jogging prior to and during pregnancy. Med Sci Sports Exerc 1987; 19:124–130.
8. Abrams RM, Caton D, Clapp JF, Barron DH. Thermal and metabolic feature of life in utero. Clin Obstet Gynecol 1970; 13:549–564.
9. Clapp JF, Seaward BL, Sleamaker RM, Hiser J. Maternal physiological adaptations to early human pregnancy. Am J Obstet Gynecol 1988; 159:1456–1460.
10. Clapp JF. Oxygen consumption during treadmill exercise before, during and after pregnancy. Am J Obstet Gynecol 1989; 16:1458–1464.
11. Metcalfe J, Stock MK, Barron DH. Maternal physiology during gestation. In: Knobil E, Neil J, eds. The physiology of reproduction. New York, Raven Press, 1988, p. 2145–2176.
12. Dale E, Mullinax KM, Bryan DH. Exercise during pregnancy: effects on the fetus. Can J Appl Sports Sci 1982; 7:98–102.
13. Clapp JF, Dickstein S. Endurance exercise and pregnancy outcome. Med Sci Sports Exerc 1984; 16:556–562.
14. Clapp JF, Wesley M. Selective aspects of pregnancy outcome in recreational runners. Proc Soc Gynecol Invest Abst no. 129, 1987.
15. Clapp JF. The effects of maternal exercise on early pregnancy outcome. Am J Obstet Gynecol 1989; 161:1453–1457.

18

Fetal Responses to Maternal Exercise

Raul Artal Mittelmark and Marvin D. Posner

Over recent years, recognition of various fetal heart rate (FHR) patterns has provided the obstetrician with a most valuable tool in assessing fetal well-being. Typical changes in FHR patterns are known to reflect hypoxic and nonhypoxic stress, hypoxia or asphyxia, and sympathetic and parasympathetic activity. The significance and pathophysiology of such changes are described in detail in Chapter 7.

Exercise induces significant cardiovascular changes of which the selective redistribution of blood flow to the working muscles away from the splanchnic organs has the most potentially adverse effects on the fetus. It is recognized that uterine blood flow could be compromised during exercise as reported in both human and animal studies, though reports to the contrary have also been published (1–5). Reduction of blood flow to the uterus could lead to fetal hypoxia and to asphyxia; to cause such changes, the reduction in uterine blood flow should be in excess of 50%. Such circumstances may result in decreased O_2 tension and an increase in CO_2 tension (respiratory acidosis) (6). In the normal healthy pregnant woman, such occurrences should be only rarely encountered during mild and moderate exercise, but they are more likely to occur during strenuous and prolonged exercise.

It appears that the healthy fetus can tolerate brief periods of asphyxia, such as those that may occur during limited periods of maternal exercise. Initially, the fetus will respond to such events with tachycardia and an increase in blood pressure. This appears to be a protective mechanism for the fetus to facilitate circulation of more blood, which will increase the O_2 and decrease the CO_2 tension.

As discussed in Chapter 14, maternal exercise is associated with a significant increase in circulating catecholamines. Due to a high concentration of enzymes (catechol-*o*-methyl transferase and monoamino-oxidase) the placenta metabolizes the catecholamines very efficiently and, under normal conditions, only 10–15% of the catecholamines in maternal circulation reach the fetus. Elevated catecholamines could have an additional restrictive effect on the fetal circulation. The combined effect of reduced blood flow to the uterus and vasoconstriction secondary to elevated catecholamines could lead to fetal asphyxia and bradycardia. Such a possibility is more than a theoretical consideration, but it is not currently known how often it occurs.

In Table 18.1 we have summarized the published literature on FHR responses to maternal exercise. Because of the different methodology utilized in these studies, comparison and interpretation of data must be done with great caution. It appears that, by and large, the FHR response to maternal exercise is associated with an increase of approximately 10–30 beats per minute. Our own studies (19) indicate that such changes are consistent and are independent of either gestational age or intensity of maternal exercise. Figures 18.1–18.3 illustrate schematically the changes in fetal heart rates after mild maternal exercise (approximately 2.5 METs), moderate exercise (approximately 5 METs), and strenuous exercise (approximately 8 METs) as observed in 45 patients. Immediately after and within 5 min of exercise, the FHR remained elevated in most of the subjects with every type of exercise. Within 15 min, the FHR returned to pre-exercise values in the subjects enrolled in the mild and moderate exercise studies, whereas in the strenuous exercise (V_{O_2max})group, the FHR remained elevated for at least 30 min.

To date, published data on FHR responses to maternal exercise include 546 subjects. In 49 subjects, fetal bradycardia was reported to occur during or after exercise, an incidence

Table 18.1. Fetal Heart Rate (FHR) Responses to Maternal Exercise[a]

Author	Sample Size	Population	Gestational Age (weeks)	Monitoring Device	Type of Exercise	Intensity of Exercise	FHR During Exercise	FHR After Exercise
Hon and Wohlgemuth (7)[a]	26	Mixed	34–41	Abdominal ECG	Master step test	Moderate	NA	= ↑ ↓
Soiva et al. (8)[b]	24	Mixed	28–40	Phonocardiograph	Bicycle ergometer	Mild, moderate strenuous	NA	= ↑ ↓
Hodr and Brotanek (9)[c]	56	Mixed	29–36	Phonocardiograph	Master step test	Moderate	NA	= ↑ ↓
Stembera and Hodr (10)[d]	67	Mixed	38–40	Phonocardiograph	Master step test	Moderate	NA	= ↑ ↓
Pokorny and Rous (11)[e]	14	Mixed	36–40	Phonocardiograph	Bicycle ergometer	Mild	= ↑	= →
Pomerance et al. (12)[f]	54	Normal	35–37	Auscultation	Bicycle ergometer	Moderate	NA	→ ↑
Eisenberg de Smoler et al. (13)[g]	22	Mixed	28–40	Abdominal ECG	Master step test; treadmill	Moderate	NA	= →
Pernoll et al. (14)[h]	16	Mixed	24–40	Doppler U/S[m]	Bicycle ergometer	Mild	NA	← →
Sibley et al. (15)[i]	7	Normal	17–40	Doppler U/S	Swimming	Strenuous	↑	=
Dale et al. (16)[j]	4	Normal	31–37.5	Doppler U/S	Treadmill	Strenuous	→	=
Hauth et al. (17)[k]	7	Normal	28–38	Doppler U/S	Jogging	Moderate	NA	←
Collings et al. (18)[l]	20	Normal	22–34 ±	Doppler U/S	Bicycle ergometer	Strenuous	↑	←
Artal et al. (19)	15	Normal	35.1 ± 5.65	Doppler U/S	Treadmill	Mild	↑	←
Artal et al. (19)	15	Normal	34.7 ± 4.31	Doppler U/S	Treadmill	Moderate	↑ →	← →
Artal et al. (19)	15	Normal	34.1 ± 6.85	Doppler U/S	Treadmill	V_{O_2max}	↑	← →

Study	n	Status	Gestational age	Method	Exercise	Intensity	Response	FHR
Pipers et al. (20)	28	Normal	35.6	Doppler U/S	Semirecumbent cycling	Moderate	NA	=
Clapp (21)	6	Normal	20 and 32	Doppler U/S	Treadmill	Moderate-Strenuous	NA	↑
Jovanovic et al. (22)	6	Normal	36–38.5	Doppler U/S	Cycling	Moderate	↓	↑
Veille et al. (23)	10	Normal	33 ± 3	Doppler U/S	Walking	Moderate-Strenuous	NA	↑
Veille et al. (23)	10	Normal	37 ± 1	Doppler U/S	Cycling	Mild-moderate	=	=
Rauramo (24)	61	Mixed	32–40	Doppler U/S	Bicycle ergometer	Mild	NA	↓
Paolone et al. (25)	4	Normal	28–34	M-Mode echo-cardiograph	Bicycle ergometer and treadmill	Mild-moderate	=	=
Carpenter et al. (26)	45	Normal	20–34	Linear array 2-dimension U/S	Bicycle ergometer	Mild, moderate-strenuous	=	↓ =
Wolfe et al. (27)	12	Normal	37.8 ± 0.6	Doppler U/S	Isometric hand grip	Mild-moderate	=	=
Artal et al. (unpublished)	2	Normal	40 (labor)	Direct fetal scalp monitoring	Bicycle ergometer	Moderate	=	=

a ↑ Increase in FHR baseline; =, minimum or no change in FHR; ↓ bradycardia; PIH, pregnancy-induced hypertension; DM, Diabetes mellitus; NA, not available.
a 10 healthy pregnant, five PIH, two essential hypertension, two DM.
b 13 healthy pregnant, five postdates, 11 PIH (pregnancy-induced hypertension).
c 50 healthy pregnant, six premature labor.
d 15 healthy pregnant, 52 (unspecified number of PIH, postdates, DM, poor OB history).
e 12 healthy pregnant, one PIH, one DM.
f 54 healthy pregnant.
g 18 healthy pregnant, two severe PIH, two fetal CNS anomalies.
h Eight healthy pregnant, one twins, one heart disease, one drug addict, five obese.
i Seven healthy pregnant.
j Four healthy pregnant athletes.
k Seven healthy pregnant athletes.
l 20 healthy pregnant.
m U/S, ultrasound.

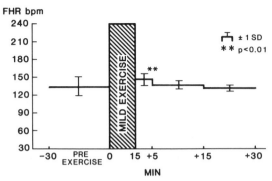

Figure 18.1. Fetal heart rate responses to mild maternal exercise. (From Artal R, et al. Fetal heart responses to maternal exercise. Am J Obstet Gynecol 1986; 155(4):729–733.)

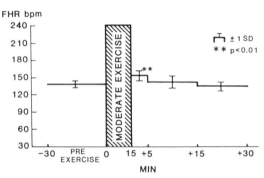

Figure 18.2. Fetal heart rate responses to moderate maternal exercise. (From Artal R, et al. Fetal heart responses to maternal exercise. Am J Obstet Gynecol 1986; 155(4):729–733.)

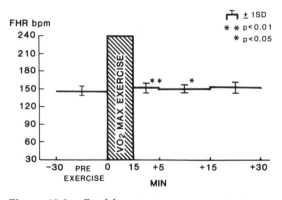

Figure 18.3. Fetal heart rate responses to strenous (Vo_2) maternal exercise. (From Artal R, et al. Fetal heart responses to maternal exercise. Am J Obstet Gynecol 1986; 155(4):729–733.)

of 8.9%. Although 11 of the subjects who experienced bradycardia had an abnormal pregnancy (pregnancy-induced hypertension and premature labor), the other subjects were normal.

Recording of FHR during exercise is technically very difficult. Nevertheless, there are a few reports of such recordings (11, 15, 16, 18, 22, 25–28). By and large, the recordings obtained during exercise indicate an increase in FHR over the pre-exercise baseline. In 151 recorded cases obtained during exercise, fetal bradycardia was recorded in only 29 cases (an incidence of 19.2%). Six of the 29 cases were normal patients and completed their pregnancy successfully.

Figures 18.4–18.6 illustrate FHR recordings with episodes of bradycardia during and immediately after maternal exercise (28). These recordings, although not continuous during the exercise testing, have been chosen for publication because they illustrate unique and confirmatory information obtained in our laboratory, such as fetal bradycardia emerging from the exercise period and continuing into the recovery period (28). The FHR tracing in these cases remained identical during and after exercise. It is not yet clear whether brief episodes of fetal bradycardia are common during maternal exercise and the mechanism by which they are triggered can only be a subject of speculation.

It appears very likely that a reduction in uterine blood flow, accompanied by elevated catecholamines, leads to brief periods of fetal asphyxia that are generally well tolerated by the majority of fetuses. The initial response is tachycardia, but with prolonged hypoxia and vagal stimulation, it results in bradycardia.

Another possibility is that such occurrences are within the realm of normal fetal reflex responses to major maternal hemodynamic and hormonal events. This latter explanation could explain those cases in which fetal bradycardia occurs as soon as the subject begins to exercise.

Fetal bradycardia is a relatively rare event that by and large reflects fetal distress. Fetal bradycardia has been linked to cord compres-

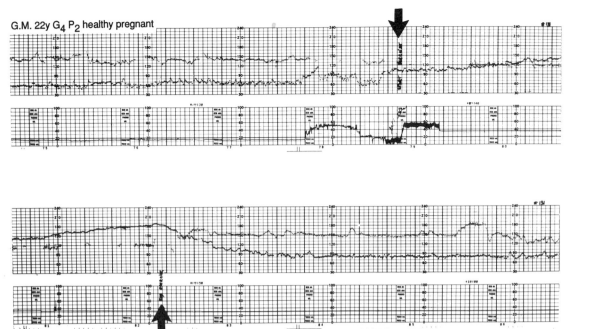

Figure 18.4.   Case 1: Fetal bradycardia during and after strenuous maternal exercise (panels 79–82). In panels 75–77 and 83–86, the upper tracings are fetal heart rates and the lower tracings are maternal heart rates. In panels 79–82, the upper tracings are maternal heart rates, the lower tracings are fetal heart rates.

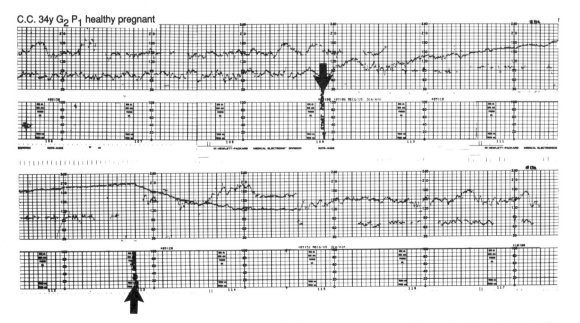

Figure 18.5.   Case 2: Fetal bradycardia during and after strenuous maternal exercise (panels 109–113). In panels 106–109 and 115–117, the upper tracings are fetal heart rates and the lower tracings are maternal heart rates. In panels 110–113, the upper tracings are maternal heart rates, the lower tracings are fetal heart rates.

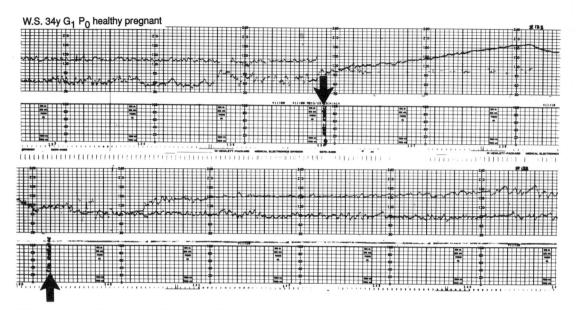

Figure 18.6. Case 3: Fetal bradycardia after strenuous maternal exercise (panels 137–139). In panels 133–136 and 141–145, the *upper tracings* are fetal heart rates, *lower tracings* are maternal heart rates. In panels 137–139, the *upper tracings* are maternal heart rates, the *lower tracings* are fetal heart rates.

sion, uterine hyperactivity and tetany, and congenital cardiac lesions and arrhythmias. A variety of other rare causes have been described such as paracervical anesthesia or other drug administration to the mother. In most of the cases in which fetal bradycardia was recorded in conjunction with maternal exercise, the bradycardia was moderate—100–119 bpm. Such bradycardia in labor has been described as a physiological response to a continuous stimulus with no association to fetal or neonatal hypoxia (29). One suggested mechanism is head compression due to cephalopelvic disproportion with malposition. Certainly exercise may lead to temporary malposition of the fetal head. It remains to be determined whether this is the case and, if so, does cephalic or breech presentation have a higher incidence of this transient event during exercise. No linkage has been reported between fetal bradycardia and maternal exercise. Some of the reported cases of fetal bradycardia may be erroneous and linked to artifacts (25, 28). The new generation of FHR monitors use autocorrelation methods; though they often produce excellent FHR tracings, such devices can be deceptive as they sometimes record other periodic movements that could be generated during walk-

ing or jogging. Nevertheless, the reality is that fetal bradycardia occurs with an unknown frequency, and it is important to point out that severe bradycardia (fetal heart rates below 100 bpm) were reported to occur after maternal exercise in 16.2% of subjects enrolled in one maximal exertion study (26). These reports have generated significant concerns, primarily because of the inability to predict when and who may experience an adverse fetal event and what may be the consequences. The major concern is that maternal exercise could compromise uterine blood flow and result in fetal hypoxia, as reflected in the typical fetal heart rate changes. Due to the inaccessibility of the fetus, validation of such events could ultimately be obtained only with direct internal fetal heart rate monitoring (unpublished data) or two dimensional ultrasound (25, 26). In a pilot study (unpublished), we have obtained such recordings during maternal exercise in labor (Figs. 18.7 and 18.8). The subjects were tested while in labor and volunteered to perform a submaximal exercise test. At cervical dilatation of 4 cm, amniorexis was performed and fetal scalp electrodes were applied for continuous and direct FHR monitoring. The patients engaged in a bicycle ergometry incremental exercise

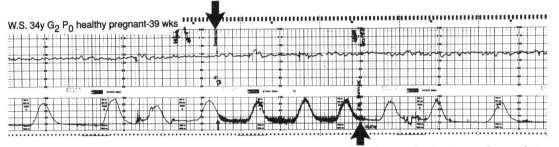

Figure 18.7.   Intrapartum recordings of FHR and uterine activity. *Arrows,* beginning and completion of exercise.

to approximately 60% of their last known maximal aerobic capacity. The exercises lasted 3.4 and 3.8 min. The FHR patterns before, during, and after the exercise routine did not change in these two cases. It is important to note that both mothers were athletes and engaged throughout pregnancy in frequent and strenuous physical activities. One subject averaged 20–30 miles of cycling a day, and the second individual was a physical educator who also engaged in strenuous activities. During their pregnancies they benefited from close obstetrical supervision and frequent fetal monitoring, and they had uncomplicated pregnancies. Both delivered spontaneously and vaginally at term and the birthweights were 2660 and 2950 g, respectively. The low birthweights are probably a reflection of impaired transplacental transfer of nutrients due to strenuous maternal exercise through pregnancy. At follow-up at 1 and 4 years of age, both infants were developing well. Though these observations involve two cases only, they are unique. They are the first known direct recordings of fetal heart rates during exercise in labor. One could expect that the combined effect of uterine activity during labor with maternal exertion would limit uterine perfusion and expose pla-

cental reserves, or lack of placental reserves. The observation made during this pilot study is that healthy infants of healthy mothers can tolerate intermittent periods of maternal exercise through pregnancy and even short periods of exertion during labor. It is conceivable that these fetuses were well conditioned and adapted to periods of exercise-induced hemodynamic shifts and did not respond with the obvious signs of distress reflected in heart rate patterns. It may also be that brief submaximal exercise has little effect on placental blood flow as demonstrated in a study that measured placental blood flow with the xenon technique during a submaximal exercise routine (30).

This finding is supported by studies indicating that the fetus is capable of maintaining aortic blood flow during moderate bradycardia (31). Similar interactions between fetus and mother are discussed in the next sections.

Doppler Velocimetry During Maternal Exercise

Doppler velocimetry has been used for a number of years now as a noninvasive technique to evaluate placental resistance. The majority of studies have described the effect

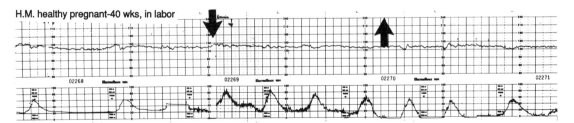

Figure 18.8.   Intrapartum recordings of FHR and uterine activity. *Arrows,* beginning and completion of exercise.

of various clinical conditions during pregnancy on the velocity-time waveform.

The principles of Doppler velocimetry involve the frequency shift of a known sound wave caused by a stream of moving particles. Red blood cells moving toward the transducer beam are recorded as higher frequencies, and red blood cells moving away from the transducer are recorded as lower frequencies as compared with the original beam. The frequency shift or difference (Fd) is expressed according to the following equation:

$$Fd = 2 \, (foV \, Cos \, O/c)$$

where fo is the frequency of the insonated beam, V is the velocity of the red blood cells, O is the angle of insonation, and c is the speed of sound in tissue (a constant of 1540 m/sec). If we rearrange the equation to solve for V:

$$V = c \, Fd/2 \, fo \, Cos \, 0.$$

The results of the calculations are dependent on the angle of insonation. The true velocity is, therefore, not measured without knowledge of the angle between the blood vessel and the sound beam (i.e., pulsed wave Doppler).

From the practical point of view, we limit our examination to the velocity-time waveform. The relationship most widely analyzed is the peak systolic to peak end diastolic ratio (S:D or A:B) (Fig. 18.9). In most cases (i.e., continuous wave Doppler), the angle is unknown. Being a ratio, this term is independent of the angle of insonated sound waves. Because each artery has its own characteristic appearance, the velocity-time waveform can be obtained without an actual B-mode image of the artery.

Doppler velocimetry has been used in several studies to describe the effects of maternal exercise on the maternal uterine artery and the fetal umbilical artery blood flow resistance. Comparison of the S:D ratio derived from the maternal uterine artery velocity waveform pre- and 3 min postmoderate exercise did not differ. Eleven patients at 16 to 26 weeks' gestation (32) exercised on a stationary bicycle to achieve a maternal heart rate of 60–75% of maximal heart rate. None of the women became exhausted during the exercise routine. It was concluded that moderate, nonstrenuous bicycle exercise is not associated with changes in uterine artery waveforms as measured by continuous wave Doppler ultrasound.

In another study performed near term (36–41 weeks) the ratio of S:D before and within 2 min after exercise did, however, differ (33). In this study, pregnant women exercised at

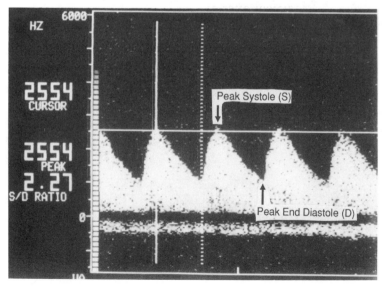

Figure 18.9.   Normal blood flow velocity wave form at term gestation obtained from the umbilical artery.

20 watts for 5 min. Two minutes after the exercise the S:D ratios did return to pre-exercise values.

The same study also evaluated waveforms from the fetal umbilical artery and reported an elevation in fetal heart rate in the postexercise phase coupled with no significant changes in umbilical S:D ratio. This lack of change was observed for 20 min postexercise.

Similar findings were reported in other studies in which measurements of S:D ratios from the fetal descending aorta were not significantly altered by a mild exercise at 25 watts (20).

In another study, 18 women in the last half of gestation were evaluated with Doppler velocimetry of the umbilical artery after exercise to 85% of their maximal heart rate (34). The results indicated no significant change in S:D ratio after the exercise. Of note, however, was a significant increase in the S:D ratio in three of the women for the first 1 min after exercise. The authors attributed the change to an increase in fetal heart rate in two fetuses and, in the third, in whom the increase lasted 5 min, no explanation could be given.

The major shortcoming of all studies using Doppler velocimetry to evaluate the effect of maternal exercise on arterial waveforms is the fact that all measurements are taken either immediately before or immediately after an exercise routine. Due to obvious technical restrictions, recordings are difficult, if not impossible, to obtain during the actual exercise periods. Any resistance changes within the various vessels during maternal exercise may return to pre-exercise baseline values immediately after exercise, and thus the changes, if any, could be missed. Furthermore, fetal activity (i.e., body and breathing movements), which produce difficult waveforms for analysis, presents another problem with this research tool.

FETAL ACTIVITY AND MATERNAL EXERCISE

The interactions between the fetus and mother compose a fascinating, but often poorly understood, relationship. The introduction of additional indexes to assess fetal well-being constitutes a further refinement of this process.

Fetal behavior, movements, and breathing have been extensively researched in recent years. Such parameters have been incorporated into a fetal biophysical profile that appears to identify accurately more than 85% of anomalous factors leading to fetal asphyxia, distress, and death (35).

Hypoxia appears to affect significantly, i.e., to reduce, the frequency of fetal breathing and body movements. Fetal breathing movements (FBM) are episodic and occur approximately 30% of the time during the last trimester of pregnancy. FBM occurrence appears to be related to the stage in gestation, time of day, and maternal plasma glucose and catecholamine levels. Some investigators have suggested that measurements of FBM may be a more sensitive indicator of fetal state than is FHR (36). Furthermore, it has been suggested that irregular FBM occur during increased long-term FHR variability and regular FBM occur during decreased long-term FHR variability (37).

Another component of the fetal biophysical profile is fetal movements (FM). FM also appear to reflect fetal conditions closely and, as such, are utilized for both research and clinical surveillance (38, 39). FM occur on an average of 5–20% of each hour.

Fetal activity during and after maternal exercise has been studied very little. One study reported a transient increase in the incidence of FBM after brief moderate maternal exercise. In addition, the same study demonstrated a greater responsiveness of FBM to exercise when compared with FHR (40).

Recognizing the existence of significant responses by the maternal sympathoadrenal system to exercise in pregnancy (41), we have studied its interactions with FBM and FM (42). The results of this study are illustrated in Figure 14.7. In this study, we have demonstrated a direct relationship between the level of sympathetic activity in the mother and the incidence of FBM and FM after maternal exercise. The results suggest that catecholamine levels may alter glucose levels and, as such, lead to an increase or decrease in FBM; such correlations have been previously recognized (43). In addition, the data also suggest fetal well-being and, as such, could be readily utilized to confirm such status. Fetuses of hypertensive mothers suspected to be distressed have a decrease in FBM after maternal exercise and so do hypoxic fetuses and fetuses monitored immediately before and during labor.

LONG-TERM EFFECTS OF MATERNAL EXERCISE ON THE FETUS

The existing published data suggest that maternal exercise may have brief or lasting effects on the fetus. Although most of the interactions between maternal exercise and the fetus may be transitory, questions remain as to the long-lasting effects on the fetus.

Of much relevance and concern is the fact that with exercise the body core temperature may increase to levels that could have teratogenic effects. Such effects have to be evaluated with extreme caution since it appears that maternal body temperature is modulating the fetal temperature (44), and most of the fetal heat is transferred across the placenta to the mother (45) and, as such, could reach significant elevations in the fetus. The data derived from studies conducted in research animals strongly indicate that exposure in early gestation to temperatures in excess of 39°C is teratogenic and frequently results in neurotubal defects (46–48). The published information in the human is less convincing since it has been collected among individuals at risk for malformations (49–51) and the only prospective study conducted among 165 women exposed to first trimester fever has failed to confirm such findings (52). Nevertheless, until a confirmatory study is done, we must exercise caution and limit exposure to hyperthermia in the first trimester of pregnancy. For additional information see Chapter 23.

Though most of the time it is very difficult to distinguish between the various parameters leading to reduced birthweight and intrauterine growth retardation (IUGR), strenuous exercise in pregnancy could have such an adverse effect on the fetus. It has been recognized for a long time that infants of

working mothers do have decreased birthweight by as much as 400 g (53–55). It also appears that pregnant laboratory animals that are forced to exercise strenuously also deliver smaller offspring (56, 57).

Anecdotal reports of similar effect have been reported in the human, and a larger study has determined that women who continued strenuous exercise through pregnancy gained less weight and delivered earlier (by 8 days), and their infants had a consistently reduced birthweight (by approximately 500 g) (58). These reports must be interpreted with caution, yet they alert us to the possible complications.

Consequently, pregnant women who do engage in strenuous exercise should be carefully monitored for developing complications and should exercise only under medical supervision. Monitoring the interactions between mother and fetus during and after exercise could serve not only as a research tool but also may be incorporated as a clinical aid for fetal surveillance.

REFERENCES

1. Lotgering KR, Gilbert RD, Longo LD. Exercise responses in pregnant sheep: oxygen consumption, uterine blood flow and blood volume. J Appl Physiol 1983; 55:834.
2. Chandler JCD, Bell AW. Effects of maternal exercise on fetal and maternal respiration and nutrient metabolism in the pregnant ewe. J Dev Physiol 1981; 31:161.
3. Clapp JF. Acute exercise stress in the pregnant ewe. Am J Obstet Gynecol 1980; 136:489.
4. Curret LB, Ott JA, Rankin JHG, Ungerer T. Effect of exercise on cardiac output and distribution of uterine blood flow in pregnant ewes. J Appl Physiol 1976; 40:725.
5. Morris N, Osborn SB, Wright HP, Hart A. Effective uterine blood flow during exercise and normal and pre-eclamptic pregnancies. Lancet 1956; 2:481.
6. Wilkening RB, Meschia G. Fetal oxygen uptake, oxygenation and acid-base balance as a function of uterine blood flow. Am J Physiol 1983; 244:H749.
7. Hon EH, Wohlgemuth R. The electronic evaluation of fetal heart rate. Am J Obstet Gynecol 1961; 81:361.
8. Soiva K, Salmi A, Gronroos M, Peltonen T. Physical working capacity during pregnancy and effect of physical tests on foetal heart rate. Ann Chir Gynaecol 1963; 53:187.
9. Hodr J, Brotanek Y. Changes of actography and foetal heart rates in premature deliveries. In: Horsky J, Stembera ZK, eds. Intra-uterine dangers to the foetus. Amsterdam: Excerpta Medica Foundation, 1967, p. 343.
10. Stembera ZK, Hodr J. The exercise test as an early

diagnostic aid for foetal distress. In: Horksy J, Stembera ZK, eds. Intra-uterine dangers to the foetus. Amsterdam: Excerpta Medica Foundation, 1967, p. 349.

11. Pokorny J, Rous J. The effect of mother's work on foetal heart sounds. In: Horsky J, Stembera ZK, eds. Intra-uterine dangers to the foetus. Amsterdam: Excerpta Medica Foundation, 1967, p. 359.
12. Pomerance JJ, Gluck L, Lynch VA. Maternal exercise as a screening test for uteroplacental insufficiency. Obstet Gynecol 1974; 44:383.
13. Eisenberg de Smoler P, Krachmer SK, Ayala LC, Dominguez JA. El electrocardiograma fetal durante el ejercicio materno. Ginecol obstet Mex 1974; 35:521.
14. Pernoll ML, Metcalf J, Paul M. Fetal cardiac response to maternal exercise. In: Longo LD, Reneau DD, eds. Fetal and newborn cardiovascular physiology. New York: Garland Press, 1978, vol. 2, p. 389.
15. Sibley L, Ruhling RO, Cameron-Foster J, Christensen C, Bolen T. Swimming and physical fitness during pregnancy. J Nurse-Midwifery 1981; 26:3.
16. Dale E, Mullinax KM, Bryan DH. Exercise during pregnancy: effects on the fetus. Can J Appl Sport Sci 1982; 7:98.
17. Hauth JC, Gilstrap LC, Widmer K. Fetal heart rate reactivity before and after maternal jogging during the third trimester. Am J Obstet Gynecol 1983; 142:545.
18. Collings CA, Curet LB, Mullin JP. Maternal and fetal responses to a maternal aerobic exercise program. Am J Obstet Gynecol 1983; 145:702.
19. Artal R, Romem Y, Wiswell R. Fetal heart responses to maternal exercise. Am J Obstet Gynecol 1986; 155(4):729–733.
20. Pijpers L, Wladimiroff JW, McGhie J. Effect of short-term maternal exercise on maternal and fetal cardiovascular dynamics. Br J Obstet Gynaecol 1984; 91:1081.
21. Clapp JF III. Fetal heart rate response to running in midpregnancy and late pregnancy. Am J Obstet Gynecol 1985; 153:251–252.
22. Jovanovic L, Kessler A, Peterson CM. Human maternal and fetal responses to graded exercise. J Appl Physiol 1985; 58:1719–1722.
23. Veille JC, Hohimer AR, Burry K, Speroff L. The effect of exercise on uterine activity in the last eight weeks of pregnancy. Am J Obstet Gynecol 1985; 151:727–730.
24. Rauramo I. Effect of short-term physical exercise on foetal heart rate and uterine activity in normal and abnormal pregnancies. Ann Chir Gynaecol 1987; 76:1–6.
25. Paolone AM, Shangold M, Paul D, Minnitti J, Weiner S. Fetal heart rate measurements during maternal exercise—avoidance of artifact. Med Sci Sports Exerc 1987; 19(6):605–609.
26. Carpenter MW, Sady SS, Hoegsberg B, Sady MA, Haydon B, Cullinane EM, Coustan DR, Thompson PD. Fetal heart rate response to maternal exertion. JAMA 1988; 259(20):3006–3009.
27. Wolfe LA, Lowe-Wylde SJ, Tranmer JE, McGrath MJ. Fetal heart rate during maternal static exercise. Can J Spt Sci 1988; 13(3):95–96P.
28. Artal R, Romem Y, Paul RH, Wiswell R. Fetal bradycardia induced by maternal exercise. Lancet 1984; 2:258.
29. Young BK and Weinstein HM. Moderate fetal bradycardia. Am J Obstet Gynecol 1977; 126:271–275.
30. Rauramo I, Forss M. Effect of exercise on maternal hemodynamics and placental blood flow in healthy women. Acta Obstet Gynaecol Scand 1988; 67:21.
31. Tonge HM, Wladimiroff JW, Noordam MY, Stewart PA. Fetal cardiac arrhythmias and their effect on volume blood flow in descending aorta of human fetus. J Clin Ultrasound 1986; 14:607–612.
32. Moore DH, Jarrett JC, Bendick PJ. Exercise induced changes in uterine artery blood flow, as measured by Doppler ultrasound, in pregnant subjects. Am J Perinatol 1989; 5:94.
33. Morrow RJ, Ritchie WK, Bull SB. Fetal and maternal hemodynamic responses to exercise in pregnancy assessed by Doppler ultrasonography. Am J Obstet Gynecol 1989; 160:138.
34. Veille JC, Bacevice AE, Wilson B, Janos J, Hellerstein HK. Umbilical artery waveform during bicycle exercise in normal pregnancy. Obstet Gynecol 1989; 73:957.
35. Manning FA, Morrison I, Lange IR. Antepartum determination of fetal health: composite biophysical profile scoring. Clin Perinatol 1982; 9:285.
36. Boddy K, Dawes GS. Fetal breathing. Br Med Bull 1975; 31:3.
37. Timor-Tritsh J, Zador I, Hertz RH, Rosen MG. Human fetal respiratory arrhythmia. Am J Obstet Gynecol 1977; 127:661.
38. Manning FA, Platt LD, Sipos L. Fetal movements in humans in the third trimester. Obstet Gynecol 1977; 54:699.
39. Sadovsky E, Yaffe H. Daily fetal movement recording and fetal diagnosis. Obstet Gynecol 1973; 41:845.
40. Marsal K, Lofgren O, Gewnser G. Fetal breathing movements and maternal exercise. Acta Obstet Gynaecol Scand 1979; 58:197.
41. Artal R, Platt LD, Sperling M, Kammula R, Jilek J, Nakamura RM. Maternal exercise: cardiovascular and metabolic responses in normal pregnancy. Am J Obstet Gynecol 1981; 140:123.
42. Platt LD, Artal R, Semel J, Sipos L, Kammula RK. Exercise in pregnancy. II. Fetal responses. Am J Obstet Gynecol 1983; 147:487.
43. Lewis PJ, Trudinger BJ, Mangez J. Effect of maternal glucose on fetal breathing and body movements in late pregnancy. Br J Obstet Gynaecol 1979; 85:586.
44. Schroder H, Gilbert RD, Power GG. Fetal heat dissipation: a computer model and some preliminary experimental results from fetal sheep. Proceedings of the Society for Gynecologic Investigation, Dallas, Texas, 1982, p. 113.
45. Abrams R, Caton D, Clapp J, Barron DH. Thermal and metabolic features of life in utero. Clin Obstet Gynecol 1970; 13:549.
46. Edwards MJ. Congenital defects in guinea pigs: fetal resorptions, abortions and malformations following induced hyperthermia during early gestation. Teratology 1969; 2:313.
47. Skreb N, Frank Z. Developmental abnormalities in the rat induced by heat shock. J Embryol Exp Morphol 1983; 11:445.
48. Kilham L, Ferm VH. Exencephaly in fetal hamsters exposed to hyperthermia. Teratology 1976; 14:323.
49. Miller P, Smith DW, Shepard TH. Maternal hyperthermia as a possible cause of anencephaly. Lancet 1978; 1:519.
50. Smith DW, Clarren SK, Harvey MAS. Hyperthermia

as a possible teratogenic agent. J Pediatr 1978; 92:878.

51. Fraser FC, Skelton J. Possible teratogenicity of maternal fever. Lancet 1978; 2:634.

52. Clarren SK, Smith DW, Harvey MAS, Ward RH. Myrianthopoulos NC. Hyperthermia—a prospective evaluation of a possible teratogenic agent in man. J Pediatr 1979; 95:81.

53. Fox ME, Harris RE, Brekken AL. The active-duty military pregnancy: a new high-risk category. Am J Obstet Gynecol 1984; 129:705.

54. Taferi N, Naey RL, Gobzie A. Effects of maternal undernutrition and heavy physical work during pregnancy on birth weight. Br J Obstet Gynaecol 1980; 87:222.

55. Naeye RL, Peters E. Working during pregnancy, effects on the fetus. Pediatrics 1982; 69:721.

56. Terada M. Effect of physical activity before pregnancy on fetuses of mice exercised forcibly during pregnancy. Teratology 1974; 10:141.

57. Nelson PS, Gilbert RD, Longo L. Fetal growth and placental diffusing capacity in guinea pigs following long-term maternal exercise. J Dev Physiol 1983; 5:1.

58. Clapp, JF, Dickstein S. Endurance exercise and pregnancy outcome. Med Sci Sports Exerc 1984; 16:556.

19

Effect of Maternal Exercise on Pregnancy Outcome

Raul Artal Mittelmark, Fred J. Dorey, and Thomas H. Kirschbaum

In recent years numerous articles and case reports have addressed issues concerning maternal exercise and its potential effects on the mother and her fetus. The essential question asked throughout this text is: "Does continuation of physical activity in pregnancy affect the course and outcome of the pregnancy?" In this chapter we will attempt to evaluate critically the pertinent published literature in order to assess whether it can be used to answer that question. The theoretical potential pregnancy outcome variables that could be related in any way to maternal exercise are listed in Table 19.1. They cover the prenatal intrapartum and neonatal period. A review of the literature does not establish an association between the listed complications and maternal exercise, nor can it refute an association. We arrived at this conclusion after establishing that all published reports suffer from major design flaws, in particular: (*a*)

Table 19.1. Theoretical Outcome Variables of Pregnancy That Could Be Related to Maternal Exercise

1. Spontaneous abortion
2. Uterine bleeding
3. Abruptio placentae
4. Premature labor and premature rupture of membranes
5. Cord prolapse
6. Malpresentation
7. Operative or instrumental delivery
8. Pregnancy-induced hypertension
9. Congenital anomalies
10. Intrauterine growth retardation
11. Fetal distress
12. Meconium aspiration
13. Stillbirth
14. Low Apgar scores
15. Neonatal adaptation difficulties
16. Length of labor
17. Postpartum recovery

lack of randomization, (*b*) small sample size, (*c*) lack of appropriate analysis, and (*d*) failure to consider prepregnancy fitness level when evaluating the results (Table 19.2).

A study by Clapp and Dickstein (1) illustrates the appropriate study design to assess the relationship between maternal exercise and pregnancy outcome. The study evaluates the prepregnancy fitness level and, at the same time, recognizes the decline in activity level as pregnancy progresses that could lead to inadequate adherence to the exercise protocols. Unfortunately the sample size was too small to draw any definitive conclusions about pregnancy outcomes.

Most published studies have a subject selection bias with most subjects being athletically inclined, which limits the applications of the results to active women. There are no published studies evaluating whether sedentary subjects have a higher or lower incidence of complications in pregnancy than those with average or greater activity levels.

These and other inadequacies are well illustrated in a relatively large sample size study published by Kulpa et al. (2). A total of 141 low-risk pregnant subjects who had an interest in recreational sports were randomized into a "control" group or exercise group, but there was no control group since all subjects were exercising. The subjects kept a log of their activities, but no objective quantification of their exercise activities was reported. Their fitness levels were predicted from heart rate during a submaximal exercise test (note that the relationship between V_{O_2} and heart rates may be altered in pregnancy). Of the 141 original subjects, only 85 (60.2%) completed the study. Twenty-six subjects (18.4%) were excluded from the study because of obstetric complications, a relatively high incidence of complications for a low-risk population.

Table 19.2.   Review of Studies on Complications and Maternal Exercise

Authors	Purpose	Study Design	Groups Compared
Clapp and Dickstein (1)	Evaluate endurance exercise and outcome	Sample survey, prospective, all antepartum registrants interviewed, n=336	1. Sedentary women before and during pregnancy; n=152 2. Exercised before pregnancy but reduced level during; n=47 3. Maintained exercise level at or near prepregnancy level; n=29
Kulpa et al. (2)	Determine effect of outcome on a conditioned athlete and whether training effect can be demonstrated	Random prospective study	Random-prospective of 141 studied; 85 completed the study
South-Paul et al. (4)	Determine whether pregnancy affects physical fitness	Pre- and postcomparison of independent sample means	n=23; subjects assigned at random to exercise versus nonexercise; 7 non- and 10 exercise subjects completed study
Dibblee and Graham (5)	Evaluate fitness during and after delivery	Sample survey, physicians referral, n=19	Results at end of 1st, 2nd, 3rd trimester and postpartum compared; "fit" versus "unfit" compared; n=8, n=8
Morton et al. (6)	Compare heart rate stroke volume during exercise	Pre- and postcomparison	23 volunteers referred from community exercise classes; 10 identified as fit
Berkowitz et al. (7)	Evaluate risk factors for preterm delivery	Case control study	Cases (women who delivered singleton live term infants before 37 weeks' gestation: n=175; controls (drawn from random sample of singleton term births): n=313
Jarrett and Spellacy (8)	Assess relationship between jogging during pregnancy and outcome	Retrospective, sample survey	67 questionnaires returned
Tafari, et al. (9)	Determine whether physical activity with limited caloric intake affects fetal growth	Prospective, survey	Survey questions to assess work levels: hard work group, n=64; light work group, n=66; survey diet habit on 2-day basis
Collings et al. (10)	Investigate effects of exercise on pregnancy and fetus	Pre- and postcomparison of independent means	20 patients: exercise not randomized n=12; control, n=8
Hall and Kaufmann (11)	Compare effect of physical conditioning program on outcome	Sample survey	Control group, n=393; low exercise, n=82; moderate exercise, n=309; strenuous exercise, H=61
Erkkola and Makeb (13)	Correlate physical fitness with heart volume	Partly randomized	Exercise group, n=393; control group, n=82; second control group (not randomized)
Pomerance et al. (14)	Determine whether physical fitness is related to outcome	Pre- and postpregnancy comparison	54 women given a physical fitness score; 41 completed the study

[a]ANOVA, analysis of variance.

Statistics[a]	Covariates	Conclusions	Comments
ANOVA; Chi-square	Yes; matched analysis	Group 3 gained less weight, delivered earlier, had lighter offspring. These women also had lower preconception weight.	No prepregnancy information; No compliance information if in an exercise group
Chi-square	No	Exercise not associated with increased morbidity; high percentage subjects removed during study	Exclusive group completed study; difficult to get basic information; data poorly presented
Students *t* tests			Very small sample
Not indicated (probably multiple *t* tests)	No	No difference between fit and unfit except higher Apgar scores at 1 min. $V_{O_{2max}}$ declined during pregnancy and rose after delivery	Small sample size
Unpaired *t* tests; ANOVA	No	Response different during pregnancy; no postpartum data	Sample too small to compare fit with unfit; repeated measure ANOVA should be utilized
Cases and controls not matched, questionnaire to obtain data; Chi-square, *t* test, log linear, logistic regression	Yes	Subjects were younger, more likely unmarried, black, and of low socioeconomic status, high gravidity, but similar parity. History of previous preterm delivery most important risk factor, suggests limited but not exaggerated activity was beneficial	Sample of women who exercise during pregnancy but not prepregnancy was small: $n = 26$; not clear what analysis was done for results in this paper versus an earlier one
Student's *t* test and correlation	No	Number of miles jogged during pregnancy decreased; low incidence of complications; jogging in healthy women not harmful	Obvious possible bias in sample survey; small sample size; not used multivariates
Probably *t* tests; no covariate adjustments	No	Hard physical labor group: lower than recommended caloric intake, lower pregnancy loading weights, and smaller newborn	
Repeated measures; ANOVA	No	No difference in labor duration, Apgar scores, or growth	Sample size far too small; nonrandomized
ANOVA with multiple test adjustments	No	Lower cesarean-section in exercise group; pregnancy outcomes more favorable in exercise group	Biased results from patient selection to groups; not randomized; no prepregnancy evaluation
Multiple *t* tests	No	Heart volume related to physical fitness; can improve physical fitness with training	Small sample size; no prepregnancy evaluation
Linear regression analysis		Prepregnancy weight and weight gain correlated to birth-weight; few outcomes related to physical fitness	Small sample size

[a] ANOVA, analysis of variance.

Twenty subjects (14.1%) dropped out, eight (5.6%) aborted spontaneously, and two did not comply. Based on this report, one might have made the argument that having 39.8% subjects disqualified from the study implies that exercise in either form, mild or intense, is not desirable during pregnancy. However, this study is frequently quoted in the literature as evidence that exercising pregnant women do well and have favorable outcomes. Investigators must consider the incidence of individual complications in the general population in determining sample size. To conclude as Kulpa et al. did in the abstract of the article that exercise had no associated obstetric complication, the number of subjects enrolled should have been between 200 and 500 depending on the particular complication rate (3).

There are no reports in the literature to answer the question of whether changing exercise patterns during pregnancy is either beneficial or harmful to the outcome of pregnancy. Furthermore, we are in no position to answer the questions: Do sedentary women have a better pregnancy outcome than active women? Does physical activity improve pregnancy outcome?

There are a number of study design problems that make it difficult to compare results from different studies. One significant difficulty in evaluating the literature is that there is no uniform reporting of the level of fitness of the subjects enrolled. Very often fitness is predicted from submaximal tests using prediction equations based on the performance of nonpregnant women. Another problem is the lack of uniform objective quantification of the different exercise routines. Some studies report statistically significant differences that are meaningless from the clinical point of view when evaluating exercise and pregnancy outcome. Furthermore, there are no reports in pregnancy on exercise-related injuries. None of the studies utilizes a multivariate analysis adjusted for covariates such as age, weight, parity, and fitness. In assessing such complex issues in which so many covariates could interfere, utilizing a *t*-test or Chi-square analysis is not enough.

Due to the relatively low incidence of obstetrical complications in a low-risk population, significant information could be obtained only from large, randomized prospective studies that include prepregnancy information and covariates and that monitor objectively the subject's compliance. A summary of the articles evaluating the effect of exercise on pregnancy outcome is listed in Table 19.2. Consistent findings in these studies include the following:

1. Women who exercised before pregnancy and continued to do so during pregnancy tended to weigh less, gain less weight, and deliver smaller babies than controls.
2. All women, regardless of initial level of physical activity, decrease their activity as pregnancy progresses.
3. No information is available to assess whether active women have better pregnancy outcome than their sedentary counterparts. No information is available on sedentary women.
4. Physically active women appear to tolerate labor pain better.

Due to inadequate study sample size, all of the above findings should be considered only as trends and will have to be validated by larger studies. Results that are inconsistent from study to study are listed in Table 19.3. It is impossible at this time to assess the relative increase or decrease in complication rates among women who exercise in pregnancy. To detect a two-fold increase in ad-

Table 19.3. Conflicting Reported Risks of Exercise in Pregnancy

	Not Altered by Exercise	Altered by Exercise
Maternal		
Musculoskeletal injuries	No reports	No reports
Cardiovascular complication	No reports	No reports
Spontaneous abortion	Ref. 17	Refs. 1, 15, 16
Premature labor	Refs. 14, 18	Ref. 1
Fetal		
Fetal distress	Refs. 1, 18	Ref. 19
Intrauterine growth retardation	Refs. 5, 14, 18	Ref. 1
Fetal malformations	No reports	No reports

Table 19.4.   Sample Size Required to Detect Twofold Increase in Adverse Reproductive Outcomes[a,b]

Outcome	Sample Size[c]
Pregnancy loss	
Spontaneous abortion (<20 weeks' gestation) Stillbirths	322 pregnancies
Birth/developmental defect	
Low birthweight	586 live births
Major birth defects (all)	631 live births
Neural tube defects	1819 live births
Severe mental retardation	8986 live births
Infant (<1 year) death	1856 live births

[a]From Rosenberg MJ, Kuller LH. Reproductive Health Policies in the Workplace, 1983: p. 201–226.
[b]Alpha—0.05; beta—0.20.
[c]Divided evenly between exposed and unexposed groups.

verse reproductive outcomes, studies will have to include a large sample size (Table 19.4 (20)).

In summary, future studies will have to control for the following essential factors: appropriate sample size considering incidence of complications; exercise history, type, intensity, and duration during pregnancy and its relation to $V_{O_{2max}}$ changes in weight and body composition; and a proper population to allow application of the data obtained to the general population.

Based on the present published literature, it is not possible to conclude in a scientific way whether maternal exercise is beneficial or detrimental to pregnancy. Nevertheless, these studies have contributed significantly to the understanding of maternal and fetal responses to exercise in pregnancy.

REFERENCES

1. Clapp JF, Dickstein S. Endurance exercise and pregnancy outcome. Med Sci Sports Exer 1984; 16(6):556–562.
2. Kulpa PJ, White BM, Visscher R. Aerobic exercise in pregnancy. Am J Obstet Gynecol 1987; 156(6):1395–1403.
3. Aleong J, Bartlett DE. Improved graphs for calculating sample sizes when comparing two independent binomial distributions. Biometrics 1979; 35:875–881.
4. South-Paul JE, Rajagopal KR, Tenholder MF. The effect of participation in a regular exercise program aerobic capacity during pregnancy. Obstet Gynecol 1988; 71(2):175–179.
5. Dibblee L, Graham TE. A longitudinal study of changes in aerobic fitness, body composition, and energy intake in primigravid patients. Am J Obstet Gynecol 1983; 147(8):908–914.
6. Morton MJ, Paul MS, Campos GR, Hart MV, Metcalf G. Exercise dynamics in late gestation: effects of physical training. Am J Obstet Gynecol 1985; 152(1):91–97.
7. Berkowitz GS, Kelsey JL, Holford TR, Berkowitz RC. Physical activity and the risk of spontaneous preterm delivery. J Reprod Med 1983; 28(9):581–588.
8. Jarrett CJ, Spellacy WN. Jogging during pregnancy: an improved outcome? Obstet Gynecol 1983; 61(6):705–709.
9. Tafari N, Naeye RL, Gobezie H. Effects of maternal undernutrition and heavy physical work during pregnancy on birth weight. Br J Obstet Gynaecol 1980; 87:222–226.
10. Collings CA, Curet LB, Mullin JP. Maternal and fetal responses to a maternal aerobic exercise program. Am J Obstet Gynecol 1983; 145(6):702–707.
11. Hall DC, Kaufmann DA. Effects of aerobic and strength conditioning on pregnancy outcomes. Am J Obstet Gynecol 1987; 157(5):1199–1203.
12. Erkkola R. The physical work capacity of the expectant mother and its effect on pregnancy, labor and the newborn. Int J Gynaecol Obstet 1976; 14:153–159.
13. Erkkola R, Makeb M. Heart volume and physical fitness of parturients. Am J Clin Res 1976; 8:15–21.
14. Pomerance JJ, Gluck L, Lynch VA. Physical fitness in pregnancy: its effect on pregnancy outcome. Am J Obstet Gynecol 1974; 119(7):867–876.
15. Clapp JF. The effects of maternal exercise during pregnancy on uterine blood flow and pregnancy outcome. In: Moawad AH, Lindheimer MD, eds. Uterine and placental blood flow. New York, Masson, 1982, p. 171–176.
16. Clapp JF, Wesley M, Sleamaker RH. Thermoregulatory and metabolic responses to jogging prior to and during pregnancy. Med Sci Sports Exer 1987; 19:124–130.
17. Clapp JF. The effects of maternal exercise on early pregnancy outcome. Am J Obstet Gynecol 1989; 161:1453–1457.
18. Wong SC, McKinzie DC. Cardiorespiratory fitness during pregnancy and its effect on outcome. Int J Sport Med 1987; 8:79–83.
19. Erkkola R, Rauramo L. Correlation of maternal physical fitness during pregnancy with maternal and fetal pH and lactic acid at delivery. Acta Obstet Gynaecol 1976; 55:441–446.
20. Seabrook EC, Parkinson DK. Reproductive Health Policies in the Workplace, 1983. Published by Family Health Council of Western Pennsylvania, Inc.

20

Pregnancy in the Elite and Professional Athlete— A Stepwise Clinical Approach

Ralph W. Hale and Raul Artal Mittelmark

Sports for women have developed rapidly in the last few years. The number of elite female athletes competing in Olympic and World Championships has shown a dramatic increase as has the number of women participating in professional sports. With this added interest, there has been an increase in professional women's sports. Although the number of these sports is still limited, they have placed increased emphasis on elitism. Currently, there are professional women's teams in volleyball, basketball, and softball. Individual professional sports include tennis, golf, cycling, auto racing, horse racing, long-distance swimming, and others. In some nonprofessional sports, such as track and field, the financial incentive is often equivalent to that of a "professional sport." As a result of personal goals and financial incentives, the elite female athlete must continue her intense training throughout what historically has been referred to as the "child-bearing years." Many of these women defer any pregnancy planning during this time. Should they become pregnant, some women attempt to integrate their training and competition schedules with pregnancy and childbearing. Although the numbers are still small, the physician will find more of these patients in the future. Because the need for intensive and strenuous training, often on a year-round basis, is not always compatible with pregnancy, the physician will need to be aware of the problems that may be encountered. Pregnant athletes who intend to continue training at a high level of intensity could lessen the risks by seeking closer medical supervision. Very little information is available on the course and complications of pregnancy in the professional or elite athletes who elect to continue training during pregnancy. Being accustomed to training at a high intensity level before pregnancy, professional and elite athletes may place themselves at increased risk for overuse injuries, not realizing there are pregnancy-related changes in joints and ligaments.

Uncontrolled studies by Erdelyi (1) and Zaharieva (2) report on their personal experience and information obtained from 172 elite Hungarian and 150 Bulgarian athletes. Despite these reports being incomplete and lacking in design and format, they do provide some interesting information. Both authors conclude that continuous physical training in pregnancy may carry very little risk. Erdelyi reported a decreased incidence of complications in the pregnant athlete population (lower incidence of pregnancy-induced hypertension and cesarean sections—probably due to the skewed population, at low risk for these complications). Zaharieva (2) concludes that elite Olympic athletes have normal pregnancies, however, the information recorded in the paper may indicate otherwise (see Table 20.1).

Zaharieva (2) reports on a number of minor and other unspecified complications, but most significantly she indicates that the number of newborn babies of Olympian mothers weighing between 2600 and 3000 g (potentially growth retarded or prematurely born) was greater than the number weighing 3500 g. This information concurs with more recent published literature (3) indicating that babies of mothers exercising strenuously are weigh-

Table 20.1.   Effect of Exercise on Pregnancy(%)[a]

	Olympians	Masters of Sports	Elite Athletes
n	27	59	64
Pregnancy			
Minor complications	29.6	44.1	35.9
Unspecified complications	3.7	10.2	17.2
Physical activity-related bleeding		8.5	1.6
Delivery			
Cesarean section		4.7	1.6
Vaginal lacerations	44.4	67.8	45.3
Episiotomy	7.4	6.8	3.1
Newborn			
Intrauterine growth retardation	↑	?	?

[a]Modified from Zaharieva E. Olympic participation by women, effects on pregnancy and childbirth. JAMA 1972; 221(9):992–995.

ing less at birth. This could also explain the reported shorter first and second phase of labor in some of these subjects. It is interesting to see the very low cesarean section rate.

Physicians should be alert to the fact that elite athletes may disregard body signals and continue to exercise despite discomfort. However, the physician should also keep in mind that they are accustomed to higher intensity training than the recreational athlete and are better able to withstand heat stress. Because most of the elite and professional athletes will benefit from closer medical supervision, guidelines for their physical activities could be individualized and adapted to their professional needs. Nevertheless, the potential maternal and fetal risks are similar for the general population. Thus, the recommendations included in this chapter are a clinical approach based on the authors' experience. This approach could be modified in the future should additional and definitive studies become available.

PRECONCEPTUAL CARE AND EVALUATION

Because professional athletes usually have a fixed precompetition and competition schedule, they can often identify the time span during which they wish to be pregnant. This gives the physician an opportunity to evaluate the athlete as well as counsel her.

Professional athletes are required, by virtue of their level of competition, to maintain a rigorous exercise schedule during the competitive season. Even in the off-season for their particular athletic discipline, they need to continue a modified exercise and fitness program. If they desire pregnancy, they may try to integrate pregnancy into such a period of time.

Foremost among the concerns of most elite and professional athletes is weight control. Frequently, the nutritional status of the athlete may be inadequate. One of the first procedures for the physician to follow is to assess the intake of vitamins and other nutritional elements.

The athletes' prepregnancy evaluation should include adequate intake of vitamins and other nutrients. In the face of perceived weight gain, many athletes will significantly reduce their intake of fats, carbohydrates, and even protein (4). The physiological and medical aspects of this topic are discussed at length in Chapter 9.

Counseling of the pregnant athlete should not be limited to the importance of a balanced diet but should include specific recommendations. Most athletes, like the general population, have limited knowledge of what constitutes a balanced diet (5). It is important then to recognize that there is a tendency in athletes to overcompensate for poor nutrition by excessive intake of vitamins and other "health food" preparations (6).

Inadequate nutrition or failure to gain weight in pregnancy has been frequently associated with intrauterine growth retardation, a likely result of combined strenuous activities and deficient diet. Inappropriate dietary patterns can significantly affect a pregnancy. Deficient, but more often excessive, intake of vitamins prenatally can result in an increased incidence of human congenital malformations. Massive ingestion of vitamin D could result in a neonatal syndrome consisting of supravalvular aortic stenosis, elfin facies, and mental retardation (7). There are reports of congenital malformations in humans associated with large vitamin A ingestion during pregnancy. Vitamin A in the form of retinoic acid is a potent teratogen that may cause urogenital anomalies, ear malformations, cleft palate, and neural tube defects (8). Conversely, vitamin deficiency such as folic acid deficiency could result in increased neural tube defects (9). Furthermore, the iron status of those subjects has to be carefully assessed, since many of them may have preexisting depleted stores (10). The consequence of such anemia is fatigue and decreased exercise tolerance.

Other than poor nutrition, the professional athlete seldom will have preexisting medical conditions that would have an impact on pregnancy. These individuals are usually healthy adults who have experienced a myriad of orthopaedic injuries and problems but very few medical illnesses.

EARLY PREGNANCY

Once pregnancy occurs, the professional athlete is faced with an obvious dilemma and conflict between her professional needs and the potential restrictions imposed by the pregnancy. For financial and other reasons, the solution is rarely easy. If she has been seen for preconceptual care and has planned the pregnancy to occur during an off season, pregnancy is approached with enthusiasm. Anecdotal information indicates that some athletes may elect to terminate their pregnancy rather than face a professional setback. Statistics are hard to obtain, but some reports indicate a very high incidence of intentional abortions among elite athletes (2). It is our impression that most of the athletes whom we have met have tried to reach a compromise between a demanding career and pregnancy. One approach certainly is continuous

training under strict obstetrical observation. This is not without its drawbacks. We know of at least two world class athletes who had to interrupt their rigorous athletic training because of complications of pregnancy.

One very controversial aspect of pregnancy in the professional athlete that has been much publicized was the attempt of a few elite athletes to improve their performance by becoming pregnant and then aborting. The exact reason could only be speculated on since no valid physiological explanation could be given, though the assumption was that early pregnancy could improve performance (11). Such an approach is without scientific basis, is unethical, and should be strongly discouraged.

One other related aspect is the use of anabolic steroids in pregnancy. Though the vast majority of such individuals will have amenorrhea and will not ovulate, there is still a chance they could ovulate and become pregnant. In those rare occasions, the fetal effects include significant masculinization of the female fetus.

There is some reason for concern, however, with strenuous exercise in early pregnancy. It has been suggested that exercise-induced hyperthermia in female athletes may result in congenital anomalies, especially neural tube defects (12) (also see Chapter 23). Dehydration must be prevented because this is the leading cause of an elevated core temperature. Many athletes and coaches still harbor the myth that fluids are bad for an athlete during training. This myth must be addressed and dismissed. Pregnant women should be instructed to take a minimum of one glass of fluid for every 15 min of workout or competition and to avoid elevation in body core temperature above 38.5°C. Patients are also instructed to observe their urine color. It if appears dark, the specific gravity of the urine is tested. In this way, the patient not only becomes aware of the problem but also actively participates in the prevention of heat injuries.

The most common of the first questions that the athlete asks is, "Can physical activity cause a spontaneous abortion?" There are no data to suggest that any level of physical activity can induce a spontaneous abortion. There are many reports of patients having engaged in extremely strenuous exercise programs without incurring pregnancy loss. On the other hand, the incidence of spontaneous abortions is approximately 16% or higher in the United States. There is no conclusive evidence to suggest that athletes have a lower or higher rate (see Chapter 17). Because threatened or subsequent incomplete abortion is a contraindication to physical activity, it is important to try to plan the pregnancy so that it occurs during the off-season. However, if the length of the season necessitates that conception occur during the competitive season, first trimester bleeding, nausea, and vomiting can have a serious impact on the athlete's ability to continue to compete.

Except for the above, during the first few months of pregnancy, there are few physiological changes in the female athlete that will affect her exercise program. Most studies conclude that patients in early pregnancy can perform at or near their peak level of performance. We have treated 22 professional athletes (tennis, volleyball, basketball, golf, swimming, and softball) as well as elite athletes (track and long-distance running) who have become pregnant (R. W. Hale, unpublished observation). Our studies to date reveal no difference in their ability to train or participate, and none of the athletes has had a spontaneous abortion after the sixth week of gestation. Only three have had spontaneous abortions before this time, and two of those had documented genetic anomalies. This uncontrolled study compares favorably with our experience with nonathletes.

One potential impediment for continuing training and competing during pregnancy are the changes that occur in joints and ligaments that could lead to total physical disability. Such changes are best illustrated in the separation that may occur in the symphysis pubis. Such separation or laxity can range from a few millimeters to greater than 2 cm in the most severe cases (13). However, such occurrences will differ significantly from one individual to another; the degree of laxity will dictate the degree of disability. Training

could then be modified to maintain some degree of aerobic fitness and at the same time prevent injury. Swimming is usually the best alternative.

LATE PREGNANCY

Although the athlete may wish to continue to train and compete, it becomes extremely difficult for the professional or elite athlete to maintain a level of fitness that will allow her to continue beyond the 20th week. For some sports this may even be earlier. Participation on the professional level with the physiological changes that occur in late pregnancy are counterproductive for most athletes. The anatomical changes in posture, weight, and center of gravity also affect the athlete's performance.

We recommend that all professional or elite athletes plan to stop active competition between 16 and 20 weeks or earlier if they notice they are experiencing difficulty. Because this timing may coincide with their competitive season, some athletes may try to continue. Recently, a professional volleyball player continued to play into her 18th week of gestation. By the 20th week, her inability to dig and spike forced her to stop playing. Had she been a setter, perhaps she could have continued longer into the pregnancy.

The risk of direct fetal injury as pregnancy progresses is of significant concern. The only reported injuries are those associated with a penetrating wound, unlikely in any professional sport practiced by women, and those associated with blunt trauma, which are more likely to occur. It is well recognized that seat belts can cause a compression of the uterus that results in premature separation of the placenta after car accidents with sudden deceleration or stopping and secondary shear forces. For this reason professional automobile racers should be leary of any racing activity in pregnancy after the 24th week. Most other sports have at least the potential for blunt injury, e.g., dives in volleyball, charges and other fouls in basketball, falls in horse racing and cycling, etc. Although there are no current data due to the small number of

Table 20.2. Risks of Exercise in Pregnancy for the Elite Athlete

Risks	Guidelines
Maternal	
1. Musculoskeletal injuries	With evidence of joint and ligament laxity, individualize and modify training.
2. Cardiovascular complications	Could exceed 140 bpm, but only after medical clearance. Warning signs: palpitations and tachycardia at rest, any signs of orthostatic hypotension.
3. Threatened abortion or premature labor	Stop training
4. Hypoglycemia	Prevent hypoglycemia by following proper nutrition.
Fetal	
1. Fetal distress	Be alert to fetal activity. In the presence of any complication, stop training and resume after medical clearance.
2. Intrauterine growth retardation	Stop training
3. Fetal malformations	Avoid hyperthermia and dehydration immediately after conception and weeks thereafter.
4. Fetal injuries	Avoid sports in which there is a higher probability of blunt trauma after 16–20 weeks' gestation.

exposures, blunt trauma should remain a concern for the physician.

The female professional athlete should expect to have the same pregnancy outcome as any other woman. Nevertheless, some real and theoretical concerns should be considered when counseling a pregnant athlete (Table 20.2). Clapp and Dickstein (3) suggest that endurance exercise resulted in less weight gain by the mother (4.6 kg), earlier deliveries (−8 days), and smaller babies (by 500 g). We do not know the exact frequency of occurrence for intrauterine growth retardation, but certainly the combination of strenuous training combined with a deficient diet could result in fetal growth retardation. We often read in lay publications about success stories of exceptional athletes, but it is only rarely that we learn about failures and exercise-related complications. In our own clinical practice, we know of at least one individual who missed the Olympic trials because of premature labor and inability to continue to train for her event.

A frequently asked question is, "In the absence of complications, can pregnant women maintain an intensive training program and, if so, can they maintain their aerobic fitness through pregnancy?" The cardiovascular load associated with pregnancy could precipitate cardiovascular complications during intense training. Nevertheless, one has to recognize that professional and elite athletes are accustomed to train at a high heart rate. After proper medical clearance such athletes could probably continue to exercise above the 140 heart rate limit recommended for the general pregnant population. However, we should point out that rare cardiovascular complications can also occur in athletes. Warning signs could be the appearance of palpitations and tachycardia at rest.

In an unpublished report, R. Artal studied three professional athletes through pregnancy and performed V_{O_2max} testing on several occasions. The results are listed in Table 20.3. The impression from this preliminary study is that physiologically these subjects can sustain their prepregnancy V_{O_2max} if able to train, though larger studies may prove

Table 20.3. V_{O_2max} (ml/kg/min)

Weeks' Gestation	10	14	29	38	Post-partum
Subject 1	40.9	43.7	29.9	26.6	31.9[a]
Subject 2		44.0	45.0	44.9	53.4
Subject 3			38.8		37.3

[a]The decline in V_{O_2max} in this individual is a reflection of a decrease in the intensity of training to a complete stop by 38 weeks.

otherwise. Recent case reports reflect an increased interest within the scientific community to elucidate the physiological responses of pregnant elite athletes to exercise (15).

POSTPARTUM

A return to full physical activity to overcome the detraining process that occurred during pregnancy is the primary concern of the athlete after delivery. Most want to start training immediately.

There are few sources of data to indicate the optimal time to resume physical activity, and it should be individualized. It appears that any activity before the second postpartum week adds little to the ability of the patient to return to her previous V_{O_2max} and resume her competitive activities. This is especially so if a degree of coordination is required. The relaxation of ligaments and joints does not disappear significantly before the second postpartum week and, in most instances, only 4–6 weeks' postpartum. As a result, we have been routinely recommending that the patient not consider a return to a training exercise routine until after a 2-week checkup, and then she can restart her conditioning program. Weight training should probably be delayed for 6–8 weeks and gradually be rebuilt to avoid potential injuries.

Because most athletes are very oriented toward their bodies and natural events, breastfeeding is the usual method preferred by athletes. There is no known contraindication to nursing and exercise, though the quality of the milk may differ after exercise. It does, however, require preplanning and adequate hydration. The exercising woman who is also lactating requires 12–16 8-ounce glasses of fluid a day and an additional 400–600 calories per day. If her exercise program is prolonged and strenuous, she may need even more. This is necessary to prevent dehydration and subsequent "drying" of the breast milk. Zaharieva (2) reports that a decrease in lactation has occurred in 18.5% of the training athletes. She also reported an unusually high incidence (22%) of mastitis. We are unaware of any mechanical problems that exercise causes for the breast, though for the athlete a leakage of fluid can be troublesome during competition. Nursing pads may alleviate most of the problems.

SUMMARY

As more women enter professional competitive sports, the physician will encounter an increasing number of patients who are either professional or elite athletes.

The professional elite athlete can consider becoming pregnant during her competing season. She should, however, avail herself of preconceptual counseling. This should include a dietary evaluation and a review of desired pregnancy dates and counseling on potential limitations of pregnancy. If necessary, ovulation induction should be considered.

Once pregnant, the professional and elite athlete does not appear to face any problems specific to her professional status. Although actual studies are minimal, our available data indicate that these individuals are at no greater risk. The maternal risks are predominantly overuse injuries, and the fetal risks are related to hyperthermia, dehydration, and premature labor. Intrauterine growth retardation may occur with a higher frequency.

After pregnancy, the athletes may return to competition as soon as they feel ready. Generally, they could resume conditioning activities within 2–4 weeks of delivery. Pregnancy for the elite athlete, like the general population, should not be a state of confinement; however, unrestricted or even restricted physical activity involves a certain degree of risk that must be recognized. Acceptance of the various risks then becomes a personal choice.

REFERENCES

1. Erdelyi GJ. Gynecological survey of female athletes. J Sports Med Phys Fitness 1962; 2:174–175.
2. Zaharieva E. Olympic participation by women, effects on pregnancy and childbirth. JAMA 1972; 221(9):992–995.
3. Clapp JF, Dickstein S. Endurance exercise and pregnancy outcome. Med Sci Sports Exer 1984; 16:556–562.
4. Chen JD, Wang JF, Li KJ, et al. Nutritional problems and measures in elite and amateur athletes. Am J Clin Nutr 1989; 49:1084.
5. Heinemann L, Zerbes H. Physical activity, fitness

and diet: behavior in the population compared with elite athletes in the GDR. Am J Clin Nutr 1989; 49:1007.

6. van Erp-Baart AMJ, Saris WM, Binkhorst RA, et al. Nationwide survey on nutritional habits of elite athletes. Part II—Mineral and vitamin intake. Int J Sports Med 1989; 10:511.

7. Garcia RE, Friedman WF, Kabacr MM, et al. Idiopathic hypercalcemia and supravalvular stenosis: documentation of a new syndrome. N Engl J Med 1964; 271:117–120.

8. Bernhardt IB, Dorsey DJ. Hypervitaminosis A and congenital renal anomalies in a human infant. Obstet Gynecol 1974; 43:750–755.

9. Lawrence KM, James N, Miller MH, et al. Double-blind randomized controlled trial of folate treatment before conception to prevent recurrence of neural tube defects. Br Med J 1981; 282:1509–1511.

10. Newhouse IJ, Clement DB. Iron status in athletes, an update. Sports Medicine 1988; 5:337.

11. Strobel E. Pregnancy as a doping measure? Dangerous development in high performance sports. Fortschr-Med 1988; 106(29):14.

12. Hale RW. Exercise and pregnancy: how each affects the other. Post Grad Med 1987; 82:61.

13. Bruser M. Sporting activities during pregnancy. Obstet Gynecol 1968; 32:721–725.

14. Bung P, Spatling L, Huch R, Huch A. Performance training in pregnancy. Geburtshilfe-Franenheilkd 1988; 48(7):500–511.

21

Amenorrheic Athlete and Conception

Barbara L. Drinkwater and Val Davajan

It became evident in the early 1970s that a number of women participating in competitive athletics had ceased having monthly menstrual periods. As a result, there has been concern that the new opportunities for women in sports might have long-term negative consequences for their future reproductive success. Those concerns lessened when it became evident from numerous anecdotal reports that women who had retired from active competition and resumed normal menses had conceived and delivered healthy babies. As a result, many female athletes have come to regard the amenorrhea associated with exercise as a benign event and to welcome the absence of monthly periods. Only those who are aware that the hypoestrogenic amenorrheic athlete is at risk for premature bone loss (1–5) and those who want to conceive are likely to seek a physician's advice on how to return to normal ovulatory cycles.

The extent of menstrual irregularities among active women in the general population is unknown. Among those women who are exercising solely for fun and fitness, the incidence of secondary amenorrhea is probably not much above that reported for average, nonathletic women (2–3%). This condition occurs most frequently among women participating in activities that involve strenuous training and/or where the emphasis on low body weight may result in poor nutrition and/or an inadequate caloric intake (Table 21.1).

Table 21.1. Prevalence of Secondary Amenorrhea[a]

Population	Number	%	Definition
Controls			
College	500	2.3	> 2 months with no periods
Swedes	2000	3.3	< 3 periods/year
Runners			
Cross-country	128	24.0	< 3 periods/year
Cross-country	38	44.7	No periods for the last 3 months
> 30 mi/wk	89	24.0	0–5 periods/year
5–30 mi/wk	22	14.0	0–5 periods/year
NY Marathon	270	1.0	< 1 period for the last 10 months
Joggers	885	6.0	No definition provided
Marathon	237	25.7	< 3 periods/year
Ballet dancers			
Students	69	18.8	At least 3 months with no period
Professional (29) + Students (5)	34	44.0	At least 3 months with no period
Athletes			
College varsity	140	12.1	No periods for the last 3 months or < 4 periods/year
Swimmers	197	12.3	< 3 periods/year
Cyclists	33	12.1	< 3 periods/year

[a]Adapted from Sanborn CC. Menstrual dysfunction in the female athlete. In: Teitz CC, ed. Scientific foundations of sports medicine. Philadelphia: BC Decker, Inc., 1989; p. 117–134.

Part of the difficulty in determining the prevalence of secondary amenorrhea among active women is the lack of a standard definition of amenorrhea (absence of menses) and oligomenorrhea (infrequent menses) (6). Amenorrhea, for example, may be defined in one study as 3 months without menses and in another study as 12 months without a period. As a result, the estimate of the occurrence of amenorrhea among active women varies from 1–44% (Table 21.1). Often, there is no evidence presented in these surveys that exercise is implicated in the amenorrheic condition. Women with eating disorders, for example, may exercise strenuously to burn calories, yet the source of their problem goes far beyond exercise per se. Unless the onset of amenorrhea follows either the initiation of an exercise program or an increase in the intensity of training, the disruption of menses may be unrelated to exercise.

MECHANISMS

The mechanisms underlying the menstrual irregularities experienced by female athletes (delayed menarche, secondary amenorrhea, oligomenorrhea, and an inadequate luteal phase) have not yet been identified. There is general agreement that the secondary amenorrhea associated with exercise, the so-called athletic amenorrhea, can be classified as hypothalamic chronic anovulation and has no underlying pathology such as premature ovarian failure, hyperandrogenism, or hyperprolactinemia (7). However, it cannot be assumed that exercise is the precipitating factor when an athlete presents with amenorrhea. Only a clinical workup (p. 244) can determine if the amenorrhea is related to exercise or to an underlying pathological condition.

Current research is concentrating on the gonadotropin-releasing hormone (GnRH) and what factors associated with strenuous physical activity may be affecting the GnRH pulse generator (8–10). Complicating the search for the precipitating factor is the possibility that the etiology underlying these menstrual irregularities may be multifactorial, that these factors may vary from one woman to another, and that disruption of the hypothalamic-pituitary-ovarian (HPO) cycle may occur only in those women predisposed to cyclic irregularity (9).

Although disruptions of the normal menstrual cycle may originate at the hypothalamus, the mechanism for the disruption is unknown. A number of hypotheses have been advanced to explain why some athletes experience menstrual irregularities and others do not. Some theories relate to individual characteristics of the athlete that cannot be modified, such as age, parity, previous menstrual irregularities, and age of menarche. Others point to factors that the athlete can control, such as diet, body fat, and her training program. Because only the latter factors can be modified, the physician must rely upon changing these factors to reestablish the ovulatory cycle in these amenorrheic athletes if they wish to conceive.

Body Fat

The low body weight/body fat hypothesis proposed by Frisch and colleagues (11–13) has been popularized by the media but discredited by other investigators. The technique Frisch used to predict the percentage of body fat from an estimate of total body water has been strongly criticized by Trussell (14) and Reeves (15); and a number of other studies have failed to find a significant difference in body weight or percentage of body fat between amenorrheic and eumenorrheic athletes (2, 16–18). In some instances, normal menses resumes without an appreciable gain in body weight (19, 20). However, body composition may play a role in a multifactorial explanation of exercise-associated amenorrhea. Some women may be more sensitive than others to decreased fat stores or to the abrupt loss of such stores. Certainly the extremely low-weight amenorrheic athlete concerned with her fertility should be encouraged to gain weight. Apart from the additional metabolic demands on her energy stores during pregnancy, these women are more at risk for decreased bone density (21).

Diet

Theories that dietary intake plays a role in menstrual dysfunction focus on two aspects of the daily diet: (*a*) caloric intake relative to energy expenditure; and (*b*) nutrient content of the food. Several studies (2, 4, 5, 22) have reported that amenorrheic athletes consume fewer calories than their eumenorrheic peers, whereas others have reported no significant difference (23, 24). However, in all but one of these studies, the caloric intake of the athletes was less than their predicted daily energy expenditure. In individual cases, this energy deficit might be severe enough to initiate hormonal responses, such as elevated cortisol and depressed thyroid function, similar to those observed in cachexia and starvation. The resultant effect on the hypothalamic-pituitary adrenal (HPA) axis may be sufficient to disrupt the normal reproductive cycle (8).

Dietary protein, fat, fiber, and zinc have all been reported to discriminate between amenorrheic and eumenorrheic athletes (22–24). Theoretically, an inadequate nutrient intake could affect neurotransmitter synthesis, which could have a significant effect on hypothalamic function. However, there is no evidence that the dietary difference between menstrual groups has had that effect. Until there are more definitive data to support a link between nutrients and menstrual dysfunction, no specific dietary advice can be given to the amenorrheic woman that will assure her a return to normal menses.

Exercise

Research into the etiology of athletic amenorrhea has begun to move away from the purely descriptive study and delve more deeply into the endocrine basis of the proposed mechanisms. Although a number of studies evaluating the acute and chronic effects of exercise on hormonal concentrations have been published, the data are often conflicting and difficult to interpret. An excellent critical review of the literature in this area has been compiled by Loucks and Horvath (7).

The response of the endocrine system to acute exercise is determined by measuring the concentration of circulating hormones before and after a single exercise bout. Unfortunately, increases in the peripheral concentration of hormones are difficult to interpret. They may not represent changes at the hypothalamic level and cannot be assumed to reflect increased biological activity. It is also uncertain whether the elevated levels are a result of hemoconcentration, increased secretion, or decreased clearance (25). However, the more practical question is whether intermittent elevated levels of specific hormones for relatively short periods of time can interfere with the normal functioning of the HPO axis.

The chronic effects of exercise can be observed in the adaptations of physiological systems after a prolonged training period. In some cases, such as the decrease in resting heart rate, these adaptations can be observed at rest. Other chronic effects, such as an increase in muscular strength after weeks of weight training, are evident only when a demand is placed on the system. A number of investigators have compared basal, or resting, levels of hormones in amenorrheic and eumenorrheic athletes. Others have examined the responses of trained and untrained women or eumenorrheic and amenorrheic athletes to a standard exercise. A few longitudinal studies have followed women throughout a strenuous conditioning program to observe how endocrine responses change during the training program.

Although studies of both acute and chronic exercise have failed to identify a specific mechanism that might disrupt reproductive function, a number of potential mechanisms have been postulated. Some of these, such as hyperandrogenism and hyperprolactinemia, have been eliminated from consideration (9), while others discussed below are still under investigation.

Effect of Exercise on Neurotransmitter-Hypothalamic Function

Because many athletes with menstrual dysfunction have demonstrated an exaggerated response of gonadotropins after administration of GnRH, it has been suggested that the condition is mediated at the hypothalamic level (26). Endogenous opioid peptides are known to inhibit pulsatile gonadotropin release (27) and have been implicated by Bullen et al. (28) and Howlett et al. (29) as a major contributing factor in exercise-related menstrual irregularities. This same group of investigators (30) had shown previously that β-endorphins rise in response to acute exercise in nonathletes and that this response is augmented after training (Fig. 21.1). In addition to the rise in β-endorphins, Howlett et al. (29) also reported a rise in met-enkephalin concentration after acute exercise. Presumably the increase in β-endorphin is the result of its release from the anterior pituitary and occurs in conjunction with release of adrenocorticotropic hormone (ACTH), a known stress hormone. The source of the met-enkephalin remains unknown although Howlett et al. postulate that it may be released from the adrenal medulla, sympathetic nerve endings, or gut. The increase may also be related to a decreased rate of degradation or release of an immunoreactive met-enkephalin from its precursor in plasma (31).

Russell et al. (32) reported an interesting study in which catechol estrogens as well as β-endorphins were monitored in five female swimmers during two training periods. Both hormones were elevated during a strenuous training period (100,000 yards/week) in the five competitive swimmers who became oligomenorreic (Fig. 21.2). Hormonal levels decreased during moderate training (60,000 yards/week) and normal menses resumed. Russell et al. (32) suggest that the two hormones may indirectly suppress GnRH release via their effect on catecholamine degradation and activity. Catechol estrogens are thought to reduce the rate of catecholamine metabolism leaving more dopamine available as a potential GnRH suppressor, while β-endorphins compete with norepinephrine (a GnRH stimulator) for receptor sites in the median eminence of the hypothalamus (32). The resultant inhibition of the pulsatile release of GnRH would lead to a suppression of LH and FSH and eventually to the menstrual disturbances seen in athletes. The observation of Russell et al. (32) that only five of 13 swimmers became oligomenorrheic although all 13 women underwent the same training lends support to Loucks' (9) theory that individual variability in response to stressors explains why some women athletes experience menstrual irregularities and others do not.

Because opioid receptors in the median eminence of the hypothalamus are known to exist and opioids have been reported to inhibit pulsatile release of GnRH, it is tempting to suggest that release of exercise-induced opiates into plasma contributes to the men-

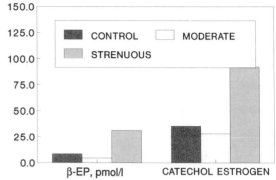

Figure 21.2. β-Endorphin (β-EP) and catechol estrogens for swimmers during periods of moderate training (60,000 yards/wk) and strenuous training (100,000 yards/wk). Samples were obtained before exercise and compared to data obtained from inactive controls. (Adapted from Russell et al. The role of β-endorphins and catechol estrogens on the hypothalamic-pituitary axis in female athletes. Fertil Steril 1984; 42:690–695.)

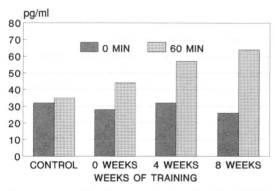

Figure 21.1. The changes in β-endorphin (β-EP) + β-lipotrophin (β-LPH) during a 60-min exercise session. Venous blood samples were taken before exercise (0 min) and after cycling (60 min) before (0 weeks) and after 4 weeks and 8 weeks of training. Control values were obtained before and after sitting on the cycle ergometer for 60 min. (Adapted from Carr et al. Physical conditioning facilitates the exercise induced secretion of β-endorphins and β-lipotrophin in women. N Engl J Med 1981; 305:560–563.)

strual irregularities seen in some athletes. However, Carr et al. (30) question whether the observed increase in endogenous opiates during exercise is large enough to play a physiological role in the etiology of athletic amenorrhea.

Several recent reports (8, 33, 34) have suggested that the HPA response to exercise might affect the normal function of the hypothalamic-pituitary-ovarian (HPO) axis. Loucks et al. (8) assessed the functional integrity of the HPO and HPA axes in eumenorrheic and amenorrheic athletes and sedentary controls by measuring pulsatile luteinizing hormone (LH), ACTH, and cortisol secretion over a 24-hour period under varying conditions. LH pulse frequency was markedly reduced in the amenorrheic women (Fig. 21.3) whereas the LH response to GnRH stimulation was increased. There was no difference in ACTH response, but cortisol levels were elevated in the amenorrheic group throughout the 24-hour period.

Perhaps the most interesting observation in this study was the alteration in HPO response in the eumenorrheic athletes. These women had a reduced LH frequency, increased LH pulse amplitude, a reduction in FSH response to GnRH stimulation, and a decrease in luteal function. Although the menstrual patterns of these women were normal in all respects, the apparent decrease in secretory activity of the corpus luteum suggests that fertility might be compromised in some cyclic athletes. Because both groups of athletes had maintained the same menstrual status over several years, Loucks et al. (8) concluded that diminished luteal function was not part of a continuum leading to amenorrhea but a separate condition. They suggest that individual characteristics may make some women more susceptible to the observed alterations in the hormonal response to strenuous exercise training and that it is these women who will become amenorrheic.

Additional support for the role of the HPA axis in athletic amenorrhea was provided by Ding et al. (34). Basal cortisol levels were higher in amenorrheic athletes (585 nmol/ liter) than in eumenorrheic athletes (411 nmol/ liter) or nonactive women (397 nmol/liter).

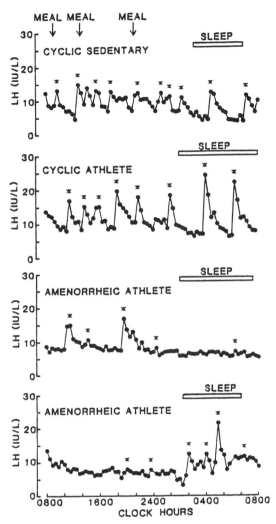

Figure 21.3. Serum LH levels at 20-min intervals for 24 hours in a cyclic sedentary subject, a cyclic athlete, and two amenorrheic athletes. A range of patterns was found in amenorrheic women. The *asterisks* indicate pulses, as identified by the cluster pulse analysis program using a 2 × 1 cluster size and balanced T criteria of 2.1. (Reprinted from Loucks et al. Alterations in the hypothalamic-pituitary-ovarian and the hypothalamic-pituitary-adrenal axes in athletic women. J Clin Endocrinol Metab 1989; 68:402–411.)

Seven women who had been amenorrheic at least 12 months before entering the study resumed menses within 6 months. All cortisol levels for these women and the nonactive women were within the normal range. None of the women whose cortisol levels exceeded the upper range of normal resumed menses in the 6-month period.

The mechanisms underlying athletic amenorrhea are still not fully defined. Most investigators believe that the amenorrhea is a neurotransmitter-hypothalamic-induced phenomenon precipitated by several factors operating synergistically. These factors may be a combination of personal characteristics, life-style, and hormonal responses to strenuous exercise. There is no specific amount of training, weight loss, or body fat that appears to cause menstrual irregularities in all women. Women react differently to exercise and appear to have individual thresholds, which when crossed, lead to oligomenorrhea or amenorrhea. Fortunately, this endocrinopathy is reversible. Most athletes resume normal cycles within 2 or 3 months after the intensity of the training program and frequency and duration of the training sessions are moderated.

CLINICAL WORKUP

In establishing a protocol for the workup of women who develop menstrual abnormalities related to exercise, the major factors to be dealt with include establishing the degree of hypoestrogenicity that may exist and determining whether there is an undetected pathological state independent of exercise that may be the major etiological factor. With these two points in mind, the following protocol is suggested for working up women with oligomenorrhea/amenorrhea associated with exercise (Table 21.2). The initial step after a complete history and physical is to obtain a serum prolactin (PRL). If the PRL level is less than 20 ng/ml, the status of the sella turcica is not evaluated. However, if the woman has hyperprolactinemia she should have a serum thyroid-stimulating hormone (TSH) evalua-

Table 21.2.   Workup of Exercise-Induced Oligomenorrhea/Amenorrhea

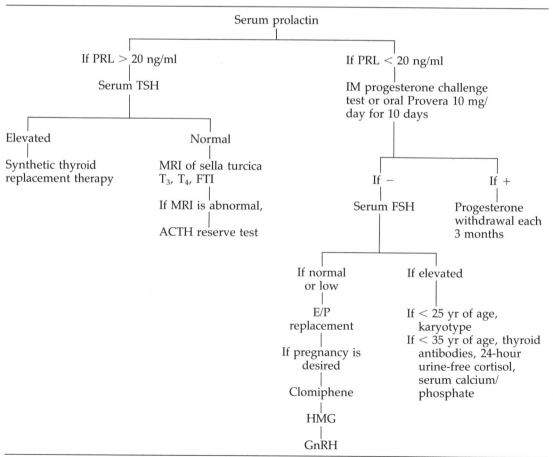

tion to rule out hypothyroidism. If the TSH is normal, she should then have a complete endocrinological evaluation in order to determine whether or not she has a prolactin-secreting adenoma. This workup should include magnetic resonance imaging (MRI) and serum T_4, T_3, and a free thyroxin index (FTI). If the MRI is abnormal, a test for ACTH reserve should be done.

If the amenorrheic woman has a normal serum PRL, her estrogen status should be determined as it has been reported that the hypoestrogenic status can be associated with a decreased vertebral bone density (1–5) in these young women. An intramuscular (IM) injection of progesterone-in-oil (100–200 mg/ml) is given as a challenge test. If the woman has any uterine bleeding, it can be assumed that her serum estradiol (E_2) level is above 40 pg/ml and no estrogen replacement is required. However, if she does not have withdrawal bleeding after 200 mg of progestrone IM, a serum E_2 level should be obtained. If the level is below 40 pg/ml, an estrogen/progestin (E/P) replacement therapy should be instituted. A conjugated estrogen replacement of 0.625 mg/day is given from days 1–25 of the month. On days 14–25 of the month, 5 mg of medroxyprogesterone acetate (Provera) should be given in order to avoid an unopposed estrogen effect on the endometrium. In is not clear at what age replacement therapy should be started, but age 17 seems appropriate because most young women have gone through menarche by that age. This rather vigorous and early start of E/P replacement therapy is based on concern for the risk of premature osteopenia in hypoestrogenic athletes.

If an athlete with hypoestrogenic amenorrhea decides not to accept E/P replacement therapy, she should be advised of the potential for developing premature osteoporosis and be willing to take full responsibility for not taking the recommended therapy. Finally, if an amenorrheic athlete has a negative withdrawal to the progesterone challenge and an elevated serum follicle-stimulating hormone (FSH) level, the diagnosis is premature ovarian failure. These women should be evaluated for a possible gonadal dysgenesis or multiglandular autoimmune disease (Table 21.2).

The amenorrheic athlete with no underlying pathology who wishes to conceive should be advised to make moderate changes in her exercise regimen and dietary habits to encourage resumption of normal menses. Previous studies (36, 37) have found that reducing running mileage and slightly increasing body weight (~5%) result in a return to regular menstrual periods and normal endogenous estrogen levels. If the amenorrhea persists, ovulation can usually be induced by administration of clomiphene citrate. If the amenorrhea is associated with a hypoestrogenic state, then either human menopausal gonadotropin HMG or GnRH should be administered. In conclusion, amenorrheic athletes should be encouraged to continue their physical activity as they vary their training and diet to encourage resumption of normal menses. If menses does not return, they should be evaluated periodically as to their estrogen and prolactin status.

REFERENCES

1. Cann CE, Martin MC, Genant HK, Jaffe RB. Decreased spinal mineral content in amenorrheic women. JAMA 1984; 251:626–629.
2. Drinkwater BL, Nilson K, Chesnut CH III, Bremmer W, Shainholtz S, Southworth M. Bone mineral content of amenorrheic and eumenorrheic athletes. N Engl J Med 1984; 311:277–281.
3. Lindberg JS, Fears WB, Hunt MM, Powell MR, Boll D, Wade CE. Exercise-induced amenorrhea and bone density. Ann Intern Med 1984; 101:647–648.
4. Marcus R, Cann C, Madvig P, Minkoff J, Goddard M, Bayer M, Martin M, Gaudini L, Haskell W, Genant H. Menstrual function and bone mass in elite women distance runners. Ann Intern Med 1985; 102:158–163.
5. Nelson ME, Fisher EC, Catsos PD, Meredith CN, Turksoy RN, Evans WJ. Diet and bone status in amenorrheic runners. Am J Clin Nutr 1986; 43:910–916.
6. Drinkwater BL. Athletic amenorrhea: a review. In: Exercise and health. Champaign, IL: Human Kinetics Publishers, Inc. 1984, p. 120–131.
7. Loucks AB, Horvath SM. Athletic amenorrhea: a review. Med Sci Sports Exerc 1985; 17:56–72.
8. Loucks AB, Mortola JF, Girton L, Yen SSC. Alterations in the hypothalamic-pituitary-ovarian and the hypothalamic-pituitary-adrenal axes in athletic women. J Clin Endocrinol Metab 1989; 68:402–411.
9. Loucks AB. Effects of exercise training on the menstrual cycle: existence and mechanisms. Med Sci Sports Exerc (In press).
10. Veldhuis JD, Evans WS, Dmers LM, Thorner MO, Wakat D, Rogol AD. Altered neuroendocrine regu-

lation of gonadotropin secretion in women distance runners. J Clin Endocrinol Metab 1985; 61:557–563.

11. Frisch RE. Fatness and fertility. Scientif Am 1988; 258:88–95.

12. Frisch RE, McArthur JW. Menstrual cycles: Fatness as a determinant of minimum weight for height necessary for the maintenance or onset. Science 1974; 185:949–951.

13. Frisch RE, Revelle R. Height and weight at menarche and a hypothesis of critical body weights and adolescent events. Science 1970; 169:397–398.

14. Trussell J. Menarche and fatness: Reexamination of the critical body composition hypothesis. Science 1978; 200:1506–1509.

15. Reeves J. Estimating fatness. Science 1979; 204:881.

16. Wakat DK, Sweeney KA, Rogol AD. Reproductive function in women cross-country runners. Med Sci Sports Exerc 1982; 14:263–269.

17. Baker ER, Mathus RS, Kirk RF, Williamson HO. Female runners and secondary amenorrhea: correlation with age, parity, mileage, and plasma hormonal and sex-hormone-binding globulin concentrations. Fertil Steril 1981; 36:183–187.

18. Sanborn CF, Albrecht BH, Wagner WW Jr. Athletic amenorrhea: lack of association with body fat. Med Sci Sports Exerc 1987; 19:207–212.

19. Abraham SF, Beumont PJV, Fraser IS, Llewellyn-Jones D. Body weight, exercise and menstrual status among ballet dancers in training. Br J Obstet Gynaecol 1982; 89:507–510.

20. Warren MP. The effects of exercise on pubertal progression and reproductive function in girls. J Clin Endocrinol Metab 1980; 51:1150–1151.

21. Drinkwater BL, Bruemner B, Chesnut CH, III. Menstrual history as a determinant of current bone density in young athletes. JAMA 1990; 263:545–548.

22. Bruemner B, Drinkwater BL. Nutrient intake in amenorrheic and eumenorrheic athletes. Med Sci Sports Exerc 1986; 18:S37.

23. Deuster PA, Kyle SB, Moser PB, Vigersky RA, Singh A, Schoomaker EB. Nutritional intakes and status of highly trained amenorrheic and eumenorrheic women runners. Fertil Steril 1986; 46:636–643.

24. Lloyd T, Buchanan JR, Bitzer S, Waldman CJ, Myers C, Ford BG. Interrelationships of diet, athletic activity, menstrual status, and bone density in collegiate women. Am J Clin Nutr 1987; 46:681–684.

25. Keizer HA, Kuipers H, Verstapper FTJ, Janssen E. Limitations of concentration measurement for evaluation of endocrine status of exercising women. Can J Appl Sport Sci 1982; 7:79–84.

26. McArthur JW, Bullen BA, Bettins IZ, Pagane M, Bader TM, Klianski A. Hypothalamic amenorrhea in runners of normal body distribution. Endocr Res Commun 1980; 7:13–25.

27. Moult PA, Grossman A, Evans JM, Reese LH, Beser GM. The effect of naloxone on pulsatile gonadotropin release in normal subjects. Clin Endocrinol 1981; 14:321–324.

28. Bullen BA, Skrinar GS, Beitins IZ, et al. Endurance training effects on plasma hormonal responsiveness and sex hormone excretion. J Appl Physiol 1984; 56:1453–1463.

29. Howlett TA, Tomlin S, Ngahfoong L, Rees LH, Bullen BA, Skrinar GS, McArthur JW. Release of B-endorphin and metenkephalin during exercise in normal women: response to training. Br Med J 1984; 288:1950–1952.

30. Carr DB, Bullen BA, Skrinar GS. Physical conditioning facilitates the exercise-induced secretion of β-endorphins and B-lipotrophin in women. N Engl J Med 1981; 305:560–563.

31. Smith R, Grossman A, Gaillard R, et al. Studies on circulating met-enkephalin and B-endorphin. Normal subjects and patients with renal and adrenal disease. Clin Endocrinol 1981; 15:291–308.

32. Russell JB, Mitchell DE, Musey PI, Collins DC. The role of B-endorphins and catechol estrogens on the hypothalamic-pituitary axis in female athletes. Fertil Steril 1984; 42:690–695.

33. Loucks AB, Horvath SM. Exercise-induced stress responses of amenorrheic and eumenorrheic runners. J Clin Endocrinol Metab 1984; 59:1109–1120.

34. Ding JH, Sheckter CB, Drinkwater BL, Soules MR, Bremner WJ. High serum cortisol levels in exercise-associated amenorrhea. Ann Intern Med 1988; 108:530–534.

35. Sanborn CC. Menstrual dysfunction in the female athlete. In: Teitz CC, ed. Scientific foundations of sports medicine. Philadelphia: BC Decker Inc., 1989; p. 117–134.

36. Drinkwater BL, Nilson K, Ott S, Chesnut CH III. Bone mineral density after resumption of menses in amenorrheic athletes. JAMA 1986; 256:380–382.

37. Lindberg JS, Powell MR, Hunt MM, Ducey DE, Wade CE. Increased vertebral bone mineral in response to reduced exercise in amenorrheic runners. West J Med 1987; 146:39–42.

22

Pregnancy and Altitude: Physical Activity at High Altitude

Renate Huch

For those who reside permanently at high altitudes as well as for those from lower regions who ascend to such altitudes, the reduced O_2 availability must be met with compensatory physiological alterations that assure the balance between O_2 demand and supply. This adaptive capability is greater in states of physical rest than during exercise. It seems reasonable to assume that during pregnancy, when important circulatory and ventilatory alterations necessitated by physiological factors have already occurred, the adaptive capabilities at altitudes would be further limited, possibly with negative effects on the course of pregnancy and the development of the child in utero. The aim of this chapter is to review the known facts and the related studies that have been carried out on this topic. First, the nonpregnant organism will be considered with a description pertaining to the extent and frequency of altitude exposure, the lack of oxygen at various altitudes, and the physiological compensatory reactions—their types, extent, and time of occurrence.

EXTENT OF REDUCED O_2 AVAILABILITY

There are about 40 million people throughout the world who live at altitudes over 8000 ft (2438 m). It is estimated that about the same number of people from lower regions visit such high-altitude areas each year (1). For Colorado, it is estimated that approximately 2% of the yearly visitors are pregnant women (1). Once the province of the fit and few (1), these high-altitude areas are today accessible to nearly everyone via modern modes of transportation, including cable cars and planes—physical limitations and risks are no longer factors naturally preventing access to altitude. Flying itself, with its flight-specific conditions, carries millions of people per year to a similar exposure. At the normal cruise levels of commercial airliners, the cabin pressure corresponds to altitudes between sea level and 2400–2500 m (approximately 8000 ft) (2) Thus, many pregnant women and their fetuses can be either chronically or acutely exposed to the special effects of altitude.

What is common to both chronic and acute altitude exposure is that, with increasing altitude, the absolute quantity of oxygen available in the atmosphere decreases. How well a living organism can cope with life at high altitudes depends first of all on its ability to adapt to the decreased O_2 content, that is, the reduced O_2 partial pressure. Table 22.1 shows the decrease in the partial pressure as a function of the altitude. One differentiates between low, moderate, and high altitudes, although the borders between these are rather pragmatic and not uniformly defined. For example, the point where high altitude is said to begin varies between 2500 and 3000 m (approximately 8000–10000 ft) (3, 4).

Table 22.1. Decrease of Barometric and Oxygen Partial Pressure with Increasing Altitude[a]

Altitude		Barometric Pressure (mm Hg)	Oxygen Partial Pressure (mm Hg)
m	feet		
0	0	760.00	159
1000	3,280	674.13	141
2000	6,560	596.31	125
3000	9,840	525.95	110
4000	13,100	462.49	97
5000	16,400	405.39	85
6000	19,700	354.16	74

[a]Modified from Gilbert DL. Cosmic and geophysical aspects of the respiratory gases. In: Fenn WO, Rahn H, eds. Respiration. Baltimore: Williams & Wilkins, 1964; p. 153–176.

CHRONIC AND ACUTE ALTITUDE EXPOSURE

Two important differences, however, distinguish chronic from acute altitude exposure and require a separate analysis of the various effects. The first difference is due to the fact that, at ever higher altitudes, not only are there changes in oxygen partial pressure but in environmental factors as well—climatic conditions, cosmic radiation, terrain, sanitation, nutritional status, and so forth—and these help determine the form and quality of life for the people who live year-round at high altitudes. The limits inherently posed by altitude exposure are thus determined by the ability of the individual person to adapt to these factors. It will be shown that immediately or within a short time after acute exposure, such an acclimatization (at best) is only partial. For the optimum, days, or weeks, if not generations are required. That is the second important difference between the effects of chronic or acute exposure at high altitude.

LIMITATIONS FOR PERMANENT LIFE AT AND ACUTE EXPOSURE TO HIGH ALTITUDE

The highest altitudes where human settlements are known are in Asia (Himalayas, 4930 m, approximately 16,000 ft; Tibet (4600 m, approximately 15,000 ft); and in South America (in the Andes; mines in the Aucanquilcha (6180 m, approximately 20,000 ft; and the camp for the workers at 5180 m, approximately 17,000 ft). The highest altitude settlements in North America and Europe are at lower altitudes (Colorado plateau, 3000 m, approximately 10,000 ft and the Oetztaler Alps, 2300 m, approximately 7700 ft) (5). Temporary exposure seems to have no particular limits if the will and exceptional physiological prerequisites, training, and proper planning are present (6, 7); the spectacular ascents without oxygen by Messner and Habeler in 1978 of Mount Everest (8) (8848 m, approximately 29,000 ft) have shown that. For the average person, however, a discussion of the effects of altitudes of between 2500 and 4000 m (approximately 8000–13,000 ft) is more re-alistic: altitudes that are common for recreational activities, sports (skiing), and mountain climbing. Thus, these altitudes are also those that should be discussed as a possible risk factor for the woman who is pregnant.

PHYSIOLOGICAL REACTIONS TO ALTITUDE EXPOSURE

The human organism has various adaptation mechanisms to compensate for the decreasing P_{O_2}, that is, for the reduced quantity of O_2 when ascending to heights or residing there. Changes take place at all levels of oxygen transport, from inspiration down to the level of the mitochondria, i.e., in ventilation, diffusion, circulation, in the oxygen transport properties of the blood, microcirculation, and at the cell level. Due to the acclimatization processes, the symptoms related to hypoxia are modified during rest, and the capacity for work and exercise increases.

Table 22.2 lists the main physiological reactions to altitude. The order given corresponds approximately to the chronological order of occurrence of the reactions, beginning with the immediate functional alterations, continuing to medium-term alterations in the composition of the blood or new physiological steady-states, and finally to morphological alterations that may first be observable after many years or generations.

Table 22.2.   Physiological Reactions to Altitude Hypoxic Stress

	Time necessary for acclimatization	
Increase in minute ventilation; tidal volume > rate		minutes
Increase in cardiac output; heart rate > stroke volume		
Increase in blood pressure; systolic > diastolic		
Increase in pulmonary artery pressure and perfusion		
Decrease in Hb oxygen affinity		
Increase in hemoglobin and hematocrit		
Blood volume expansion		
Increase in arteriovenous difference		
Morphological alterations (e.g., chest form, capillary density)		
Increase in mitochondria and cell enzyme concentrations		generations
Blunted hypoxic response		
Increase in Hb oxygen affinity		

The immediate alterations are those of the cardiorespiratory system. Above approximately 3000 m (approximately 10,000 ft), the minute ventilation starts to rapidly increase, first linearly, and then, above 5000 m (approximately 16,500 ft) increasingly exponentially and more as the result of an increase in the tidal volume (9). The increase in the first few minutes after ascent is the greatest because the maximal initial hypoxic stimulation of the peripheral chemoreceptors is reduced through the hypocapnia-induced decrease of the central respiratory drive (10). Cardiac output also increases immediately after altitude exposure as a result of sympathetic activity induced by hypoxic stress. Most researchers describe this as a result of the increased heart rate rather than stroke volume (4, 11, 12, 13). Between 2000 and 6000 m (approximately 6500 and 20,000 ft), the heart rate increases linearly, above 6000 m, exponentially. The systolic blood pressure rises, while there is usually a slight decrease in diastolic pressure (4, 9), especially above 5000 m (approximately 16,500 ft) (9). There is general agreement that after the initial increase in minute ventilation and cardiac output, these return to original values within 1–4 days at medium altitudes, and in higher regions they at least drop from the maximum that had been reached (4, 11, 13). According to Lenfant (11), this decrease in cardiac output is a definite result of the stroke volume decrease, possibly, in fact, as a direct depressing action of hypoxia on the myocardium. Little is known about the important aspect of a blood flow redistribution in humans at high altitudes, although such a redistribution is known to be important for the adaptation to chronic hypoxia. Pulmonary arterial pressure always rises, possibly resulting from both an increase in lung perfusion through redistribution and an increased pulmonary vasoconstriction (13, 14).

With respect to an improvement in oxygen transport, the adaptive alterations in the blood are most efficient. On the one hand, there is an absolute increase in the oxygen-carrying capacity, and short-term a relative increase as well because the plasma volume decreases and hematocrit increases. Approximately 6–12 hours after high altitude exposure, a clear increase in erythropoietin is measured in the serum and urine with subsequent hemoglobin synthesis (15, 16). The extent of this adaptive mechanism diminishes within a few days (11), having attained its maximum on the 3rd day (16). A hemoglobin concentration that is higher than that at sea level continues to be a factor found at higher elevations. On the other hand, there is also a change in oxygen affinity. As soon as 3 hours at only 1800 m (6000 ft), the intraerythrocyte 2,3-DPG concentration significantly increases (17), shifting the hemoglobin dissociation curve to the right, thus compensating the in vivo affinity increase by hyperventilation alkalosis.

It is known that many other adaptation processes need a very long period of time to establish themselves and, in some cases, reach the optimum only after many generations. Among these are morphological alterations in the lungs, an improved lung diffusion capacity, changes in the respiratory pattern, and the development of a specific chest form (18). On the cell and tissue levels, an increased capillary density, an increased mitochondrial density, the role of myoglobin for facilitated oxygen diffusion, and a larger cytochrome concentration at altitude are mechanisms that have been discussed (11, 19–21). A final point is a change that, at first, seems paradoxical: for native highland populations and for those who have lived in such regions for decades, there is a decrease in the sensitivity to react to hypoxia with an increase in ventilation, that is, blunted hypoxic response is observed (11, 22–24). This adaptation is described as irreversible, although as discussed later, this does not seem to be the case for pregnant women and is understood as an appropriate mechanism to stimulate the synthesis of hemoglobin constantly.

There are some studies on record that have investigated the adaptation processes in relation to gender. It has been shown that, at least during rest, women seem to adapt better than men to high altitudes in terms of, for example, hemoconcentration, hyperventilation, and acid-base balance (25). Symptoms of altitude sickness occur less often in women.

In summary, the human organism experiences both functional and morphological reactions to altitude exposure. Some of the adaptations are only temporary, yet crucial for avoiding impairments and damage caused by hypoxia. For certain of the mechanisms mentioned, it is very difficult to recognize the physiological benefit. An example is the change in oxygen affinity mentioned; although a shift to the right of the dissociation curve is beneficial for the unloading of O_2 in tissues, at higher altitudes, the disadvantage for the loading of O_2 by the pulmonary capillaries outweighs the advantage of oxygen release at the cell level (26). With certain physical reactions, there is an inherent risk of overcompensation. Examples are excessive hyperventilation and increasing blood viscosity.

Maladaptation can result in the so-called acute mountain sickness (AMS), or high-altitude deterioration. In extreme cases, all the signs of central hypoxia and the occurrence of lung edema are observed. Typical symptoms of AMS are euphoria or fatigue, severe headaches, dyspnea, dizziness, vomiting, and loss of appetite (1, 5, 26, 27), occurring between 12 and 96 hours after acute and continuing exposure. These symptoms, according to investigations by Hackett et al. (28) and Johnson and Rock (27), were experienced in 42–67% of those ascending to 14,000 ft (4268 m), and in 30% at 3000 m (10,000 ft), respectively. A most recent systematic investigation in the Swiss Alps showed the correlation of AMS to altitude: at 2850 m (9500 ft), the prevalence was 9%; at 3050 m (10,000 ft), 13%; at 3650 m (12,000 ft), 34%; and at 4559 m (15,000 ft), 54% (29).

EXERCISE AT ALTITUDE

When physical work or sport are engaged in at high altitudes, there are even more demands placed on the organism. From numerous reports on expeditions at high altitudes, it is only too well known that the actual physical limits at altitude are seen in the combination of high altitude and physical work (7, 8, 13). The same holds for those with no special training in sports and mountain climbing at altitudes above 2500 m (approximately 8000 ft).

There are crucial differences at altitudes between the situation during rest and when physical work is being performed:

—Similar to the situation at sea level: Exercise itself requires an increase in the cardiorespiratory function due to an increased O_2 demand during physical exertion.

—This exercise-induced increase is greater in the first few days than later after acclimatization.

—Different from the situation at sea level and making physical work at high altitude extra difficult: at sea level, exercise increases the lung diffusion capacity. With altitude hypoxia, the diffusion capacity of the lungs (and probably that of the tissues as well) is impaired (30). Oxygen saturation at high altitude is thus decreased in relation to the altitude and the amount of exercise in spite of sharply increased ventilation and the increase of the alveolar P_{O_2}, documenting the clear widening of the alveolar-arterial difference when exercising at altitude (30–33).

The decrease in cardiopulmonary performance during exercise at high altitude or the increased demand on the biological reserves is well documented. For a given submaximal work load, the oxygen uptake is indeed described as independent of altitude but the stress to the cardiorespiratory system is greater (7, 11, 25, 34–36). At every level of altitude, the increase in heart rate, cardiac output, ventilation, lactate, catecholamine, cortisol, and the decrease in plasma insulin is greater, whereas the buffer capacity of the blood is lower than at sea level for equivalent physical stress. Figure 22.1 shows that, with exercise, the ventilation increases much more at altitude than at sea level and that this increase is much greater in one not acclimatized to altitude. The apparent advantages in the adaptation processes previously mentioned for women (compared with men) during rest were not observed during exercise (25). There is agreement that the maximum oxygen uptake, that is, the aerobic work capacity, relative to the altitude, decreases sharply, thus limiting the performance capacity (25, 30, 32, 35, 36–39). There is no improvement in $\dot{V}_{O_2max}$

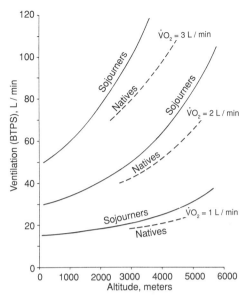

Figure 22.1. Minute ventilation as a function of the altitude at three levels of exercise. With permission from Lenfant C, Sullivan K. Adaption to high altitude. N Eng J Med 1971; 284:1298–1309.

through acclimatization (37). Most of the works cited come to the conclusion that the crucial limitations posed by the combination of exercise and altitude are not primarily due to cardiocirculatory factors but the increasingly less efficient ventilation found with increasing altitude. Due to the relatively slow onset and full development of certain adaptation processes, it must be assumed that the combined effects of high altitude and exercise produce the greatest stress to the organism in the first 3–4 days after acute (and continuing) exposure to altitude.

REPRODUCTION AND ALTITUDE

It is certainly legitimate to interpret survival and continuity of a particular population at altitude as THE indicator for the tolerance of the organism for all types of stress, including that of reproduction and pregnancy. On the other hand, failures in the reproduction process would clearly indicate certain limits that altitude exposure might pose. This must not necessarily be only the result of a chronic lack of oxygen. Specific effects of the social, cultural, and natural environment (40) in highland regions might

also play a role. Special points of interest are the pregnancy-specific physiological alterations at high altitudes in comparison with those at lower elevations.

Reproductive problems at high altitudes were noted even several centuries ago (41, 42). Since then, many investigations on the specific characteristics of reproduction and pregnancy and about the newborn at high altitudes have been made (1, 40, 42–63). Usually these studies concern inhabited areas above 3000 m (10,000 ft); most of them, in fact, areas above 4000 m (13,000 ft). Table 22.3 lists special reproductive characteristics that have been studied at these altitudes.

The physiological course of the gametogenesis does not seem to be influenced by altitude. The vast majority of studies on animals show that altitude exposure has a surprisingly small influence on oogenesis and spermatogenesis. The decrease in sperm motility and the increase of abnormal forms that have been observed in the human are temporary phenomena, as are the changes in the reproductive endocrinology, which have been investigated to a good extent in man (41).

Since the time of the menarche can be relatively easily determined, many data are available on this (41). On an average, the menarche occurs 2 years later than at lower altitudes. Puberty in boys also seems to be delayed. As for the changes caused by altitude in fertilization and implantation, only results from studies on animals can be ref-

Table 22.3. Special Reproductive Characteristics in Female Residents at High Altitude

No evidence for damage to gametogenesis
Delay in menarche
Normal fecundity
Low fertility (=low number of offspring per woman)
Repeated miscarriages (early?, late?)
High incidence of pregnancy-induced hypertension
High incidence of placenta praevia
Reduced birthweight
 High incidence of growth retardation
 Unaltered gestational length
Increase in malformation rate (?)
High neonatal and infant mortality

erenced because of the very nature of the problem. It has been found that the egg cell, whether fertilized or not, is very sensitive to acute hypoxia (41). The loss of fertilized ova is related to the degree of hypoxia, and thus, to altitude (41). It remains an open question as to what degree these findings are applicable to humans. In humans, an increased occurrence of placenta previa has been ascertained (53), which, similar to the situation for smoking during pregnancy (64), might imply an implantation impairment due to hypoxia. There is no direct evidence in humans that there is a loss of the fertilized egg in early stages.

If one takes the average number of offspring per woman as the definition of fertility (65), then fertility is definitely lower at high altitudes. As to the causes, however, the discussions are quite controversial. Factors that can lower the statistical number of offspring per woman in a given population include the already mentioned late menarche, and then culturally-dictated late marriages, the frequent absence of men away on expeditions, the inclusion of nuns in the statistical data, and the high infant mortality rate (42, 43), which can be as high as 25% in the first year of life (42). On the other hand, it is also pointed out that contraceptive methods are not practiced in these areas (66) and that the fecundity itself does not appear to be greatly affected. Ignoring the high infant mortality rate and assuming a normal fecundity, one must come to the conclusion that there is a higher percentage of miscarriages, either early or late. In addition to the effect of oxygen, iodine deficiency, typical for high altitudes, has also been discussed as a possible cause of the lower fertility rate and, the higher rate of miscarriages (63). There is a known connection between hypothyroidism and reproductive failure and spontaneous abortions.

Concerning the course of pregnancy and delivery at high altitudes, Sobrevilla and colleagues (60) compared the estrogen excretion in pregnant women in the last 2 weeks before delivery at 4200 m (approximately 14,000 ft) with that in pregnant women at sea level. They found that the estrogen excretion, especially that of estriol as a sensitive indicator of the functioning of the fetal-placental unit, to be significantly reduced at high altitudes, and that it correlated well with the birthweight, and the weight of the placenta. The lower the estriol value, the lower the birth weight, and the weight of the placenta was. Moore and colleagues (55) tested both prospectively and retrospectively the interesting hypothesis that the occurrence of pregnancy-induced hypertension (PIH) is related to hypoxia. At 3100 m (approximately 10,000 ft), they found that there was indeed more PIH, proteinuria and edema of the upper extremities, and higher blood pressure, and that this was definitely related to the altitude. The correlation of arterial pressure and altitude in pregnant women at 1600, 2400, and 3100 m (approximately 5000, 8000, and 10,000 ft, respectively) is clearly demonstrated in the data of Moore et al. (55). Although the mechanism is not fully understood, it appears to operate inversely to arterial oxygen saturation. It seems that there is only one systematic investigation on record that was taken during delivery at high altitudes. Sobrevilla et al. (59) studied maternal and fetal blood gases in humans at 4200 m (approximately 14,000 ft). In a later section, we shall refer to these investigations again due to their clear indication that the fetus also is capable of adaptation to higher altitudes.

Numerous studies have concentrated on the birthweight of infants from pregnancies at high altitudes (15, 47, 48, 51–54, 60, 64, 67). Studies where sex, parity, maternal stature, and nutritional status were carefully controlled show beyond any doubt that birthweight is reduced in humans at highland regions, meaning that it is inversely proportional to the altitude. The data of Moore et al. (56) also show clearly the correlation between altitude and birthweight, 100 g/1000 m (approximately 3000 ft) elevation. That this reduction is specific to altitude was well documented by Howard et al. (68). For women who first gave birth at low altitude and then later at 3100 m, the second child weighed, on an average, 380 g less than the first one.

All signs indicate that this weight reduction is a result of intrauterine growth retardation and not the result of a shortened period of pregnancy. Most reviews of the etiology of birth weight reduction identify oxygen insufficiency as a possible cause. This viewpoint is also supported by data from Moore et al. (58). They noted that maternal smoking at 3100 m (approximately 10,000 ft) was associated with a reduction in birthweight two or three times greater than that reported for sea level. Meyer (64) also proposes an interesting hypothesis linking maternal smoking and the effects of altitude. That the etiology of growth retardation is due to a reduced oxygen supply at altitude seems quite plausible when noting a similar growth retardation in infants whose mothers have heart disease (69). The findings described an increased incidence of PIH; the known association between this and growth retardation also fit well into the picture. The noteworthy acclimatization of native highland populations to high altitude stress is also reflected in the birthweight. Haas et al (47) found a significant ethnic difference in birthweight and length.

In animal studies, it has been proved that hypoxia is a teratogenic factor (41). For humans, however, there are very little data available; the losses already mentioned in the pre- or early implantation phase would camouflage such an effect. Alzamora et al. (70) found a striking number of persons in the highlands of Peru with certain cardiac defects, vaguely indicating a possible connection.

Moreover, it is certain that newborn and infant mortality is high at high altitudes, even though there are indications that improved living standards in these areas in recent years have led to a substantial drop in the mortality rate (1). Neonatal mortality increases in a linear fashion with decreasing barometric pressure, seeming to suggest that lack of oxygen is the principal cause. Cosmic radiation is possibly another influencing factor (41).

ADAPTATION TO THE STRESS OF PREGNANCY AT HIGH ALTITUDE

Besides the basic facts about the course of pregnancy and outcome, many studies have focused on the biological mechanisms that meet the combined strain resulting from altitude and pregnancy. According to the data available, three of the main mechanisms are: a further increase in the pregnancy-induced cardiopulmonary functions; functional and morphological alterations in the placenta; and adaptations of the fetus in utero (51, 55, 56, 49, 71). Similar observations have also been made in animals (61, 72–74).

Maternal Ventilation

It is known that the pregnant woman hyperventilates even at sea level, lowering the P_{CO_2} to 30 mm Hg already in early stages of pregnancy without, however, increasing the P_{O_2} much above the nonpregnant value (75). At high altitudes, however, this hyperventilation results in an impressive increase in the arterial P_{O_2} over and above that of the nonpregnant human. While at an altitude of about 4000 m (approximately 13,000 ft), the range of the mean arterial P_{O_2} of the nonpregnant native highlander is only 45–50 mm Hg (59); pregnant women at 4200 m (approximately 14,000 ft) were found to have a mean P_{O_2} of 60.8 mm Hg (59). The mean arterial P_{CO_2} in the pregnant women was 24.5 mm Hg. Hellegers and colleagues (71) compared the end-expiratory O_2 and CO_2 values in both pregnant and nonpregnant women at 14,500 ft (approximately 4500 m) and found a similar increase in the P_{O_2}. While the mean P_{O_2} and P_{CO_2} values for nonpregnant persons were, respectively, 51 and 28 mm Hg, the mean values for pregnant women were, respectively, 59 and 23 mm Hg. Moore et al. (54) found that at 4300 m (approximately 14,000 ft), the ventilation of pregnant women was approximately 25% higher than that of nonpregnant women, the reason being an increase in tidal volume. The alveolar P_{O_2} increased from 58 to 63 mm Hg, corresponding to a saturation increase from 83 to 87%, and the P_{CO_2} decreased from 31 to 26 mm Hg.

It is clear from such data that the pregnant woman can increase her ventilation over and above the normal hyperventilation typical at high altitudes. According to the studies by Moore et al. (54), this ability evidently is related to an increased ventilatory responsiveness to hypoxia with pregnancy, yet the underlying causes have not yet been discovered (54). The data of Moore et al., however, very impressively show that the blunted hypoxic response in natives or long-term residents at high altitude that was previously described is not irreversible but, during pregnancy, can reoccur. Their data also give convincing evidence that this ability to increase the maternal ventilation favors fetal growth, and is one of THE decisive adaptive mechanisms to the combination of altitude AND pregnancy. Figure 22.2 shows that the birth weight increases with increasing minute ventilation. These data thus also support the assumption that hypoxia must be one of the main factors responsible for the reduced birth weight at high altitudes.

Alterations in Placental Structures and Function at High Altitude

Morphological changes and their implications for alterations in the placental function in pregnancies at high altitude have been investigated in numerous studies on both humans and animals (49, 53, 59, 61, 66, 76). Adaptive alterations facilitating oxygen diffusion would theoretically imply an improvement in the diffusion capacity by increasing the surface area, decreasing the thickness of

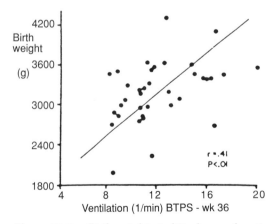

Figure 22.2. Birthweight at altitude as a function of maternal ventilation. From Moore LG, Jahnigen D, Rounds SS, Reeves JT, Grover RF. Maternal hyperventilation helps preserve arterial oxygenation during high-altitude pregnancy. J Appl Phys Resp Env Exerc Physiol 1982; 53:690–694.

the layers separating maternal and fetal erythrocytes, and increasing blood flow on one or both sides of the placenta.

There is no particular agreement among the various results reported on the relatively easy to measure placental weight and it is difficult to find a common denominator among them (49, 51, 53, 59). Yet the differences compared to lowland placentas are minimal. There is no doubt, however, but that the ratio of placental weight to newborn weight is higher and that this ratio also increases with increasing altitude, basically reflecting the decreasing birth weight at high altitudes. Some of the morphometric studies show a clearly enlarged intervillous surface area with a decrease of the intervillous space, increased vascularization, and a larger total surface area when considered macroscopically. There is a closer approximation of the fetal vessels to the trophoblast surface (49). As a result, the maternal-fetal barrier becomes thinner. Meschia et al. (76) also found an enlarged diffusion area in the placenta of the llama, an animal that is most well-adapted to high altitudes. This must be qualified, however, by the fact that some of the morphological alterations reported in the placenta at high altitudes are of questionable functional value or even disadvantageous for oxygen transport. A high percentage of placental infarct, which is detrimental to placental function, was seen to occur at high altitudes (53). Purely functional investigations on the placenta at high altitudes have only taken place in animals. In pregnant ewes adapted to altitude, uterine blood flow was found to be higher than at sea level (77).

Evidence for Fetal Acclimatization to High Altitude

Although there is no doubt that the development of the fetus in utero is dependent upon the previously described maternal adaptations, it might also be expected that the fetus itself is capable of adaptation to the reduced oxygen tension. This assumption is based on our general knowledge about the fetal reaction to hypoxia at sea level. The very nature of certain acute and chronic fetal compensatory reactions, e.g., blood flow redistribution with certain organ systems being favored for blood flow, has so far precluded studies being made on them at high altitude. And there are only few data on the human fetus that would allow, either directly or indirectly, any conclusions to be drawn about a possible long-term compensatory mechanism (59, 78, 79). Assessments of blood gases in the human fetus exist so far only for the time of birth. Sobrevilla et al. (59) measured a mean P_{O_2} of 19 mm Hg in fetal scalp blood at 4200 m (approximately 14,000 ft), compared with a value of 21.5 mm Hg at sea level, a difference that is not significant. Likewise, there was no difference seen in the fetal pH. This stands in contrast to the difference of 30 mm Hg in the maternal P_{O_2} values between sea level and at high altitudes. Compensatory increases, albeit only slight, of hemoglobin, hematocrit, and the percentage of HbF were seen by Ballew and Haas (78) at 3600 m. Sobrevilla et al. (59) saw no changes in the hematocrit at 4200 m (approximately 14,000 ft). On the balance, these few investigations do provide evidence that the human fetus at high altitude is not hypoxic. Knowing the degree of maternal hypoxemia and the extent of the placental adaptation, the assumption is justified that the fetus itself has resources aiding it to adapt to the reduced oxygen availability. Results from animal studies are in agreement with this general statement (72).

In summary, reproductive efficiency is impaired at high altitude and is dependent on the altitude itself. There are numerous direct and indirect indicators that lack of oxygen is evidently the major factor. Quite noteworthy are the findings that show that the pregnant woman can meet the additional O_2 demand over and above what is necessary for the altitude-specific acclimatization. Hyperventilation has been shown to be one of the decisive adaptations to high altitude AND pregnancy, an adaptation that, as the first historical reports on the Spanish newcomers to the New World in the 17th century in the Andes show, can only be acquired over a very long time period (41).

EFFECTS ON PREGNANT WOMEN OF ACUTE HIGH ALTITUDE EXPOSURE

Because not all of the physiological adaptive mechanisms set in at once, the tolerance limits for those living permanently at high altitudes cannot be used in comparison. Numerous pregnant women use modern modes of transportation to reach high altitudes within a very short time span or are acutely exposed to the height of 2000–2500 m (6500–8000 feet) in commercial airplanes after pressurization (2, 80). Pregnancy-specific alterations in oxygen consumption and lung function, resulting in a lower oxygen reserve than in the nonpregnant state, pose theoretically a particular risk for hypoxia in the pregnant woman who is acutely exposed to altitude. Makowski et al. (74) saw that in mother and fetus— these were, however, studies with animals and at much higher altitudes (14,260 ft, 4345 m)—days went by before the oxygen content and saturation improved. The lowest saturation in the umbilical vein was observed between the 2nd and 4th day after altitude exposure. From these data, we may assume that the altitudes that can be recommended as safe are lower for the pregnant woman with acute altitude exposure than for native highlanders. Possible limits even for moderate altitude exposure should also be discussed because these exposures are normally combined with physical activity and exercise. Today people go hiking, climbing, or skiing in the mountains, and this may involve great physical strain. For those who fly, there is less concern for the seated passenger, but more for the working stewardess (2, 81).

For pregnancy, the possible risks of an acute altitude exposure, with or without physical work, have been discussed only theoretically (82–84) or on the basis of studies with animals. We, therefore, decided to run a study on mother and fetus with respect to their physiological reactions under real or simulated altitude exposure (2, 85, 86). It should be emphasized that our studies were not structured to allow an analysis of the limits of stress at extremely high altitudes during pregnancy, but rather to investigate whether the altitudes experienced as a routine matter by many women were tolerable for mother and fetus.

Flying During Pregnancy

There are four situations in which a pregnant woman might be exposed to flight-specific influences: as a passenger, as a stewardess (with additional physical stress due to flight duties), as a patient being transported in a rescue plane, or as a pilot. The last two situations are relatively rare; in rescue flights, moreover, additional oxygen is on hand. Flights as a pregnant passenger or as a pregnant stewardess are, of course, quite common. Airlines allow pregnant women to fly except in the last weeks of pregnancy. Certain airlines also allow a stewardess who is pregnant to continue to work during the early months of pregnancy (87).

Among the flight-specific influences, the relative hypoxemia and flight anxiety have long been discussed as risks for the pregnant woman. Analogue to findings from animal studies (88, 89), which showed a significant reduction of the uterine blood flow with a sharp increase in noradrenalin when the mother animal was under psychic stress, fear of flying can be disadvantageous for the human fetus.

Both of these risks were investigated by our group in real situations, noting the effect on mother and fetus during 20 inner European commercial flights (2). In Table 22.4, further details on the study are shown, and Table 22.5 summarizes the results. The maternal organism showed significant reactions, analogous to those observed in the nonpregnant organism. The first compensatory reaction to altitude and the P_{O_2} decrease was a significant increase in the heart rate and a slight rise in blood pressure. During the entire flight, there was no change observed in the P_{CO_2} or in the respiratory rate, so that one can assume that the tidal volume also remained constant. At this altitude therefore, there is not yet an increase in the hyperventilation that already exists in the pregnant woman; this fact is in agreement with observations of the changes in ventilation in nonpregnant women under 3000 m (approxi-

Table 22.4. Characteristics of the Women Studied and the Variables Measured[a]

Pregnant volunteers	
Total number	10
Mean age (yr)	28
Primiparous	7
Smoker	2
Length of gestation (wk)	32–38

Parameter monitored (continuously and noninvasively)
  Maternal transcutaneous P_{O_2}
  Maternal transcutaneous P_{CO_2}
  Maternal respiratory rate
  Maternal heart rate (from electrocardiogram)
  Maternal blood pressure, systolic
  Maternal blood pressure, diastolic
  Maternal uterine pressure (external)
  Fetal heart rate (ultrasound Doppler)
  Cabin pressure (electronic barometer)

[a]From Huch R, Baumann H, Fallenstein F, Schneider KTM, Holdener F, Huch A. Physiologic changes in pregnant women and their fetuses during jet air travel. Am J Obstet Gynecol 1986; 154:996–1000.

mately 10,000 ft) that was described earlier in this chapter.

The baseline and the other variables that were evaluated from the recording of the fetal heart rate were in the normal range in all of the flight phases. There was no indication of reduced fetal heart rate variability. Only three times during take-off and ascent and once at cruising altitude (three fetuses were involved) were there marked accelerations (three of short duration and one of 8 min). Because the fetal accelerations were not accompanied

Table 22.5. Results of the Zurich Flight Study.

For a pregnant woman during flight
  The maternal P_{O_2} decreases by 25%;
  The P_{CO_2} remains constant throughout the flight;
  The maternal heart rate increases significantly;
  The blood pressure rises slightly at cruising altitude;
  The respiratory rate remains constant in spite of the decrease in P_{O_2};
  The mean fetal heart rate and the fetal heart rate pattern remain normal in all flight phases;
  In individual cases, the fetal heart rate accelerates;
  In no flight phase are there any signs in the fetal cardiogram of insufficient oxygen supply.

by maternal heart rate accelerations, which we would have interpreted as an indicator of maternal anxiety, we interpreted them as reactions to the vibrations and acceleration of the plane. In summary, our investigations indicate that the relative hypoxemia and flight anxiety are not so severe that they pose a risk to either mother or fetus while in flight during pregnancy. Flying in modern commercial aircraft should not be considered harmful to the pregnant woman and her fetus if additional risk factors (e.g., smoking, anemia) are excluded.

In the pregnant stewardess, a possible risk results from the combination of moderate altitude and physical work. Wahley (90) quoted calculations that make it appear that the physical work of a flight attendant is not inconsiderable. Yoshioka et al. (81) compared the heart rate increase and energy expenditure in four nonpregnant stewardesses under actual flight conditions (although only at 1500 m, approximately 5000 ft) with that from the same work under simulated cabin conditions, but at ground level with normal atmospheric pressure. They found the extent of physical stress to be clearly higher in flight. Simply walking uphill or pushing the beverage cart, which can weigh up to 85 kg, resulted in heart rates up to 120 bpm in their investigations.

ACUTE ALTITUDE EXPOSURE AND PHYSICAL STRESS DURING PREGNANCY

We, therefore, studied the combination of acute altitude exposure and physical stress in 12 volunteers with normal pregnancies and mean gestational age of 36 weeks under real conditions in the mountains in Laax, Switzerland (85). The lower cable car station was at 1080 m (approximately 3500 ft), the upper station at 2228 m (approximately 7300 ft). Before and after the 10-min ascent, a 3-min ergometry test at 25 watts was run (at 1080 m and 2228 m). The same maternal and fetal variables as in the flight study were measured. With six other pregnant women (mean gestational age of 34 weeks), the same investigation was simulated in a low pressure chamber, the only difference being that for

each 3-min period of stress 50 watts was used.

The maternal physiological reactions observed in the mountain study correspond both in behavior and in degree to the data from the flight study. Between the lower and upper stations, the transcutaneous P_{O_2} fell 18 mm Hg, whereas the transcutaneous P_{CO_2} remained constant, as did the respiratory rate. During the ascent covering an altitude difference of 1100 m (approximately 3500 ft), the maternal heart rate scarcely showed any changes; during rest, the mean value was 101 bpm. During exercise, only the maternal respiratory rate and heart rate showed clear changes: the respiratory rate increased on the average by 8 breaths per min, and the heart rate increased by a mean of 25 bpm at 1080 m and at 2228 m (approximately 3500 and 7200 ft). The maternal variables of the six women in the low pressure chamber showed similar changes. The maternal heart rate increase with 50 watts was, however, 17 bpm on the average. For further details, the reader is referred to the original reports (85, 86).

The 18 fetal cardiograms were analyzed during and immediately after the maternal exercise (Table 22.6). Registrations that could be evaluated, and only a few exist for the

Table 22.6. Fetal Heart Rate Patterns During and After Maternal Exercise.[a]

Fetal Heart Rate Patterns	Exercise 2200 m		Exercise 1100 m	
	During	After	During	After
	Maternal Stress: 25 watts (n = 12)			
Analysis (technically feasible) (n)	6	11	4	12
With tachycardia	2 (165/170)	0	0	0
With bradycardia	0	1[b]	0	0
	Maternal Stress: 50 watts (n = 6)			
Analysis possible (n) of these	2	6	3	6
With tachycardia	1 (180)	0	1 (185)	0
Decreased variability	0	1	0	0

[a]From Bung et al. Fetale Herzfrequenz bei mütterlicher Höhenexposition und körperlicher Belastung. Gynakol Prax 1987; 11:217–226.

phases of maternal exercise, were assessed as either normal or suspect with respect to baseline, variability, presence of accelerations, or absence of late decelerations. Even without considering the three cases of tachycardia during maternal exercise—two slight, one more pronounced—it is still to be noted that there were two fetuses (one in the mountain test, one in the pressure chamber test) with abnormal heart rate patterns after maternal exercise at the higher altitude.

In summary, findings from most of the 18 mothers and fetuses in the study show that at moderate altitude and with moderate exercise the combined stress is tolerable for healthy women; at least, the compensatory capabilities are sufficient. However, based on two observations of suspect fetal heart rate behavior after maternal exercise at the higher elevation it may be concluded that caution is justified, particularly when additional risks are present (nicotine consumption, growth retardation, anemia). As indicated in Table 22.6, in one of the cases with a suspect fetal heart rate the mother was a heavy smoker.

PRACTICAL CONCLUSIONS

Based on physiological facts and the previously described observations, Table 22.7 attempts to summarize possible limitations for acute altitude exposure and exercise during pregnancy and to provide a rationale for counseling pregnant women. By their very nature, these guidelines may include a wide margin of safety because of the immense

Table 22.7.   Recommendations for Acute Altitude Exposure and Exercise During Pregnancy

---

Avoid acute exposure >3000 m (approximately 10,000 ft)

Avoid exercise >2500 m (approximately 8000 ft)

Avoid intense exercise during the first 3–4 days after exposure >2000 m (approximately 6500 ft)

Reduce exercise as elevation increases

Be aware of symptoms of acute mountain sickness starting 12 hours after exposure

Be aware of additional maternal and fetal risk factors (e.g., anemia, smoking, growth retardation)

---

adaptive capabilities to altitude stress of both the mother and the fetus.

REFERENCES

1. Moore LG. Altitude-aggravated illness: examples from pregnancy and prenatal life. Ann Emerg Med 1987; 16:965–973.
2. Huch R, Baumann H, Fallenstein F, Schneider KTM, Holdener F, Huch A. Physiologic changes in pregnant women and their fetuses during jet air travel. Am J Obstet Gynecol 1986; 154:966–1000.
3. Pawson IG, Jest C. The high-altitude areas of the world and their cultures. In: Baker PT, ed. The biology of high-altitude peoples. Cambridge: Cambridge University Press, 1978: p. 17–45.
4. Schwarz A, Hüllemann KD, Metz J. Höhenanpassung. In: Hüllemann KD, ed. Sportmedizin. New York: Georg Thieme Verlag, 1983; p. 59–72.
5. Grimsehl R, Ulmer HV. Grenzen des Höhenaufenthaltes für den Menschen: Oekologische und physiologische Faktoren. Mat Med Nordm 1978; 30:144–156.
6. Riley RL, Otis AB, Houston CS. Respiratory Features of Acclimatization to Altitude. In Boothby WM, ed. Respiratory physiology in aviation. Randolph Field, TX: USAF School of Aviation Medicine, 1954; p. 143–57.
7. Sutton JR, Jones NL, Griffith L, Pugh CE. Exercise at altitude. Ann Rev Physiol 1983; 45:427–437.
8. West JB. Human physiology at extreme altitudes on Mount Everest. Science 1984; 223:784–788.
9. Laciga P, Koller EA. Respiratory, circulatory, and ECG changes during acute exposure to high altitude. J Appl Physiol 1976; 41:159–167.
10. Rahn H, Otis AB. Alveolar air during simulated flights to high altitude. Am J Physiol 1947; 150:202–221.
11. Lenfant C, Sullivan K. Adaptation to high altitude. N Engl J Med 1971; 284:1298–1309.
12. Vogel JA, Harris CW. Cardiopulmonary responses of resting man during early exposure to high altitude. J Appl Physiol 1967; 22:1123–1128.
13. West JB. Respiratory and circulatory control at high altitudes. J Exp Biol 1982; 100:147–157.
14. Lockhart A, Saiag B. Altitude and the human pulmonary circulation. Clin Sci 1981; 60:599–605.
15. Faura J, Ramos J, Reynafarje C, English E, Finne P, Finch CA. Effect of altitude on erythropoiesis. Blood 1969; 33:668–676.
16. Siri WE, Dyke DCV, Winchell HS, Pollycove M, Parker HG, Cleveland AS. Early erythropoietin, blood, and physiological responses to severe hypoxia in man. J Appl Physiol 1966; 21:73–80.
17. Humpeler E, Inama K, Jungmann H. Die Sauerstoffaffinität des Hämoglobins 3 Stunden nach passivem Höhenwechsel von 400 auf 1800 m. Wien Klin Wochenschr 1980; 9:326–329.
18. Mueller WH, Murillo F, Palamino H, et al. The Aymara of western Bolivia: V. Growth and development in an hypoxic environment. Hum Biol 1980; 52:529–546.
19. Ou LC, Tenney SM. Properties of mitochondria from hearts of cattle acclimatized to high altitude. Respir Physiol 1970; 8:151–159.
20. Reynafarje B. Myoglobin content and enzymatic ac-

tivity of muscle and altitude adaptation. J Appl Physiol 1962; 17:301–305.

21. Wittenberg JB. Myoglobin-facilitated diffusion of oxygen. J Gen Physiol 1965; 49:57–74.

22. Kryger M. Breathing at high altitude: lessons learned and application to hypoxemia at sea level. Adv Cardiol 1980; 27:11–16.

23. Mathew L, Gopinath PM, Purkayastha SS, Gupta JS, Nayar HS. Chemoreceptor sensitivity in adaptation to high altitude. Aviat Space Environ Med 1983; 54:121–126.

24. Sorensen S, Severinghaus J. Respiratory sensitivity to acute hypoxia in man born at sea level living at high altitude. J Appl Physiol 1968; 25:211–216.

25. Miles DS, Wagner JA, Horvath SM, Reyburn JA. Absolute and relative work capacity in women at 758, 586, and 523 torr barometric pressure. Aviat Space Environ Med 1980; 51:439–44.

26. Oelz O. Von der Wirkung der Höhe auf den Menschen. Schweiz Rundsch Med Prax 1982; 71:70–77.

27. Johnson TS, Rock PB. Acute mountain sickness. N Engl J Med 1988; 319:841–844.

28. Hackett PH, Rennie D, Levine HD. The incidence, importance and prophylaxis of acute mountain sickness. Lancet 1976; 27:1149–1155.

29. Maggiorini M. Acute mountain sickness (AMS) in the Swiss Alps. Zurich, Doctorate Thesis, Univ of Zürich. 1989.

30. Reeves JT, Halpin J, Cohn JE, Daoud F. Increased alveolar-arterial oxygen difference during simulated high-altitude exposure. J Appl Physiol 1969; 27:658–661.

31. Grover RF, Reeves JT, Grover EB, Leathers JE. Muscular exercise in young men native to 3,100 m altitude. J Appl Physiol 1967; 22:555–564.

32. Reeves JT, Groves BM, Sutton JR, et al. Oxygen transport during exercise at extreme altitude: operation Everest II. Ann Emerg Med 1987; 16:993–998.

33. West JB, Lahiri S, Gill MB, Milledge JS, Pugh LGCE, Ward MP. Arterial oxygen saturation during exercise at high altitude. J Appl Physiol 1962; 17:617–621.

34. Ceretelli P. Limiting factors to oxygen transport on Mt. Everest. J Appl Physiol 1976; 76:658–67.

35. Levitan BM, Bungo MW. Measurement of cardiopulmonary performance during acute exposure to a 2440-m equivalent atmosphere. Aviat Space Environ Med 1982; 53:639–642.

36. Stenberg J, Ekblom B, Messin R. Hemodynamic response to work at simulated altitude, 4,000 m. J Appl Physiol 1966; 5:1589–1594.

37. Boutellier U, Deriaz O, diPrampero P, Cerretelli P. Exercise at altitude: V. Aerobic performance at altitude: Effects of acclimatisation and hematocrit with reference to training. Int J Sports Med 1990; (11) Suppl. 1:S21–S26.

38. Krejci J. Sport im Gebirge—gesund und gefährlich. Selecta-Schweiz 1986; 10:395–403.

39. Niederhäuser HU. Höhenaufenthalte. DIA-GM 1988; 5:27–30.

40. Baker PT. The biology of high-altitude peoples. Cambridge: Cambridge University Press, 1978; p. 1–357.

41. Clegg EJ. Fertility and early growth. In: Baker PT, ed. The biology of high-altitude peoples. Cambridge: Cambridge University Press, 1978; p. 65–115.

42. Dutt, JS. Altitude and fertility: the confounding effect of childhood mortality—a Bolivian example. Soc Biol 1980; 27:101–113.

43. Bangham CRM. Fertility of Nepalese Sherpas at moderate altitudes: Comparison with high-altitude data. Ann Hum Biol 1980; 7:323–330.

44. Cotton EK, Grunstein MM. Effects of hypoxia on respiratory control in neonates at high altitude. J Appl Physiol 1980; 48:587–595.

45. Cotton EK, Hiestand M, Philbin GE, Simmons M. Re-evaluation of birth weights at high altitude. Study of babies born to mothers living at an altitude of 3100 meters. Am J Obstet Gynecol 1980; 138:220–222.

46. Gubhaju B. Fertility differentials in Nepal. J Biosoc Sci 1983; 15:325–331.

47. Haas JD, Frongillo EA, Stepnick CD, Beard JL, Hurtado LG. Altitude, ethnic and sex difference in birth weight and length in Bolivia. Hum Biol 1980; 52:459–477.

48. Haas JD, Moreno-Black G, Frongillo EA, et al. Altitude and infant growth in Bolivia: A Longitudinal Study. Am J Phys Anthropol 1982; 59:251–262.

49. Jackson MR, Mayhew TM, Haas JD. Morphometric studies on villi in human term placentae and the effects of altitude, ethnic grouping and sex of newborn. Placenta 1987; 8:487–495.

50. Kissane JM. Reproductive failure. A survey of pathogenic mechanisms with emphasis on mechanisms for repeated failures. In: Naeye RL, Kissane JM, Kaufman N, eds. Perinatal diseases. Baltimore/London: Williams & Wilkins, 1981; p. 369–81.

51. Krueger HJA, Arias-Stella J. The placenta and the newborn infant at high altitudes. Am J Obstet Gynecol 1970; 106:586–591.

52. Lichty JA, Ting RY, Bruns PD, Dyar E. Studies of babies born at high altitude. Am J Dis Child 1957; 93:666–678.

53. McClung J. Effects of high altitude on human birth: Cambridge: Harvard University Press, 1969.

54. Moore LG, Brodeur P, Chumbe O, D'Brot J, Hofmeister S, Monge C. Maternal hypoxic ventilatory response, ventilation, and infant birth weight at 4,300 m. J Appl Physiol 1986; 60:1401–1406.

55. Moore LG, Hershey DW, Jahnigen D, Bowes W. The incidence of pregnancy-induced hypertension is increased among Colorado residents at high altitude. Am J Obstet Gynecol 1982; 144:423–429.

56. Moore LG, Jahnigen D, Rounds SS, Reeves JT, Grover RF. Maternal hyperventilation helps preserve arterial oxygenation during high-altitude pregnancy. J Appl Phys Resp Env Exerc Physiol 1982; 53:690–694.

57. Moore, LG, McCullough RE, Weil JV. Increased HVR in pregnancy: relationship to hormonal and metabolic changes. J Appl Physiol 1987; 62:158–163.

58. Moore LG, Rounds SS, Jahnigen D, Grover RF, Reeves JT. Infant birth weight is related to maternal arterial oxygenation at high altitude. J Appl Phys Resp Env Exerc Physiol 1982; 53:695–699.

59. Sobrevilla LA, Cassinelli MT, Carcelen A, Malaga JM. Human fetal and maternal oxygen tension and acid-base status during delivery at high altitude. Am J Obstet Gynecol 1971; 111:1111–1118.

60. Sobrevilla LA, Romero I, Kruger F, Wittembury J. Low estrogen excretion during pregnancy at high altitude. Am J Obstet Gynecol 1968; 102:828–833.

61. Steven DH, Burton GJ, Sumar J, Nathanielsz PW. Ultrastructural observations on the placenta of the Alpaca (Lama pacos). Placenta 1980; 1:21–32.

62. Taylor ES. Observations on pregnancy at altitude. Am J Obstet Gynecol 1968; 102:801–802.

63. Weitz C. Fertility of Nepalese Sherpas at moderate altitudes: Comparisons with high-altitude data. Ann Hum Biol 1981; 4:383–388.

64. Meyer MB. Effects of maternal smoking and altitude on birth weight and gestation. In: Reed DM, Stanley FJ, eds. The epidemiology of prematurity. Baltimore: Urban & Schwarzenberg, 1977; p. 81–104.

65. Baker PT. The adaptive fitness of high-altitude populations. In: Baker PT, ed. The biology of high-altitude peoples. Cambridge: Cambridge University Press, 1978; p. 317–350.

66. Saco-Pollitt C. Birth in the Peruvian Andes: Physical and behavioral consequences in the neonate. Child Dev 1981; 52:839–846.

67. Henry L. Some data on natural fertility. Eugenics Quarterly 1961; 8:81–91.

68. Howard RC, Lichty JA, Bruns P. Studies of babies born at high altitude. II. Measurement of birth weight, body length, and head size. Am J Dis Child 1957; 93:670–674.

69. Ueland K, Novy MJ, Metcalfe J. Hemodynamic responses of patients with heart disease to pregnancy and exercise. Am J Obstet Gynecol 1972; 113:47–59.

70. Alzamora V, Rotta A, Battilana G, et al. On the possible influence of great altitudes on the determination of certain cardiovascular anomalies. Pediatrics 1953; 12:259–262.

71. Hellegers A, Metcalfe J, Huckabee WE, Prystowsky H, Meschia G, Barron DH. Alveolar P_{CO_2} and P_{O_2} in pregnant and nonpregnant women at high altitude. Am J Obstet Gynecol 1961; 82:241–245.

72. Blechner JN, Cotter JR, Hinkley CM, Prystowsky H. Observations on pregnancy at altitude, II. Transplacental pressure differences of oxygen and carbon dioxide. Am J Obstet Gynecol 1968; 102:794–805.

73. Cotter JR, Blechner JN, Prystowsky H. Observations on pregnancy at altitude: I. The respiratory gases in maternal arterial and uterine venous blood. Am J Obstet Gynecol 1967; 99:1–8.

74. Makowski EL, Battaglia FC, Meschia G, et al. Effect of maternal exposure to high altitude upon fetal oxygenation. Am J Obstet Gynecol 1968; 100:852–861.

75. Huch R. Maternal hyperventilation and the fetus. J Perinat Med 1985; 13:1–15.

76. Meschia G, Prystowsky H, Hellegers A, Huckabee W, Metcalfe J, Barron DH. Observations on the oxygen supply to the fetal llama. Q J Exp Physiol 1960; 45:284–291.

77. Metcalfe J, Meschia G, Hellegers A, Prystowsky H, Huckabee W, Barron DH. Observations on the placental exchange of respiratory gases in pregnant ewes at high altitude. Q J Exp Physiol 1962; 47:74–92.

78. Ballew C, Haas JD. Hematologic evidence of fetal hypoxia among newborn infants at high altitude in Bolivia. Am J Obstet Gynecol 1986; 155:166–169.

79. Naeye RL. Children at high altitude: pulmonary and renal abnormalities. Circ Res 1965; 16:33–38.

80. Aldrete JA, Aldrete LE. Oxygen concentrations in commercial aircraft flights. South Med J 1983; 1:12–14.

81. Yoshioka TM, Narusawa K, Nagami C, et al. Effects of relative metabolic rate and heart rate variation on the performance of flight attendants. Aviat Space Environ Med 1982; 53:127–132.

82. Cameron RG. Should air hostesses continue flight duty during the first trimester of pregnancy? Aerospace Med 1973; 44:552–556.

83. Parer JT. Effects of hypoxia on the mother and fetus with emphasis on maternal air transport. Am J Obstet Gynecol 1982; 142:957–961.

84. Scholten P. Pregnant stewardess—should she fly? Aviat Space Environ Med 1976; 47:77–81.

85. Baumann H, Bung P, Fallenstein F, Huch A, Huch R. Reaktion von Mutter und Fet auf die körperliche Belastung in der Höhe. Geburtshilfe Frauenheilkd 1985; 45:869–876.

86. Bung P, Baumann H, Huch R, Huch A. Fetale Herzfrequenz bei mütterlicher Höhenexposition und körperlicher Belastung. Gynäkol Prax 1987; 11:217–226.

87. Huch R. Fliegen in der Schwangerschaft. Gynakologe 1987; 20:165–170.

88. Morishima HO, Pedersen H, Finster H. The influence of maternal psychological stress on the fetus. Am J Obstet Gynecol 1978; 131:286–290.

89. Myers RE. Maternal psychological stress and fetal asphyxia: A study in the monkey. Am J Obstet Gynecol 1975; 122:47–59.

90. Whaley WH. Medical considerations regarding flight crews. JAMA 1982; 248:1834–1837.

23

Heat Stress and Pregnancy

Barbara L. Drinkwater and Raul Artal Mittelmark

The heat produced by the working muscles during vigorous exercise can quickly elevate body temperature to a dangerous level if heat transfer to the environment does not keep pace with heat production. Endurance athletes, such as runners, are at increased risk for heat injuries because of their frequent exposure to extreme environmental conditions while exercising for extended periods of time.

Even the recreational athlete can produce enough heat to raise core temperature above 39°C within minutes if heat dissipation is compromised. For example, a 60-kg woman can increase her metabolic heat production from 1.5 kcal · min^{-1} while standing quietly to 12.5 kcal · min^{-1} while running at a 8 min/ mile pace. Because it takes just 50 kcal of stored heat to raise her core temperature 1°C (0.83, specific heat of the body, × 60 kg), it will take only 8 min (50/12.5 × 2) to increase her temperature from a normal resting value of 37°C to 39°C if no heat is dissipated. Even when environmental conditions and clothing permit metabolic heat to be dissipated, heat production can easily exceed heat loss and internal temperature will rise.

This normal physiological response has served as a basis for the American College of Obstetricians and Gynecologists (ACOG) recommendation that pregnant women limit their *strenuous* exercise to 15 min. Should maternal core temperature reach 39°C or above, there may be adverse consequences for the fetus (1–3). The link between hyperthermia and congenital malformation appears to be well-established in experimental animals. These studies (1, 4) indicate that early pregnancy exposure to hyperthermia can lead to neurotube defects in the offspring. The association in the human is less certain and will be discussed later in this chapter.

THERMAL BALANCE

Women who intend to continue their exercise program during pregnancy should have a basic understanding of the relationship between exercise, environmental conditions, and thermoregulatory responses. The thermal balance equation, $S = M \pm (R + C) - E$, in its simplest form demonstrates that heat is stored (S) when metabolic heat production (M) is not offset by the transfer of heat from the body to the environment by radiation (R) and convection (C) or through evaporation (E) of sweat (Fig. 23.1). It should be pointed out that when ambient temperature exceeds skin temperature or when there is direct sunlight and a high radiant heat load, the term ($R + C$) will be positive and heat storage will increase unless evaporative heat loss can meet the additional demand for heat dissipation. When humidity is high, it may be impossible to evaporate enough sweat to offset heat gain and body temperature can quickly rise to 39°C or higher. A microenvironment of trapped air between clothing and skin can have the same result if the exercise clothing does not permit the evaporation of sweat.

If the intensity of the exercise is not too high and the ambient conditions are not too severe, it is possible to achieve thermal balance. Core temperature will rise when exercise begins as heat gain exceeds heat loss. As the thermoregulatory mechanisms come into play, heat loss will gradually match heat gain and a thermal steady state is achieved at an elevated core temperature.

PRESCRIPTIVE ZONE

The severity of environmental conditions is determined not only by the air temperature but also by the humidity, radiant heat load, and air movement. A number of investigators

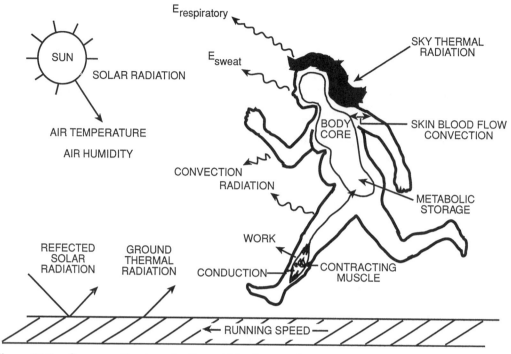

Figure 23.1. Sources of heat production within the exercising woman, avenues of heat transport from the working muscles to the skin, and heat exchange between the body and the environment. Adapted from Gisolfi CV, Wenger CB. Temperature regulation during exercise: Old concepts, new ideas. In Terjung RL, ed. Exercise and Sport Science Reviews 1984; 12:339–372.

(6–9) have attempted to integrate all these variables into a single heat stress index. The "Prescriptive Zone" goes one step further and uses one of these indexes, the Corrected Effective Temperature (CET), to describe a range of conditions where one can maintain thermal equilibrium by adjusting exercise intensity (Fig. 23.2). For example, as a runner increases her pace the range of environmental conditions where a thermal steady-state is possible becomes smaller. Exceeding the upper limit of the prescriptive zone (ULPZ) at any pace will result in a rise in core temperature (11). Understanding the relationship between running pace, the thermal environment, and core temperature can help the pregnant runner realize the importance of modifying her workout to avoid the risk of hyperthermia.

INDIVIDUAL DIFFERENCES

Not all women respond to the same degree of heat stress in identical fashion. A number of personal characteristics, such as level of physical fitness, state of acclimatization, and general health, can modify the response of the pregnant woman to the combined effect of physical activity and environmental heat stress.

Physical Fitness

The endurance athlete responds to exercise in the heat as though she were partially acclimatized (12, 13). Her cardiovascular system is more likely to meet the challenge of providing blood to the working muscles and to the peripheral blood vessels for transfer of heat to the skin without compromising cardiac output. She begins to sweat sooner and sweats more than the untrained woman. This improved sweating response keeps her skin cooler and aids in the dissipation of the metabolic heat produced during exercise. She will usually have a lower resting core temperature and heart rate and can tolerate a longer period of heat stress before reaching a critical core temperature.

Because heart rate and core temperature

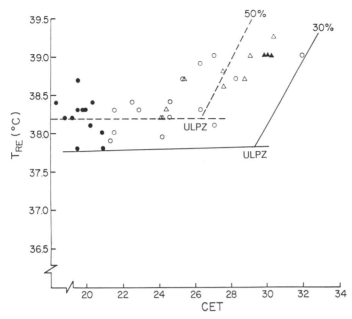

Figure 23.2. The "Prescriptive Zone" for young women walking on a treadmill at 30% and 50% of the $\dot{V}_{O_2max}$ in a wide range of ambient conditions. Note that the Upper Limit of the Prescriptive Zone (ULPZ) shifts left as relative exercise intensity increases. From Drinkwater BL, Horvath SM. Thermoregulatory response of women to intermittent work in the heat. Terminal Progress Report, National Institute for Occupational Health and Safety, 1982; 1–63.

are directly related to the relative intensity ($\%\dot{V}_{O_2max}$) of the exercise, not the absolute work load or energy expenditure (14), two women may run together at the same pace but the one with the higher aerobic power ($\dot{V}_{O_2max}$) will have the lower heart rate and the lower core temperature. As pregnancy progresses and the women's weight and metabolic requirements increase, a greater expenditure of energy would be required to maintain the prepregnancy running pace. If aerobic power has not increased, this pace now represents a higher relative exercise intensity and both core temperature and heart rate will be higher.

There is evidence that women spontaneously reduce exercise intensity as gestation proceeds (15, 16). Recreational runners who trained at 74% $\dot{V}_{O_2max}$ before pregnancy decreased their training intensity to 57% and 47% of prepregnancy $\dot{V}_{O_2max}$ at 20 and 32 weeks' gestation, respectively (15). After running for 20 min, rectal temperature increased 1.5°C before pregnancy, 0.7°C at 20 weeks', and 0.4°C at 32 weeks' gestation. While this is reassuring, it must be remembered that the

fetus appears to be most at risk when maternal hyperthermia occurs during the early stages of the first trimester. During this period, the highly trained athlete may exercise long enough and hard enough to raise her core temperature well above 39°C in all but the most benign environmental conditions.

Acclimatization to Hot Environments

A runner is at greatest risk for heat injury when there is a sudden increase in ambient temperature. Although the endurance athlete is partially adapted to heat stress, physical fitness is not a substitute for heat acclimatization and the pregnant woman who attempts to follow her usual training regimen when the weather turns warm is placing herself and the fetus at risk. Heat injury can range from mildly incapacitating, such as heat cramps, to a potentially fatal heat stroke (Table 23.1). The most effective way to avoid heat injury is reduce the intensity of the exercise, keep well-hydrated, and gradually acclimatize to the environment.

Acclimatization, the key to safe and enjoyable exercise in hot weather, is achieved by

Table 23.1.   Symptoms of Heat Disorders Listed in Order of Increasing Seriousness

Disorder	Symptoms
Heat cramp	Painful cramps in skeletal muscles due to excessive loss of fluids and minerals, primarily sodium
Heat syncope	Loss of consciousness due to blood pooling in the legs, hypotension, and inadequate oxygen supply to the brain, usually preceded by profuse sweating and a high pulse rate
Heat exhaustion	Profuse sweating, higher than normal pulse rate and respiration, slight elevation in body temperature, 38–40°C, may include nausea, headache, fatigue, anxiety, and impaired mental state
Heat stroke	High body temperature, 41–43°C, delirium, weakness, dizziness, poor coordination

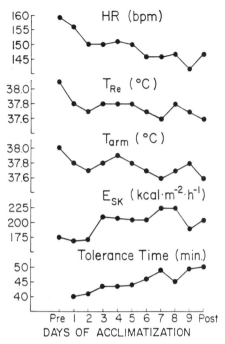

Figure 23.3.   Acclimatization of women to exercise in 48°C, 8.7 torr vapor pressure. Note decrease in heart rate and core temperature and increase in tolerance time. Reprinted with permission from Kupprat IC, Drinkwater BL, Horvath SM. Interaction of exercise and ambient environment during heat acclimatization. Hung Rev Sports Med 1980; 21:5–16.

repeated exposures to exercise in the heat and is usually achieved within 10–14 days (17). In the laboratory, the exercise period is terminated when either heart rate or core temperature reaches predetermined levels. The pregnant woman can use her usual "target heart rate" for her training regimen as her indicator of heat strain. When her heart rate exceeds that target, it is time to stop. Because the need to deliver blood to peripheral vessels as well as to the working muscles will result in a higher heart rate at any given exercise intensity in the heat, the same target heart rate will be reached earlier in the exercise period until the woman is fully acclimatized. In extremely hot conditions, neither heart rate or core temperature may reach a plateau and it is advisable to reduce both the duration and intensity of exercise. As the body becomes acclimatized, both core temperature and heart rate will decrease and the training session can be extended (Fig. 23.3).

Avoiding Hyperthemia

There are a number of precautions active women can take to avoid hyperthermia while exercising during pregnancy (19). If high thermal loads cannot be avoided, the athlete should acclimatize gradually to the ambient conditions, avoid the worst of the heat by exercising early in the morning or in an air-conditioned facility, wear appropriate clothing that will permit free evaporation of sweat, and drink plenty of fluids before, during, and after exercise. The effectiveness of fluid replacement is illustrated in Figure 23.4. Women should be cautioned not to exercise when ill and to be alert for the early symptoms of heat illness: nausea, headache, dizziness, poor coordination, and apathy. The buddy system, training with a partner, is highly recommended for women at any time as a safety measure. It is particularly important during training in hot weather when each partner can be responsible for observing early indications of heat distress in the other.

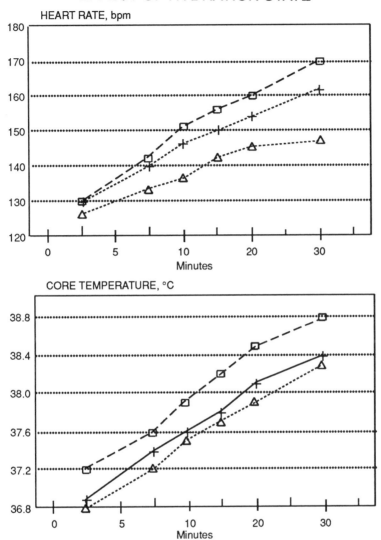

Figure 23.4. Effect of hydration state: euhydration (+), hypohydration (□), and hyperhydration (△) on core temperature and heart rate during a 30-min exercise period. Adapted from Nadel ER, Fortney SM, Wenger CB. Effect of hydration state on circulatory and thermal regulations. J Appl Physiol 1980; 49:715–721.

THERMOREGULATORY RESPONSES TO EXERCISE DURING PREGNANCY

The extent to which the thermoregulatory system can be challenged in the laboratory during pregnancy is limited because of concern for maternal and fetal well-being. For that reason, severe thermal stress has been studied only in pregnant animals (see Chapter 13). Because of the different avenues for heat dissipation and other physiological differences between species, it is not known if animal data can be extrapolated directly to pregnant women. However, the teratogenic effects observed in a number of animal species when maternal core temperature is elevated above 39°C during early gestation would suggest that pregnant women would be wise to avoid exercise-induced hyperthermia during this period (1, 4).

Maternal Responses

Only moderate exercise intensities, which mimic the running pace self-selected during their daily training runs, have been used to study thermoregulation of pregnant women (15, 16). The active women in these studies voluntarily modified their exercise program as pregnancy progressed by decreasing exercise intensity. The precise adjustments these women made relative to changes in their $\dot{V}_{O_2max}$ cannot be determined because neither study measured maximal aerobic power during pregnancy. Clapp et al. (15) observed a decrease in rectal temperature after 20 min of treadmill exercise at 20 and 32 weeks of gestation from a prepregnancy maximum of 39°C (Fig. 23.5). At the same time, exercise intensity decreased from 74% of the prepregnancy $\dot{V}_{O_2max}$ to 57% and 47%. The marked decrease in rectal temperature during exercise at 20 and 32 weeks of gestation would suggest that the decrease in relative exercise intensity was considerably greater than any decrement in $\dot{V}_{O_2max}$. If the selected training pace represented the same relative exercise intensity, one would expect core temperatures to be similar.

In contrast, Jones et al. (16) observed no change in rectal temperature during 20 min of a treadmill run for four women at 12, 24, and 32 weeks of gestation and 10 weeks postpartum. These women reduced their training pace by 20–30% by the third trimester but total energy expenditure remained the same because of the increase in maternal weight. The similarity in core temperature throughout pregnancy would suggest that these women were adjusting their exercise intensity to match the decrease in $\dot{V}_{O_2max}$.

More recently, Soultanakis (21) has found that women in the third trimester of pregnancy can maintain thermal balance as well as nonpregnant women during moderate exercise (approximately 55% $\dot{V}_{O_2max}$) for 60 min in a normal laboratory environment (Fig. 23.6). Both groups increased core temperature by approximately 0.6°C.

The results of these studies suggest that women can exercise in mild environmental conditions without danger of hyperthermia by reducing the intensity of their training as pregnancy progresses. There are no studies describing the responses of pregnant women to the combination of exercise and heat stress.

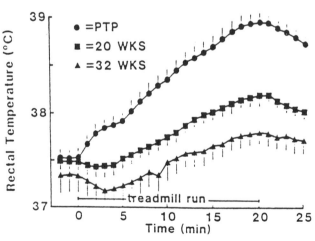

Figure 23.5.   The serial changes observed in rectal temperature before, during, and after the 20-min treadmill run prior to pregnancy *(circle)*, and at 20 *(square)* and 32 *(triangle)* weeks' gestation. Each point represents the group ± SE. Reprinted with permission from Clapp JF, Wesley M, Sleamaker RH. Thermoregulatory and metabolic responses to jogging prior to and during pregnancy. Med Sci Sports Exerc 1987; 19:124–130.

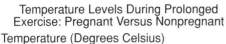

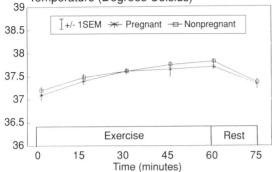

Figure 23.6. Core temperature of pregnant and nonpregnant women during 60 min of exercise at ~55% V_{O_2max}. Reprinted with permission from Soultanakis HN. Glucose homeostasis during pregnancy in response to prolonged exercise. Dissertation. University of Southern California Graduate School, 1989.

A major concern during prolonged periods of exercise in the heat would be dehydration, which could be a factor in precipitating premature labor.

Fetal Responses

The transfer of heat from one object to another depends upon a thermal gradient—a difference in temperature—between the two objects with heat flowing from the warmer to the cooler object (22). Under normal circumstances, the temperature of the fetus is about 0.5°C higher than that of the mother, facilitating the dissipation of fetal metabolic heat to the maternal circulatory system. When the maternal temperature rises, as it does during exercise, the thermal gradient may be reversed and fetal temperature will rise. Hyperthermia in the experimental animal leads to an increase in fetal umbilical circulation to facilitate dissipation of fetal heat (23). This increased circulatory demand often leads to fetal tachycardia, a symptom of fetal distress. At the same time, umbilical arteriovenous temperature and oxygen content gradients decrease. In the experimental animal, this chain of events can lead to fetal circulatory collapse.

Although there is no direct experimental evidence that fetal hyperthermia is teratogenic in humans, neither is there any evidence that the human fetus is unique among mammals in its capacity to cope with high body temperatures at vulnerable stages in its development. Considering the potential consequences to the fetus, it seems only prudent for the pregnant woman to avoid situations that might lead to hyperthermia during the first trimester of her pregnancy.

An extensive review by Edwards (1) describes the teratogenic effect of hyperthermia in a variety of species. In general, it appears that exposure to temperature elevations of only 1.5–2.5°C during specific stages of embryogenesis can be teratogenic and antimitotic with effects ranging from resorption to developmental defects. The type of defect appears to be related to the species, degree, and duration of hyperthermia, and stage of fetal development. A single short hyperthermic episode may be less dangerous than multiple or prolonged exposures, and slow increases in temperature may have less impact than an abrupt spike (1, 24). Although animal data are a useful source of corroborating evidence, species differences and comparable dosage and exposure time have to be taken into account when using these data to predict the human response.

All the human data implicating hyperthermia as teratogenic have come from case reports (1–3, 25–27), which may suggest an association but cannot prove causality. Nevertheless, one should not dismiss the case reports lightly. These reports suggest a strong association between hyperthermia and defects of the central nervous system, i.e., anencephaly, encephalocele, and spina bifida. These malformations are the result of a failure of closure of the neural tube in the phase of embryogenesis. The process of closure begins in the cervical region of the cord, caudad and cephalad, till the surface of the ectoderm becomes a continuous layer. Closure of the anterior neuropore occurs at 25 days after conception and the posterior neuropore at 27 days although the process can vary by a day or two.

In cases where the hyperthermia was secondary to an infection during pregnancy it is impossible to determine if the disease or the hyperthermia might have been responsible for the malformation (4). In the only prospective study in the literature, Clarren et al. (25) found no association between episodes of first trimester fever and occurrence of malformations.

Saunas have been suggested as a possible source of maternal hyperthermia leading to birth defects (2, 26). However, this appears unlikely under normal circumstances. Harvey et al. (28) found that nonpregnant women were unable to tolerate the extreme heat of a sauna long enough to raise their core temperature to levels presumed to be teratogenic. As Warkany (4) points out, if saunas were an important factor in hyperthermic teratogenesis, Finland would have a high incidence of neural tube defects. In fact, they have one of the lowest rates in the world (4).

Although the evidence linking hyperthermia to teratogenesis rests on animal experimentation, it does not seem unreasonable to suggest that pregnant women take precautions to avoid conditions that might lead to hyperthermia. Concern for the fetus revolves around the effect that a substantial rise in temperature might have on fetal well-being and development. Potential teratogenic effects are most likely to occur during the first 26–30 days after conception or 50 days from the last menstrual period. Once beyond that stage of embryogenesis, other theoretical side effects, such as premature labor due to dehydration, need to be considered.

Hyperthermia is a serious threat to mature healthy athletes. There is no reason to believe that it is any less a threat to the fetus. The absolute temperature threshold at which the well-being of the human fetus is threatened is unlikely to be identified because controlled laboratory experiments to determine that point would be unethical. A woman can continue to exercise during her pregnancy without placing the fetus at risk for hyperthermia by moderating her training program according to the thermoregulatory principles outlined in this chapter.

REFERENCES

1. Edwards MJ. Hyperthermia as a teratogen. Teratol Carcinog Mutagen 1986; 6:563–582.
2. Miller P, Smith DW, Shepard TH. Maternal hyperthermia as a possible cause of anencephaly. Lancet 1978; 1:519–521.
3. Shiota K. Neural tube defects and maternal hyperthermia in early pregnancy. Epidemiology in a human embryonic population. Am J Med Genet 1982; 12:281–288.
4. Warkany J. Teratogen update: Hyperthermia. Teratology 1986; 33:365–371.
5. Gisolfi CV, Wenger CB. Temperature regulation during exercise: old concepts, new ideas. In Terjung RL, ed. Exercise and Sport Sciences Reviews 1984; 12:339–372.
6. Belding HS, Hatch TF. Index for evaluating heat stress in terms of resulting physiological strains. Heat Pip Air Condit 1955; 29:129–136.
7. McArdle B, Dunham W, Hollong HE, Ladell WSS, Scott JW, Thomson ML, Weiner JS. The prediction of the physiological effects of warm and hot environments. Rep. No. RNP 47/391. London: Med Res Council, 1947.
8. Yaglou CP. Temperature, humidity, and air movement in industries: the effective temperature index. J Ind Hyg 1927; 9:297–309.
9. Yaglou CP. A method for improving the effective temperature index. Trans Am Soc Heat Vent Engrs 1947; 53:307–313.
10. Drinkwater BL, Horvath SM. Thermoregulatory response of women to intermittent work in the heat. Terminal Progress Report, National Institute for Occupational Health and Safety, 1982; 1–63.
11. Lind AR. A physiological criterion for setting thermal limits for everyday work. J Appl Physiol 1963; 18:51–56.
12. Drinkwater BL, Kupprat IC, Denton JE, Horvath SM. Heat tolerance of female distance runners. Ann NY Acad Sci 1977; 301:777–792.
13. Gisolfi CV, Cohen JS. Relationships among training, heat acclimation, and heat tolerance in men and women. Med Sci Sports 1979; 11:56–59.
14. Astrand I. Aerobic work capacity in men and women with special reference to age. Acta Physiol Scand 1960; 169 (Suppl):1–92.
15. Clapp JF III, Wesley M, Sleamaker RH. Thermoregulatory and metabolic responses to jogging prior to and during pregnancy. Med Sci Sports Exerc 1987; 19:124–130.
16. Jones RL, Botti JJ, Anderson WM, Bennett NI. Thermoregulation during aerobic exercise in pregnancy. Obstet Gynecol 1985; 65:340–345.
17. Samueloff S, Yousef MK. Adaptive physiology to stressful environments. Boca Raton, FL: CRC Press, 1987.
18. Kupprat IC, Drinkwater BL, Horvath SM. Interaction of exercise and ambient environment during heat acclimatization. Hung Rev Sports Med 1980; 21:5–16.
19. American College of Sports Medicine Position Stand. The prevention of thermal injuries during distance running. Indianapolis: American College of Sports Medicine, 1985.
20. Nadel ER, Fortney SM, Wenger CB. Effect of hydra-

tion state on circulatory and thermal regulations. J Appl Physiol 1980; 49:715–721.

21. Soultanakis HN. Glucose homeostasis during pregnancy in response to prolonged exercise. Dissertation. University of Southern California Graduate School, 1989.

22. Kerslake DM. The stress of hot environments. Cambridge: University Press, 1972.

23. Cefalo RC, Hellagers AE. The effects of maternal hyperthermia on uterine and placental blood flow. In: Moawad AH, Lindheimer DM. Uterine and placental blood flow. Masson Pub, 1982; p. 185–191.

24. Chernoff GF, Golden JA. Hyperthermia-induced ex-

encephaly in mice: effect of multiple exposures. Teratology 1988; 37:37–42.

25. Clarren SK, Smith DW, Harvey MAS, Ward RH, Myrianthopoulos NC. Hyperthermia: a prospective evaluation of a possible teratogenic agent in man. J Pediatr 1979; 95:81–84.

26. Halperin LR, Wilroy RS Jr. Maternal hyperthermia and neural tube defects. Lancet 1978; 2:212–213.

27. Smith DW, Clarren SK, Harvey MAS. Hyperthermia as a possible teratogenic agent. J Pediatr 1978; 92:878–83.

28. Harvey MAS, McRorie O, Smith DW: Suggested limits to the use of hot tubs and saunas by pregnant women. Can Med Assoc J 1981; 125:50–54.

24

Aquatic Exercise During Pregnancy

Vern L. Katz, Robert McMurray, and Robert C. Cefalo

Water aerobics is a form of exercise in which calisthenic-like exercises or aerobic dance movements occur with the individual immersed in chest deep water. Water aerobic activities have been applauded because these activities cause less stress on the joints, making exercise possible for individuals with limited mobility or ability to sustain their weight. Athletes, particularly runners, use water aerobics for rehabilitation after injury. Aerobic capacity can be sustained without undue stress on the injured appendage. Preliminary studies indicate that the hydrostatic forces of the water, concomitant with the buoyancy and improved thermoregulation of immersion, may provide advantages over land-based exercise for the pregnant woman.

This chapter begins with a review of the physiological effects of immersion, paying particular attention to the advantages for pregnant women. Then we examine the interaction of immersion and exercise, and the effects of water aerobic exercise during pregnancy. Because the physiological responses to water aerobics have not been extensively studied, inferences will be made from studies in which individuals completed leg exercises while immersed.

IMMERSION

Immersion, or hydrotherapy, is one of the oldest forms of medical prescription. Its benefits have been touted since antiquity. In mythology, the magic of the waters promised to rejuvenate the person who was immersed. However, even today, the magical rejuvenation of hot springs and spas from Callistoga, California, to Bath, England, are still sought. The magic is not a product of specific waters or the various minerals in the water. Rather, the "magic" derives from the effects of immersion. Immersion, because of its diuretic and natriuretic effects, has even been proposed as therapy for patients with some forms of renal disease and patients with cirrhosis (1–3).

The hydrostatic pressure of water exerts a force proportional to the depth of immersion (4–8). This pressure acts uniformly on the body to push extravascular fluid into the vascular space, resulting in a rapid expansion of the plasma volume (9, 10). The greater the amount of extravascular fluid, the more is transferred intravascular. The hydrostatic pressure also forces an expansion of central blood volume and a cephalad redistribution of blood (4, 5, 7, 11–13, 15, 16). The efflux occurs within seconds and, in men immersed to the neck, leads to a 700-ml intravascular expansion (7, 11, 17). The expansion bypasses the lymphatics (18), and, curiously, is less at night than during the day (19).

As the intravascular volume increases, a diuresis and natriuresis is initiated from hormonal signals from both the right atrial receptors and from the osmoreceptors (17, 20–25). Renal vascular resistance decreases resulting in an increase in blood flow and filtration. Urate excretion increases and tubular reabsorption of sodium declines (4, 5, 25, 26). The diuretic and natriuretic effects are profound and can be only partially inhibited by antidiuretic hormone (ADH) administration or dehydration (15, 27–30). The diuretic effect peaks within 1 hour and by 4 hours the urine flow begins to return to normal (4, 5, 24, 31). Conversely, the natriuresis increases steadily, peaking at about 4 hours. Thus, the two effects are independent (4, 5). The diuresis of prolonged immersion will ultimately cause the initial hemodilution of immersion to give way to a hemoconcentration (4, 5, 9, 32).

The diuresis of immersion may have positive effects on the pregnant woman who is bothered by fluid retention. We have previously shown that immersion of pregnant women in water for 20–40 min results in a 300- to 400-ml loss in fluid, while blood vol-

271

ume is maintained (33). It is possible that immersion therapy could be used to alleviate symtomatic edema in some patients.

The activity of several hormones have significant interplay with the renal responses to immersion. Plasma renin activity (PRA) and aldosterone decrease during immersion (4, 24, 27, 34). ADH generally, but not always, declines (16, 28, 30, 35). Most investigations have found that catecholamines do not change during thermoneutral immersion. However, some studies have shown a drop in norepinephrine (29, 35–39). Atrial natriuretic factor (ANF) increases, as do urinary levels of cyclic guanosine monophosphate (GMP). The ANF response does not seem to be altered with dehydration (29). Other hormonal changes include a rise in dopamine and methionine-enkephalin, as well as a drop in prolactin (40). The rise in dopamine may serve a significant function during immersion because a blockade leads to a blunted natriuresis and an elevation of prolactin (23, 40). Immersion is also associated with a progressive rise in urinary prostaglandin E metabolite (4, 35).

The hydrostatic pressure has a significant effect on the cardiovascular and pulmonary systems. Central venous pressure increases, as does pulmonary capillary wedge pressure (up to 25 mm Hg in some subjects) (10–12, 26, 30). Left ventricular end-diastolic volume and end-systolic volume increases, resulting in an increase in right and left atrial size (7, 19, 26, 37, 41, 42). The increased venous return causes an increase in stroke volume by as much as 60% during immersion (7, 15, 42). Concomitantly, heart rate declines and mean arterial blood pressure drops as a result of decrements in both systolic and diastolic pressures (4, 11, 12, 15, 17, 43). In addition, the heart may be shifted upward and horizontally (10). The centralization of the blood volume causes an engorgement of the pulmonary vasculature resulting in air trapping and a small decrease in forced vital capacity (FVC). The reduced FVC is related to a decrease in the expiratory reserve volume. However, residual volume seems to remain unchanged (19, 41, 43). These changes in pulmonary function do not impose any limitation for normal men and women.

Because water has 25 times the thermal conductivity of air, changes in water temperature may lead to significant heat loss or retention (44, 45). The thermoneutral range for immersion in man ranges from 33.5–35.5°C, depending upon the size and insulation of the subject. The thermoneutral zone for women may be lower than for men (44–50). Immersion in water between 30 and 33°C leads to vasoconstriction. Exposure to water of less than 28–30°C will result in shivering to attempt to maintain core temperature. Exposure to temperatures above 36°C will cause vasodilation and can limit a person's capacity to exercise. Thus, for untrained individuals, exercise is best performed in water of 28–30°C (44, 45, 49, 51). Most swimming pools are maintained at approximately 28°C.

PREGNANCY AND IMMERSION

Many of the physiological changes of pregnancy are potentially affected by immersion. These changes include the substantial increase in total body water and vascular volume, as well as decreases in peripheral vascular resistance and ADH threshold (52). Results from studies that have examined the effects of immersion during pregnancy are categorized in Table 24.1.

Doniec-Ulman et al. (24) recently compared the physiological responses of normal pregnant women, preeclamptic women, and nonpregnant (control) women, semireclining in a bath for 2 hours. Within 1 hour, mean arterial pressure had fallen in all subjects, with the greatest decrease in the healthy pregnant women. PRA and aldosterone concentrations were reduced in all subjects. Interestingly, ADH declined only in the two groups of pregnant women. Plasma ANF rose in all groups, with the largest increase in the nonpregnant women. Mean weight loss (due to urine output) was similar for the three groups (0.5–0.8 kg). Furthermore, the blood pressure and urinary responses could not be directly related to any hormonal mechanism (24).

Millar et al. (53), used Doppler evaluation of maternal cardiovascular changes during immersion to neck level in third trimester pregnant women (53). They found a 30%

Table 24.1. Physiologic Variables During Immersion in Pregnancy

Increases
  Plasma volume
  Blood volume
  Diuresis
  Natriuresis
  Kalliuresis
  Atrial natriuretic factor
  Cardiac output
  Stroke volume

Decreases
  ADH
  PRA, aldosterone
  Heart rate
  Blood pressure
  Edema
  Hematocrit, plasma protein
  Forced vital capacity
  Expiratory reserve volume

Unchanged
  Glucose, lactate, cortisol
  Plasma osmolality
  Plasma Na^+, K^+
  Fetal heart rate, uterine tone
  MSAFP
  Tidal volume

increase in cardiac output secondary to an increase in stroke volume. Similar to the findings of Doniec-Ulman et al., mean arterial pressure declined about 8 mm Hg (24).

We conducted a series of experiments in healthy pregnant women involving 20 min of immersion in 30°C water followed by 20 min of exercise at a moderate intensity (60% $\dot{V}_{O_2max}$) (33, 54–57, McMurray et al., Unpublished data). The women were tested in four trials at 15, 25, and 35 weeks' gestation and again 8–10 weeks postpartum. The women were seated on a cycle ergometer immersed to the level of the xiphoid. This water level was chosen because it correlates with the central blood volume changes that occur in the horizontal position (7). The findings are included in Table 24.1.

During immersion in all four trials heart rate decreased from 4–8 bpm compared to the supine preimmersion rest. Systolic blood pressure dropped, while diastolic blood pressure remained unaffected (56). During immersion in the 30°C water (lower than thermoneutral), metabolic rate increased slightly.

Cortisol levels declined during the pregnancy trials, but were unchanged postpartum. Lactate and glucose levels were unchanged. β-Endorphin levels did not change during immersion (57).

Blood and plasma volume increased (4–6%) with immersion except during the postpartum period (33). Plasma protein levels and hematocrit declined while plasma sodium NA^+, K^+, and osmolarity remained clinically normal. These changes were consistent with findings from other immersion studies (15, 21, 55).

Urine was collected before and after the experiment (an interval of approximately an hour). Despite moderate exercise, mean urine output was 327, 418, and 367 ml/hr at 15, 25, and 35 weeks' gestation, compared to 208 ml/hr during the postpartum trial (33). Similar to a study by Goodlin et al. (58), the immersion diuresis seemed to be related to the degree of a subject's edema. Considerable variation in urine output existed between individuals in our study: 44 ml/hr in one individual compared to 700 ml/hr in another. Urine Na^+ and K^+ excretion was twice that seen in studies of men. However, Na^+ and K^+ excretion was similar between pregnancy and postpartum (55).

Fetal well-being was assessed during immersion with real-time underwater ultrasound (33). In the 35-week trial, fetal heart rate did not change from supine land rest to immersion. All fetuses studied appeared to be in an active state during the 20 min of immersion. All exhibited gross body movement, fetal breathing motion, and flexion and extension. Of 11 fetuses studied, seven demonstrated bladder emptying and refilling during the 20 min. This is more rapid than would be expected from baseline. Maternal serum AFP levels remained unchanged between rest and immersion. No mother reported contractions during any immersion trial.

During immersion, forced vital capacity decreased, as did forced expiratory volume (54). Maximal voluntary ventilation and expiratory reserve volume also declined. Inspiratory capacity increased during immersion as did breathing frequency. Tidal volume remained the same. These changes were found in all pregnancy trials and during the postpartum period. None of the changes compromised the subjects.

IMMERSED EXERCISE

Studies evaluating responses to immersion exercise have employed free swimming, tethered swimming, or modified cycle ergometers (38, 47). Both tethered and free swimming are predominantly upper body exercise in which the body is totally immersed in the water. However, water aerobics are predominantly leg exercises with the body only partially immersed. Because we are primarily concerned with water aerobics, a leg exercise, this review will concentrate on results obtained from cycle ergometry. Results are summarized in Table 24.2.

The preponderance of research has indicated that the heart rate in the water during moderate intensity exercise is less than on land. However, as the intensity of the exercise approaches maximal, the difference between land and water heart rates is reduced and eventually eliminated (59–61). At lower work loads, the differences in heart rate are presumably related to an increased stroke volume.

Cardiographic measurements of left ventricular dimensions demonstrate significant increase in end-diastolic and end-systolic volumes during exercise (7, 8, 41). Some studies have suggested that water exercise results in a higher cardiac output than land exercise at

the same intensity (8, 61, 62). The hydrostatic pressure of immersion may cause an increase in stroke volume that is greater than the compensatory decrease in heart rate. Thus, cardiac output is enhanced. Plasma volume shifts do continue during immersion exercise. On land, exercise may result in a decrease in plasma volume of up to 20% (39, 61, 63). Our results in nonpregnant women suggest that the hemoconcentration of immersion exercise is not as extensive as land exercise of similar intensity. The immersion-induced hemodilution somewhat compensates for the hemoconcentration of exercise.

The ability to eliminate heat is enhanced during water exercise (50, 64, McMurray et al., unpublished data). The greater the exertion, the greater the difference between the subject's temperature comparing land and water exercise (50). This lack of elevation of core temperature could be an advantage for exercising pregnant women.

Studies comparing swimming to either land-based cycling or running have found similar heart rates (60, 65, 66). However, blood pressure is usually higher during submaximal swimming. The hemoconcentration during swimming has been shown to be similar to land cycle ergometry (67). In contrast, swimming is accompanied by a larger urine output (67). Swimming also results in lower aldosterone and PRA, and possibly greater norepinephrine (65, 66).

IMMERSION, EXERCISE, AND PREGNANCY

We have conducted two studies to examine the effects of immersion and exercise on pregnant women (33, 68). Some of these results are categorized in Table 24.2. In the first, we compared water aerobics to land aerobic exercise (68). Seven women at 25 weeks of gestation cycled for 20 min at 70% $\dot{V}_{O_2max}$ on land and in 30°C water.

Both exercise regimes were well tolerated, though all women volunteered that water exercise was easier. Maternal heart rates were greater during land exercise (10–14 bpm). Mean arterial pressures were lower in water, primarily due to differences in systolic blood pressures of 20–40 mm Hg. When maternal

Table 24.2.   Water Aerobics (W) Compared with Land Aerobics (L)

Maternal heart rate	L > W
Maternal blood pressure	L > W
Hemoconcentration	L > W
Maternal temperature	L > W
Heat storage	L > W
Urine volume	L < W
Cardiac output	L < W
Peripheral resistance	L > W
PRA, aldosterone	L > W
Recovery fetal heart rates	L > W
Increased end-diastolic volume	L < W

thermoregulation was evaluated, we found that rectal temperature increased significantly more during land exercise than in water, 0.2°C compared with 0.5°C. Heat storage during land exercise was significantly greater (21.6 kcal) compared to water exercise (10.8 kcal) (McMurray et al., unpublished data). During the land exercise mean urine output was 98 cml, compared with 261 cml during water exercise. Fetal heart rates measured after 20 min of exercise were similar between water and land exercise and unchanged from resting levels. However, at 5, 10, 15, and 20 min of supine recovery, fetal heart rates (p<.1) tended to be greater after land exercise. Six of seven fetuses experienced mild tachycardia after land exercise and only one of seven fetuses experienced tachycardia after water exercise.

In a different experiment, 12 subjects exercised in the water for 20 min at 60% of maximal heart rate at 15, 25, and 35 weeks of pregnancy and 8–10 weeks postpartum (33, 55). Subjects were able to exercise at 60% $\dot{V}_{O_2max}$ without difficulty. During immersed exercise, maternal rectal temperatures did not change in any trial periods. During the postpartum period, there was a significant drop in plasma volume during exercise: approximately 7%. In contrast, during the three pregnancy trials the plasma volume did not decline from the resting supine levels during exercise (33).

Maternal heart rates on land at 60% $\dot{V}_{O_2max}$ were higher than in the water: 148, 149, 152 compared with 135, 135, and 133 at 15, 25, and 35 weeks' gestation, respectively (56). This change was also seen (as expected) in the postpartum period: 145 compared with 131. Cardiac output as measured by CO_2 rebreathing technique was higher (as expected) during pregnancy than postpartum. Peripheral resistance was also less. Stroke volume was higher (56).

Fetal heart rates were measured by real-time ultrasound at 5 and 15 min of exercise (33). No changes in fetal heart rate were seen compared to resting values. Maternal serum AFP levels were unchanged comparing rest with after 20 min of exercise, suggesting no adverse fetal trauma. After exercise, all ba-bies had normal heart rates and reactive non-stress tests within 20 min. No increase in uterine activity was seen.

During exercise, plasma sodium, potassium, and osmolarity remained unchanged (55). Cortisol and glucose declined while lactate and triglyceride levels rose in all trial periods (57). Although pregnancy increased lipid utilization during exercise, other responses to the exercise were not affected.

Goodlin et al. (58), reported on 42 pregnant women in a water aerobics program. After mild exercise, in 34°C water, these pregnant women experienced a marked diuresis and natriuresis. The volume of the diuresis seemed to correlate with the level of subjects' edema. The natriuresis was two to three times larger than reported in men (4, 5, 15).

Sibley et al. (69), in 1981, reported an investigation designed to test whether swim conditioning could affect fitness in pregnancy. Fitness did improve slightly in swimming women compared with controls. No abnormalities were noted in mothers or babies.

The effects of immersed exercise during pregnancy on heart rate may be compared with a land experiment by Swaka et al. (70). Investigators expanded intravascular volume of their subjects with intravenous fluids before land exercise. After the volume expansion, the subjects' heart rates were significantly lower during exercise than heart rates before volume expansion. Immersion during pregnancy is analogous—pregnant women have increased extravascular fluid that is mobilized by the hydrostatic forces of immersion.

Water aerobics is not totally analogous to swimming. Swimming is a supine exercise that causes a moderate central volume redistribution, but because they are atop the water, women are much less affected by hydrostatic forces than during immersion. It is unclear if pregnant swimmers obtain significant plasma volume expansion. However, many swimmers who are swimming for fitness spend time in a vertical position before, between, and after laps at different parts of a workout period. Because immersion redistribution occurs within seconds, some hydrostatic effect will be initiated during this vertical immersion. Swimming does retain the thermoregulatory advantages and buoyancy of water aerobics.

In summary, pregnant women experienced similar, but often exaggerated responses during immersion compared with nonpregnant individuals. The diuresis and natriuresis of immersion were more profound. In contrast to nonpregnant controls and men, the immersion-induced expansion of plasma volume compensated for the exercise-induced hemoconcentration. Heart rates during water exercise are lower than during land exercise.

Water aerobics in pregnancy is a non-weight bearing exercise that occurs in a "thermal-friendly" medium. The hemodynamic changes of immersion may put less strain on uterine blood flow than land exercise does. In addition, edema is decreased. Most women comment on how enjoyable the exercises are and how much "lighter" they feel. Water aerobics is a safe and beneficial form of exercise in pregnancy.

REFERENCES

1. Berlyne GM, Suton J, Brown C, Caruso C, Friedman EA. Renal handling of urate during water immersion in the nephrotic syndrome. Mineral Electrolyte Metab 1984; 10:259–262.
2. Bichet DG, Groves BG, Schrier RW. Effect of head-out water immersion on hepatorenal syndrome. Am J Kidney Dis 1984; 3:258–263.
3. Bichet DG, Groves BM, Schrier BW. Mechanisms of improvement of water and sodium excretion by immersion in decompensated cirrhotic patients. Kidney Int 1983; 24:788–794.
4. Epstein M. Water immersion and the kidney: implications for volume regulation. Undersea Biomed Res 1984; 11:113–168.
5. Epstein M. Renal, endocrine and hemodynamic effects of water immersion in man. Contr Nephrol 1984; 41:174–188.
6. Epstein M, Miller M, Schneider N. Depth of immersion as a determinant of the natriuresis of water immersion. Proc Soc Exp Biol Med 1974; 146:562–566.
7. Risch WD, Koubenec HJ, Beckmann U, Lange S, Gauer OH. The effect of graded immersion on heart volume, central venous pressure, pulmonary blood distribution, and heart rate in man. Pflugers Arch 1978; 374:115–118.
8. Sheldahl LM, Wann LS, Clifford PS, Tristani FE, Wolf LG, Kalbfleisch JH. Effect of central hypervolemia on cardiac performance during exercise. J Am Physiol 1984; 57:1662–1667.
9. Khosla SS, DuBois AB. Fluid shifts during initial phase of immersion diuresis in man. J Appl Physiol 1979; 46:703–708.
10. Kinney EL, Cortada X, Ventura R. Cardiac size and motion during water immersion: Implications for volume homeostasis. Am Heart J 1987; 113:345–349.
11. Arborelius M Jr, Balldin UI, Lilja B, Lundgren CEG. Hemodynamic changes in man during immersion with the head above water. Aerospace Med 1972; 43:592–598.
12. Behn C, Gauer OH, Kirsch K, Eckert P. Effects of sustained intrathoracic vascular distension on body fluid distribution and renal excretion in man. Pflugers Arch 1969; 313:123–135.
13. Bennett ED, Tighe D, Wegg W. Abolition, by dopamine blockade, of the natriuretic response produced by lower-body positive pressure. Clin Sci 1982; 63:361–366.
15. Greenleaf JE. Physiology of fluid and electrolyte responses during inactivity: water immersion and bed rest. Med Sci Sports Exerc 1984; 16:20–25.
16. Greenleaf JE, Morse, Barnes PR, Silver J, Keil LC. Hypervolemia and plasma vasopressin response during water immersion in men. J Appl Physiol 1983; 55:1688–1693.
17. Lin YC. Circulatory functions during immersion and breath-hold dives in humans. Undersea Biomed Res 1984; 11:123–138.
18. Miki K, Pazik MM, Krasney E, Hong SK, Krasney JA. Thoracic duct lymph flow during head-out water immersion in conscious dogs. Am J Physiol 1987; 252:R782–R785.
19. Shiraki K, Konda N, Sagawa S, Claybaugh JR, Hong SK. Cardiorenal-endocrine responses to head-out immersion at night. J Appl Physiol 1986; 60:176–183.
20. Boening D, Ulmer HV, Meier U, Skipka W, Stegemann J. Effects of a multi-hour immersion on trained and untrained subjects: I. renal function and plasma volume. Aerospace Med 1972; 43:300–305.
21. Convertino VA, Keil LC, Bernauer EM, Greenleaf JE. Plasma volume, osmolality, vasopressin, and renin activity during graded exercise in man. J Appl Physiol 1981; 50:123–128.
22. Coruzzsi P, Biggi A, Musiari L, Ravanetti C, Novarini A. Renal hemodynamics and natriuresis during water immersion in normal humans. Pflugers Arch 1986; 407:638–642.
23. Coruzzsi P, Biggi A, Musiari L, Ravanetti C, Vescovi PP, Novarini A. Dopamine blockade and natriuresis during water immersion in normal man. Clin Sci 1986; 70:523–526.
24. Doniec-Ulman I, Kokot F, Wambach G, Drab M. Water immersion-induced endocrine alterations in women with EPH gestosis. Clin Nephrol 1987; 28:51–55.
25. Epstein M, Loutzenhiser R, Friedland E, Aceto RM, Camargo MJF, Atlas SA. Relationship of increased plasma atrial natriuretic factor and renal sodium handling during immersion-induced central hypervolemia in normal humans. J Clin Invest 1987; 79:738–745.
26. Jahn H, Schmitt R, Schohn D, Dale G. Hemodynamic modifications induced by head out water immersion in nonuremic and uremic subjects. Contr Nephrol 1984; 41:189–198.
27. Harrison MH, Keil LC, Wade CA, Silver JE, Geelen G, Greenleaf JE. Effect of hydration on plasma volume and endocrine responses to water immersion. J Appl Physiol 1986; 61:1410–1417.
28. Kravik SE, Keil LC, Silver JE, Wong N, Spaul WA,

Greenleaf JE. Immersion diuresis without expected suppression of vasopressin. J Appl Physiol 1984; 57:123–128.

29. Kurasawa T, Sakamoto H, Katoh Y, Marumo F. Atrial natriuretic peptide is only a minor diuretic factor in dehydrated subjects immersed to the neck in water. Eur J Appl Physiol 1988; 57:10–14.

30. Norsk P, Bonde-Petersen F, Warberg J. Arginine vasopressin, circulation, and kidney during graded water immersion in humans. J Appl Physiol 1986; 61:565–574.

31. Epstein M, Duncan DC, Fishman LM. Characterization of the natriuresis caused in normal man by immersion in water. Clin Sci 1972; 43:275–287.

32. Khosla SS, DuBois AB. Osmoregulation and interstitial fluid pressure changes in humans during water immersion. J Appl Physiol 1981; 51:686–692.

33. Katz VL, McMurray R, Berry MJ, Cefalo RC. Fetal and uterine responses to immersion and exercise. Obstet Gynecol 1988; 72:225–230.

34. Myers BD, Peterson C, Molina C, Tomlanovich SJ, Newton LD, Nitkin R, Sandler H, Murad F. Role of cardiac atria in the human renal response to changing plasma volume. Am J Physiol 1988; 254:F562–F573.

35. O'Hare JP, Watson M, Penney MD, Hampton D, Roland JM, Corrall RJM. Urinary prostaglandin E and antiduiretic hormone during water immersion in man. Clin Sci 1985; 69:493–496.

36. Epstein M, Johnson G, Denunzio G. Effects of water immersion on plasma catecholamines in normal humans. J Appl Physiol 1983; 54:244–248.

37. Leung WM, Logan AF, Campbell PJ, et al. Role of atrial natriuretic peptide and urinary cGMP in the natriuretic and diuretic responses to central hypervolemia in normal human subjects. Can J Physiol Pharmacol 1987; 65:2076–2080.

38. Morlock JF, Dressendorfer RH. Modification of a standard bicycle ergometer for underwater use. Undersea Biomed Res 1974; 1:335–342.

39. Novosadova J. The changes in hematocrit, hemoglobin, plasma volume and proteins during and after different types of exercise. Eur J Appl Physiol 1977; 36:223–230.

40. Coruzzsi P, Ravanetti C, Musiari L, Biggi A, Vescovi PP, Novarini A. Circulating opioid peptides during water immersion in normal man. Clin Sci 1988; 74:133–136.

41. Shiraki D, Konda N, Sagawa S, Lin YC, Hong SK. Cardiac output by impedance cardiography during head-out water immersion. Undersea Biomed Res 1986; 13:247–256.

42. Weston CFM, O'Hare JP, Evans JM, Corrall RJM. Hemodynamic changes in man during immersion in water at different temperatures. Clin Sci 1987; 73:613–616.

43. Buono MJ. Effect of central vascular engorgement and immersion on various lung volumes. J Appl Physiol 1983; 54:1094–1096.

44. Craig AB Jr, Dvorak M. Thermal regulation during water immersion. J Appl Physiol 1966; 21:1577–1585.

45. Nadel ER. Energy exchanges in water. Undersea Biomed Res 1984; 11:149–158.

46. Boutelier C, Bougues L, Timbal J. Experimental study of convective heat transfer coefficient for the human body in water. J Appl Physiol 1977; 42:93–100.

47. Epstein M, Norsk P, Loutzenhiser R, Sonke P. Detailed characterization of a tank used for head-out

water immersion in humans. J Appl Physiol 1987; 63:869–871.

48. Kollias J, Barlett L, Bergsteinova V, Skinner JS, Buskirk ER, Nicholas WC. Metabolic and thermal responses of women during cooling in water. J Appl Physiol 1974; 36:577–580.

49. McArdle WD, Magel JR, Gergley TJ, Spina RJ, Toner MM. Thermal adjustment to cold-water exposure in resting men and women. J Appl Physiol 1984; 56:1565–1571.

50. Nielsen B, Davies CTM. Temperature regulation during exercise in water and air. Acta Physiol Scand 1976; 98:500–508.

51. Goff LG, Brubach HF, Specht H, Smith N. Effect of total immersion at various temperatures on oxygen uptake at rest and during exercise. J Appl Physiol 1956; 9:59–61.

52. Davison JM, Gilmore EA, Durr J, Robertson GL, Lindheimer MD. Altered osmotic thresholds for vasopressin secretion and thirst in human pregnancy. Am J Physiol 1984; 246:F105–F109.

53. Millar ND, Quinn MJ, Evans J, Norman T, Jones A, Corrall RJM, The cardiovascular effects of head-out, water immersion in normal pregnancy. Abstract presented 5th International Congress: International Society for the Study of Hypertension in Pregnancy. July 1986: Nottingham England.

54. Berry MJ, McMurray RG, Katz VL. Pulmonary and ventilatory responses to pregnancy, immersion and exercise: A longitudinal study. J Appl Physiol 1989; 66:857–862.

55. Katz VL, McMurray R, Berry MJ, Cefalo RC, Bowman C. Renal responses to immersion and exercise in pregnancy. Am J Perinat 1990; 7:118–121.

56. McMurray RG, Katz VL, Berry MJ, Cefalo RC. Cardiovascular responses of pregnant women during aerobic exercise in water: A longitudinal study. Int J Sports Med 1988; 9:443–447.

57. McMurray RG, Katz VL, Berry MJ, Cefalo RC. The effect of pregnancy on metabolic responses during rest, immersion, and aerobic exercise in the water. Am J Obstet Gynecol 1988; 158:481–486.

58. Goodlin RC, Engdahl Hoffmann KL, Williams NE, Buchan P. Shoulder-out immersion in pregnant women. J Perinat Med 1984; 12:173–177.

59. Heigenhauser GF, Boulet D, Miller B, Faulkner JA. Cardiac outputs of post-myocardial infarction patients during swimming and cycling. Med Sci Sports Exerc 1977; 9:143–147.

60. Holmer I, Stein EM, Saltin B, Ekblom B, Astrand P. Hemodynamic and respiratory responses compared in swimming and running. J Appl Physiol 1974; 37:49–54.

61. McMurray RG, Fieselman CC, Avery KE, Sheps DS. Exercise hemodynamics in water and on land in patients with coronary artery disease. J Cardiopul Rehabil 1988; 8:69–75.

62. Sheldahl LM, Tristani FE, Clifford PS, Hughes CV, Sobocinski KA, Morris RD. Effect of head-out water immersion on cardiorespiratory response to dynamic exercise. J Am Coll Cardiol 1987; 10:1254–1258.

63. Nielsen B, Sjorgaard G, Bonde-Petersen F. Cardiovascular, hormonal and body fluid changes during prolonged exercise. Eur J Appl Physiol 1984; 53:63–70.

64. Costill DL, Cahill PJ, Eddy D. Metabolic responses to submaximal exercise in three water temperatures. J Appl Physiol 1967; 22:628–632.

65. Guezennec CY, Defer G, Cazorla G, Sabathier C, Lhoste F. Plasma renin activity, aldosterone and catecholamine levels when swimming and running. Eur J Appl Physiol 1986; 54:632–637.

66. Wolf JP, Nguyen NU, Dumoulin G, Baulay A, Berthelay S. Relative effects of the supine posture and of immersion on the renin aldosterone system at rest and during exercise. Eur J Appl Physiol 1987; 56:345–349.

67. McMurray RG. Plasma volume changes during submaximal swimming. Eur J Appl Physiol 1983; 51:347–356.

68. Katz VL, McMurray R, Goodwin WE, Cefalo RC. A comparison between non-weightbearing exercise during pregnancy on land and during immersion. Am J Perinat in press.

69. Sibley L, Ruhling RO, Cameron-Foster J, Christensen C, Bolen T. Swimming and physical fitness during pregnancy. J Nurse-Midwifery 1981; 26:3–12.

70. Swaka MN, Hubbard RW, Franescioni RP, Horstman DH. Effects of acute plasma volume expansion on altering exercise-heart performance. Eur J Appl Physiol 1983; 51:303–312.

25

Work and Exercise During Pregnancy: Epidemiological Studies

Maureen C. Hatch and Zena A. Stein

Although reports exist dating back to the 1950s, there are remarkably few epidemiological studies that provide useful evidence about the effects of work during pregnancy, and even fewer about the effects of exercise. The intent of this chapter is to summarize the most informative studies and to weigh the evidence from them, as well as to suggest useful directions for future research. There are many aspects of women's work that merit attention in relation to pregnancy (e.g., physical demands, psychosocial stress, exposure to toxic agents), but in the present context the benefits and hazards of physical effort will be emphasized. We will review the epidemiological reports concerning effects of work in a standing posture; of work involving lifting or carrying; and of work requiring other forms of strenuous activity. Also considered are studies that assess the effects of continuing work up to the time of delivery. Finally, leisure-time exercise during pregnancy is briefly discussed.

Much research on work in pregnancy has evaluated work only in a global sense (1–13), drawing no distinctions between one type of work and another (although the jobs women do clearly differ a great deal in terms of their demands and compensations). Such studies compare working women as a group to housewives, in terms of pregnancy outcome, although women who do not work outside the home cannot be seen as the appropriate comparison for women who do. On the one hand, some of the circumstances that lead women to seek paid employment may also affect the pregnancy, and the fact that many early studies found poorer outcomes among women workers than housewives could reflect the reasons for working and not the work itself. Conversely, the very fact that a woman can continue to work throughout pregnancy may indicate she is somewhat advantaged. At present, this is the usual case in Western societies: women who stay at home tend to be less healthy than employed women and are at risk of poorer pregnancy outcomes—a form of selection that is comparable to the so-called "healthy worker" effect in epidemiological studies of chronic illness in men (14). In addition, the work women do within the home (sometimes called the "second shift"), often involves at least as much stress and physical effort as does work outside. [Indeed, at least one study has identified women with several children and no domestic help as at risk for premature delivery (15).] For these reasons, research comparing women workers as a group with housewives is not useful for evaluating effects of work stress and, in fact, may lead to erroneous interpretations. Therefore, in this review we have not generally considered such studies, excepting for a few reports that examine the effects of continuing to work late in gestation.

EFFECTS OF WORKING LATE IN GESTATION

Table 25.1 summarizes the results of six studies on duration of work in pregnancy—two dealing with infant birth weight and four concerned with work as a "trigger" for preterm delivery. Regarding birth weight, a study in Boston (8) found slightly higher weights in the infants of mothers who worked throughout pregnancy than in infants of mothers who left work earlier in gestation. No data were available on the reasons for stopping work, and so any apparent advantage of working to term may, in reality, be due to the healthy worker effect. The second study, in Spain, found that women workers who opted to take their maternity leave in

Table 25.1.   Effects of Work Late in Gestation[a]

Duration Work	Study Population	Pregnancy Outcome	Adverse Effect	No Effect
All 9 months (vs. 6-wk rest leave)	Spain, deliveries (low SES excluded)	BW	Alegre et al. (1)	
All 9 months (vs. 1–8 months)	Boston, deliveries	BW		Marbury et al. (8)
3rd trimester	New Haven deliveries, case-control study	Preterm		Berkowitz et al. (17)
All 9 months (vs. rest leave for fatigue)	French factory workers	Preterm	Mamelle et al. (16)	
All 9 months (vs. none or varying)	Active-duty Air Force personnel	Preterm	Fox et al. (5)	
3rd trimester	Brooklyn deliveries (blacks only), case-control study	Preterm		Terris and Gold (13) (NS trend)

[a] Abbreviations: SES = socioeconomic status; BW = birth weight; NS = not statistically significant.

the last 6 weeks of pregnancy had significantly heavier babies than women who worked up to the time of delivery (1); the 200-g increase among infants of workers taking rest leaves was maintained in an analysis that excluded women with any other factors that might affect birth weight.

For preterm delivery (that is, delivery at less than 37 completed weeks of gestation), fairly strong evidence on the beneficial effects of rest during late pregnancy comes from a study of French workers at factories whose activities were believed to cause occupational fatigue (16). Women who took a rest leave for fatigue, unaccompanied by any current or previous obstetric problem, had a rate of preterm delivery 60% lower than comparable workers who did not opt for such leaves. Consistent with this, a less well-controlled study conducted at an Air Force obstetric hospital found substantially higher preterm birth rates for women who were on active duty up to the time of delivery (5). Two studies found no association between work-

ing late in pregnancy and preterm birth (13, 17), but the definition of late duration included work at any point in the third trimester. Thus, the evidence to date suggests that if work per se is adverse, it is only so very late in gestation, and even then perhaps only in certain types of jobs.

Studies that differentiate jobs according to the nature of the work involved, and then compare pregnancy outcomes across job categories, are more informative for the issue at hand than studies that only consider working versus not working. Tables 25.2–25.4 summarize results from investigations of work in pregnancy that have dealt specifically with aspects of jobs related to physical demands.

EFFECTS OF WORK IN A STANDING POSTURE

That prolonged periods of standing—especially when continued through the third trimester—might lead to intrauterine growth retardation is a hypothesis now tested in a number of studies (Table 25.2). The effect of

Table 25.2. Effects of Work in a Standing Posture[a]

Measure of Standing	Study Population	Pregnancy Outcome	Adverse Effect	No Association
"Continuous"	Finnish workers, case-control study	SA		Taskinen et al. (19) [OR = 1.4 (0.5, 4.4)]
≥6 hr/day	Montreal, deliveries	SA		McDonald et al. (18) (adverse effect in manufacturing sector only)
Standing job (vs. sitting), 1st prenatal visit	Guatemala, low to middle class urban prenatal patients	BW (SGA)	Launer et al. (22) [OR = 1.2 (1.0, 1.4)]	
1st trimester standing (y/n)	France, national sample of births	BW (<2500 g)		Saurel-Cubizolles and Kaminski (25)
"Most of the time," after 33 wks g	U.S., prenatal patients	BW	Naeye and Peters (21) (≥150 g; placental infarcts)	
75%/day (inferred from job title)	Washington State, birth records, case-control study	BW (<2500 g)		Meyer and Daling (24) [OR = 1.2 (1.0, 1.5)]
≥8 hr/day	Montreal, deliveries	BW (<2500 g)		McDonald et al. (23)
≥8 hr/day	Montreal, deliveries	Preterm		McDonald et al. (23)
≥3 hr/day	France, Lyon, and Hagenau deliveries	Preterm	Mamelle et al. (28) [RR = 1.6 (1.1, 2.3)]	
≥3 hr/day	Lyon, France, case-control study	Preterm		Mamelle and Munoz (1987) (OR = 1.00)
"All of the time" (vs. little or none)	New Haven deliveries, case-control studies	Preterm		Berkowitz et al. (17) (chi^2 for trend = 0.15)
Standing job (vs. sitting), 1st prenatal visit	Guatemala, low to middle class urban prenatal patients	Preterm	Launer et al. (22) [(OR = 1.56 (1.0, 2.6)]	
Stand-up job (vs. sit-down job), after midgestation	U.S., prenatal patients	GA		Naeye and Peters (21) (281 vs. 280 days)

[a] Abbreviations: SA = spontaneous abortion; BW = birth weight; GA = gestational age; OR = odds ratio; RR = relative risk.

postural stress on risk of preterm delivery has also been investigated, and there are two reports in relation to spontaneous abortion.

No association was found for standing work and spontaneous abortion (19, 20); indeed there would not seem to be strong grounds for suspecting that postural strain early in pregnancy would raise a woman's risk of miscarriage. For effects on fetal growth, there is evidence from a large prospective study of prenatal patients in the United States that prolonged standing late in pregnancy, compared with sitting work or staying at home, reduces fetal weight by 150–400 g (21); placental infarcts in the mothers of affected infants suggest low uteroplacental blood flow as a likely explanation for compromised fetal growth. A prospective study in Guatemala provides only modest support for an association between standing work and growth retardation (22); however, in this case, the timing of the postural strain in pregnancy was not considered. Three other studies, all with negative findings, looked for increases in the proportion of low birth weight infants among women whose jobs involved standing (23–25); such studies would fail to detect modest amounts of growth retardation. Standing work was found to be a risk factor for preterm delivery in the Guatemala study, while the U.S. prospective study found virtually no difference in gestational age between those with standing versus sitting jobs. Nor did three other studies offer convincing evidence that postural fatigue is likely to induce premature delivery (17, 23, 26).

If there is cause for concern about prolonged standing late in pregnancy, on biological grounds one might choose to focus future research on the issue of fetal growth. The available evidence from epidemiological studies is suggestive; apparent inconsistencies could be addressed in carefully designed studies.

EFFECTS OF LIFTING

Lifting or carrying of heavy loads increases intra-abdominal pressure and, in pregnant women, may ultimately stimulate uterine contractions (Table 25.3). Research to date does appear to show that frequent heavy lifting carries a modest (20–30%) increased risk for preterm delivery (statistically significant in one study (23), not so in two others (25, 27). Infrequent lifting or carrying, and lighter loads, seem to pose no risk of preterm birth, however. A similar pattern of results is seen for lifting in relation to risk of spontaneous abortion (18, 19). In the case of low birth weight, the evidence is less consistent: two studies report modest associations with heavy lifting (23, 25), but a prospective study from Sweden, where women coming for a first prenatal visit were asked to describe their work, found no association, even with frequent lifting of very heavy loads (27). Thus, based on the evidence available at present,

lifting does not appear to affect fetal weight adversely. Future research might concentrate on confirming and quantifying the suggested associations between frequent heavy lifting in pregnancy and outcomes related to uterine contractility.

EFFECTS OF OTHER STRENUOUS ACTIVITY

A number of epidemiologic studies have examined effects of strenuous work during pregnancy (Table 25.4). Some useful research has come from France, where occupational fatigue has been linked to preterm birth (28). Using detailed histories taken at the time of delivery, an index of fatigue was constructed from scores for postural strain, physical exertion, machine work, mental stress, and physical and chemical exposure. Figure 25.1 shows rates of preterm birth rising with occupational fatigue score, and with the number of hours worked per week. The fraction of preterm births attributable to occupational fatigue in this French population was a substantial 21% (compared with only 8% for a prior preterm delivery). A similar association with a composite activity score has been found for growth-retarded preterm births in Guatemala (22). Physical exertion specifically—one component of fatigue—has not consist-

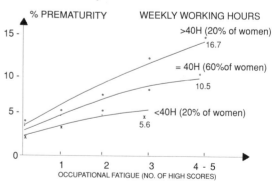

Figure 25.1. Prematurity rate among working women in Lyon and Hagenau, France (n = 1928) according to an index of occupational "fatigue" and number of hours worked per week. (From Mamelle N, Laumon B, Lazar P. Prematurity and occupational activity during pregnancy. Am J Epidemiol 1984; 119:309–322.)

Table 25.3.   Effects of Lifting[a]

Measure of Lifting	Study Population	Pregnancy Outcome	Adverse Effect	No Association
≥ 10 kg: • "Continuous" • "Seldom"	Finnish workers, case-control study	SA	Taskinen et al. (19) [OR = 3.6 (1.0, 13.7)]	(OR = 1.0)
"Heavy"	Montreal, deliveries	SA	McDonald et al. (18) (p <.01 for trend)	
"Heavy"	Sweden, laboratory workers	SA		Axelsson et al. (20) [OR = 1.4 (0.9, 2.0)]
≥ 12 kg: • 10–50 times/w • >50 times/w	Sweden, prenatal patients	SA or stillbirth		Ahlborg et al. (27) [OR = 1.11 (0.8, 1.6)] [OR = 1.06 (0.6, 1.8)]
		BW (<2500 g)		Ahlborg et al. (27) (OR <1.0)
"Heavy load carrying"	France, national sample of deliveries	BW (<2500 g)		Saurel-Cubizolles and Kaminski (25) (RR = 1.3, NS)
"Heavy, 15 times/ day"	Montreal, deliveries	BW (<2500 g)	McDonald et al. (23) (O/E = 1.26)	
		Preterm	(O/E = 1.25)	
<5 lb to 25+ lb	New Haven deliveries, case-control study	Preterm		Berkowitz et al. (17)
"Load carrying"	France, Lyon & Hagenau deliveries	Preterm		Mamelle et al. (28)
"Heavy load carrying"	France, national sample of deliveries	Preterm		Saurel-Cubizolles and Kaminski (25) (RR = 1.33 NS)
≥ 12 kg: • 10–50 times/w • >50 times/w	Sweden, prenatal patients	Preterm		Ahlborg et al. (27) (OR = 0.7, NS) (OR = 1.3, NS)

[a] Abbreviations: SA = spontaneous abortion; BW = birth weight; OR = odds ratio; O/E = observed/expected; RR = relative risk; NS = not statistically significant.

ently been found to raise the risk of preterm delivery (25, 26, 28). Nor do the findings for "physical effort" and birth weight provide convincing evidence of risk (22–25), although, again, in Guatemala a composite activity score was positively related to fetal growth retardation.

EVIDENCE FROM DEVELOPING NATIONS

In less developed countries, poor maternal nutrition must be considered an influence on fetal growth, and this needs to be weighed when interpreting the findings from the Gua-temala study, where there is evidence of some chronic malnutrition. In conditions of undernutrition, hard physical labor during pregnancy may decrease fetal weight by increasing demands on the mother. This has been seen in Ethiopia (29). Another report, from the Gambia, found adverse effects on birth weight of reduced diet and heavy work during the ploughing season, if this occurred in the third trimester (30). In Zaire, fetal growth was found to be substantially improved (for female infants especially) if women avoided heavy work in the last weeks of pregnancy, by resting in a maternity village (31). Effects

Table 25.4.   Effects of Other Strenuous Activity[a]

Measure of Strenuous Work	Study Population	Pregnancy Outcome	Adverse Effect	No Association
"Physical effort"	Montreal, deliveries	SA	McDonald et al. (18) (stronger in past than current pregnancies)	
"Active" vs. "sitting" (from job title)	Washington State birth records case-control study	BW (<2500 g)		Meyer and Daling (24) [OR = 1.14 (0.9, 1.4)]
Activity score, 1st prenatal visit	Guatemala, low to middle class urban prenatal patients	BW (SGA)	Launer et al. (22) (significant positive trend)	
"Considerable physical effort," 1st trimester	France, national sample births	BW (<2500 g)	Saurel-Cubizolles and Kaminski (25) (RR = 1.6, p <.05)	
"Great physical effort"	Montreal, deliveries	BW (<2500 g)		McDonald et al. (23) (O/E = 1.06, NS)
		Preterm		(O/E = 1.10, NS)
Activity score, 1st prenatal visit	Guatemala, low to middle class urban prenatal patients	Preterm	Launer et al. (22) (SGA and SGA preterm)	
"Considerable physical effort," 1st trimester	France, national sample births	Preterm		Saurel-Cubizolles and Kaminski (25) (RR = 1.2, NS)
"Physical effort"	France, Lyon and Hagenau deliveries	Preterm	Mamelle et al. (28) [RR = 1.6 (1.1, 2.7)]	
"Physical exertion"	France, case-control study	Preterm		Mamelle and Munoz (26) [OR = 1.1 (0.8, 1.5)]

[a] Abbreviations: SA = spontaneous abortion; BW = birth weight; SGA = small-for-gestational age; RR = relative risk; O/E = observed/expected; NS = not statistically significant.

of strenuous work late in pregnancy may vary with nutritional status of the woman, according to whether the physical demands of work disrupt energy balance.

LEISURE-TIME PHYSICAL ACTIVITY

The possibility that some physical activity in pregnancy may actually be beneficial, particularly in well-conditioned women, merits consideration. Thus far, however, there is only one epidemiological study on the effects of exercise in pregnancy: in a case-control study of preterm delivery, women who participated in sports or physical fitness exercises were found to be at decreased risk of premature birth (17), although no advantage was evident for exercise in late pregnancy (when activity-induced elevations in norepinephrine levels conceivably might trigger premature contractions). Reports from small clinical studies that compare outcomes among women who do and do not exercise in pregnancy are generally reassuring (e.g., 32), but additional research in larger populations is needed to confirm this. To date, most of the epidemiological work on exercise has focused on menstrual function and fertility rather than on pregnancy and childbirth.

CONCLUSIONS AND RECOMMENDATIONS FOR FUTURE RESEARCH

There are several problems for the epidemiologist in evaluating the available data on work and exercise in pregnancy. First, almost none of the studies reported takes account of the physical demands of work inside the home, despite the fact that household work, when considered, has been found to be influential (15, 22). Second, effects on fetal growth and length of gestation have seldom been clearly distinguished in spite of their having quite different etiologies. Third, the measures of "work" and "exercise" that have been used are imprecise and variable from study to study. Fourth, many studies have failed to account for other factors affecting pregnancy outcome that may be correlated with working or exercise (cigarette smoking is one example of such a factor). Finally, the timing of physical demands, and possible changes in these demands over the course of the pregnancy, have not often been considered.

At present among epidemiologists, there is increased interest and methodological sophistication concerning effects of occupational and leisure-time physical activity, and studies currently in progress have been designed to address the problems previously cited. For instance, our own study of 900 prenatal patients is both prospective and longitudinal: paid employment, household work, and exercise are systematically measured in each trimester of pregnancy so that their independent and joint effects at various stages of gestation can be evaluated. The pregnancy complications and birth outcomes selected for study were specified on the basis of a priori hypotheses about mechanism, and the analysis is planned so as to take account of other relevant risk factors. The latest generation of epidemiological studies on work and exercise should yield findings that are more readily interpretable than previous research.

Also useful would be additional experimental and clinical studies that define the physiological response to the types of physical demands women are likely to encounter at work, at home, and at leisure. In the meantime, the evidence for adverse effects of standing and lifting—and for beneficial effects of rest leaves in late pregnancy—seems sufficient to warrant giving the issue of physical activity in pregnancy further attention. As a prudent measure, pending results of future studies, clinicians may wish to advise their obstetric patients to avoid the following activities: repetitive heavy lifting, prolonged standing during the third trimester, and particularly in conditions of undernutrition, any strenuous work late in pregnancy.

REFERENCES

1. Alegre A, Rodriguez-Escudero FJ, Cruz E, Prada M. Influence of work during pregnancy on fetal weight. J Reproduc Med 1984; 29:334–336.
2. Baird D. The epidemiology of prematurity. J Pediatr 1964; 65:909–924.
3. Douglas JWB. Some factors associated with prematurity. J Obstet Gynaecol Br Emp, 1950; 57:143–70.
4. Drillien CM. The social and economic factors affecting the incidence of premature birth. J Obstet Gynaecol Br Emp 1957; 2:161–184.
5. Fox ME, Harris RE, Brekken AL. The active-duty military pregnancy: A new high-risk category. Am J Obstet Gynaecol 1977; 129:705–707.
6. Gofin J. The effect on birth weight of employment during pregnancy. J Biosoc Sci 1979; 11:259–267.
7. Illsley R, Billewicz WZ, Thomson AM. Prematurity and paid work during pregnancy. Br J Prev Soc Med. 1953; 8:153–156.
8. Marbury MC, Linn S, Monson RR, Wegman DH, Schoenbaum SC, Stubblefield PG, Ryan KJ. Work and pregnancy. J Occup Med 1984; 26:415–421.
9. Martin FM. Primiparae and prematurity. Med Officer 1954; 92:263–270.
10. Murphy JF, Dauncey M, Newcombe R. Employment in pregnancy: Prevalence, maternal characteristics, perinatal outcome. Lancet 1954; 1:1163–1166.
11. Murphy JF, Newcombe R, Dauncey M, Garcia J, Elbourne D. Employment in pregnancy. Lancet 1984; 1:755–756.
12. Scott EM, Thomson AM. A psychological investigation of primigravidae. J Obstet Gynaecol Br Emp 1956; 63:502–508.
13. Terris M, Gold EM. An epidemiologic study of prematurity. Am J Obstet Gynaecol 1969; 103:358–379.
14. Joffe M. Biases in research on reproduction and women's work. Int J Epidemiol 1985; 14:118–123.
15. Papiernik E, Kaminski M. Multifunctional study of risk of prematurity at 32 weeks of gestation. A study of the frequency of 30 predictive characteristics. J Perinat Med 1974; 2:30–36.
16. Mamelle N, Bertucat U, Munoz F. Pregnant women

at work: rest periods to prevent pre-term birth? Paediatr Perinatal Epidemiol 1989; 3:19–28.

17. Berkowitz GS, Kelsey JL, Holford TR, Berkowitz RL. Physical activity and the risk of spontaneous preterm delivery. J Reproduc Med 1983; 28:581–588.

18. McDonald AD, Armstrong B, Cherry NM, Delorme C, Diodati-Nolin A, McDonald C, Robert D. Spontaneous abortion and occupation. J Occup Med 1986; 28:1232–1238.

19. Taskinen H, Lindbohm ML, Hemminki K. Spontaneous abortions among women working in the pharmaceutical industry. Br J Ind Med 1986; 43:199–205.

20. Axelsson G, Lutz C, Rylander R. Exposure to solvents and outcome of pregnancy in university laboratory employees. Br J Ind Med 1984; 41:305–312.

21. Naeye RL, Peters EC. Working during pregnancy. Effects on the fetus. Pediatrics 1982; 69:724–727.

22. Launer LJ, Villar J, Kestler E, de Onis M. The effect of maternal work on fetal growth and duration of pregnancy: A prospective study. Br J Obstet Gynaecol 1990; 97:62–70.

23. McDonald AD, McDonald JC, Armstrong B, Cherry NM, Nolin AD, Robert D. Prematurity and work in pregnancy. Br J Ind Med 1988; 45:56–62.

24. Meyer BA, Daling JR. Activity level of mother's usual occupation and low infant birth weight. J Occup Med 1985; 27:841–847.

25. Saurel-Cubizolles MJ, Kaminski M. Pregnant women's working conditions and their changes during pregnancy: A national study in France. Br J Ind Med 1987; 44:236–243.

26. Mamelle N, Nunoz F. Occupational working conditions and preterm birth: A reliable scoring system. Am J Epidemiol 1987; 126:150–152.

27. Ahlborg G, Bodin L, Hogstedt C. Heavy lifting during pregnancy—a hazard to the fetus? A prospective study. Int J Epidemiol 1990; 19:90–97.

28. Mamelle N, Laumon B, Lazar P. Prematurity and occupational activity during pregnancy. Am J Epidemiol 1984; 119:309–322.

29. Tafari N, Naeye RL, Gobezie A. Effects of maternal undernutrition and heavy physical work during pregnancy on birth weight. Br J Obstet Gynaecol 1980; 87:222–226.

30. Prentice AM, Cole TJ, Foord FA, Lamb WH, Whitehead RG. Increased birthweight after prenatal dietary supplementation of rural African women. Am J Clin Nutr 1987; 46:912–925.

31. Manshande JP, Eeckels R, Manshande-Desmet V, Vlietinck R. Rest versus heavy work during the last weeks of pregnancy: influence on fetal growth. Br J Obstet Gynaecol 1987; 94:1059–1067.

32. Collings CA, Curet LB, Mullin JP. Maternal and fetal responses to a maternal aerobic exercise program. Am J Obstet Gynaecol 1983; 145:702–707.

26

Emotional Aspects of Exercise in Pregnancy

Michal Artal and Raul Artal Mittelmark

Clinical observations and reports in the literature suggest that physical activity is associated with an enhanced sense of well-being. Some authors report a correlation between regular physical exercise and a decrease in anxiety and depression (1–3). Others report that exercise conditioning during pregnancy seems to be beneficial in reducing pain perception during labor (4). One mechanism suggested for these effects is the increased secretion of plasma β-endorphin in pregnant exercisers.

Most active women desire to continue exercise during pregnancy for various reasons. Very little scientific information has been gathered concerning the psychological aspects of exercise in pregnancy. In this chapter, we will address the psychodynamics of sports and physical activity in general and those that are specific to women and to pregnant women in particular. We attempt to examine the subject from an in-depth psychoanalytic perspective.

Because of its high level of abstraction, this subject does not lend itself to examination by chemical, physical, or histological methods. Instead, different methods are employed that include clinical observations of behavior, both normal and abnormal (infant, child, and adult), and investigative exploration of ideas, feelings, fantasies, dreams, slips, and impulses. The unique advantages of the psychoanalytic method of exploring the mind are its highly intensive, in-depth and longitudinal familiarity with patients and its access to mental mechanisms that are usually inaccessible to other methods.

Why do people exercise? Our observations suggest a complex interaction of many variables rather than a unidimensional causality. From the very common and fully conscious reason "because it feels good," it is valuable to consider the underlying motives that may be conscious or partially or largely unconscious. It is the interplay of the various motives that will determine the individual attitudes and behavior.

1. *Ability to measure achievement*: A sense of achievement and accomplishment are essential for self-esteem regulation. Much of human endeavor does not lend itself to clear-cut and readily discernible results. Some endeavors require prolonged periods of time before results are clear. In other endeavors, results are equivocal, relative, subtle, mixed, and impossible to measure. Sports do offer the important psychological dimension of unequivocal results, which are readily measured, easily quantifiable, and offer some of the most dramatic and public displays of human achievement. Exercisers are able, therefore, more readily than in other areas, to measure and, thus, to experience a sense of clear-cut achievement.

2. *Externalization and diversion of conflicts*: We suggest that some of the sense of relief and well-being experienced by exercisers is due to the shifting of attention from intrapsychic conflicts causing anxiety and depression and focusing one's attention instead on external difficulties. Usually, the external difficulties are more readily solvable than the internal. It is more than avoiding one area and investing oneself in another (which is not limited only to sport). This defensive solution becomes less helpful as the element of avoidance is greater and as the area being avoided is of greater significance to the person's life. If one attempts to avoid conflicts causing depression or difficulties in interpersonal relationships, the relief attained by the avoidance is usually temporary. In the long run, the difficulties will remain unless addressed.

3. *Enhanced sense of mastery*: People feel a genuine sense of satisfaction when they engage in an activity they know is beneficial to them. Most people are aware, and the information continues to accumulate on the benefits of exercise to physical health. There is the satisfaction of taking responsibility, of actively participating in charting one's biological fu-

ture. This healthy and balanced attitude can regress to irrational sense of omnipotence—to a literal belief in mind over body and in the denial of mortality.

4. *Physical exercise as hard work*: The hard work involved in all sports, the aspect of arduous training, the sweat, and the fatigue are indispensable ingredients of physical exercise that are appropriately condensed in the term "workout." Because of the unequivocal aspects of hard work so characteristic of sport, even the demands of strict, demanding, and punitive conscience are likely to be met. Because of this aspect of physical exercise, individuals with a strong work morality and workaholics are more likely to experience that they deserve to feel good after hard workouts and such obvious deprivations. In one patient's words: "I paid my dues, I suffered enough." In people who are depressed, if guilt is an important aspect of their depression, the rigorous and, at time, painful aspect of strenuous exercise may offer some relief of their sense of guilt with lessening (temporarily) of their depression.

5. *Expression of aggression*: Pent-up anger, hostility, and tension can be discharged through vigorous use of large muscle activity. Activities such as jumping, kicking, striking, jogging, hitting, pushing, climbing, and wrestling allow such discharge. Psychological mechanisms of displacement and symbolic thinking allow even greater discharge of aggression by symbolically directing the actions and the effects toward others. Additionally, many sports are, in themselves, directly or indirectly competitive where outdoing, out-achieving, beating, and triumphing over opponents allows even more direct gratification of competitive and aggressive strivings. A clinical example for the significance of such unconscious mental mechanisms is the athlete who, because of conflicts over being number one, repeatedly slips and fails just as he/she is about to outdo the opponent or become victorious—the so-called "fear of success." Psychological mechanisms can be "shared" through the use of projection and identification. The behaviors of others can assume personal meanings for us. Spectators and onlookers may and do participate, on a psychological level, through identification with the athlete or the team and experience relief indirectly through discharge of their aggressive feelings.

6. *Physical exercise as opportunity for social interaction*: Even though there are exceptions, for the most part, physical exercise and most sports do afford and, therefore, may play an important facilitating role in social interaction. From early experiences during childhood and adolescence involving learning team work, negotiating competitive and ambitious strivings, winning and losing, cooperation and fair play, to opportunities in adult life for meaningful human interaction, sport is a significant social organizer.

In summary, we identified a number of psychological factors we believe are important in influencing the many psychological meanings of exercise for both men and women. Some of them are conscious and some are unconscious. Behaviorally, we can identify a wide spectrum of involvements and emotional attitudes: from the healthy attitude when one freely chooses to exercise and finds the activity enjoyable all the way to situations we suspect are less healthy. Like other human activities, exercise too can become a compulsive and pathological preoccupation at times with qualities similar to other addictive or compulsive behaviors, carried out as a result of, and becoming involved in emotional conflict. A clinical example for the latter is the young anorexic woman who has morbid fears of gaining weight and of succumbing to her desires to eat. This woman exercises in a manner that is extreme, compulsive, and clearly excessive as a means to achieve a sense of control she fears she is about to lose.

PSYCHODYNAMIC CONSIDERATIONS IN WOMEN AND IN PREGNANCY

In addition to the aspects previously reviewed, we believe it is helpful to consider exercise in pregnancy in the wider context of the special emotional tasks brought about by the pregnant state.

Is the pregnancy planned? Is it wanted? Is it tolerated? How much does it give rise to conflict? It is helpful to keep in mind that planned pregnancy is not necessarily free of conflict. Outward acceptance or even enthusiasm may conceal internal turmoil with anxiety and guilt. There usually is a continuum of greater or lesser ambivalence, greater or lesser conflict. Personal goals and timetables must frequently be altered. Even when the woman experiences her pregnancy as highly desirable there are unavoidable tensions between her own needs and desires as she perceives them and those of the developing fetus. Pregnancy confronts the woman with the task of resolving the conflicting needs and the changing priorities, her new responsibilities, accepting the changes in her body, the changing dietary requirements, increased fatigue, changing energy levels and sleep requirements.

The woman's feelings about herself, her femaleness, her body—all of these are involved in how she will feel about her pregnancy. Because pregnancy is an undeniable expression of her active sexuality and because it represents the fulfillment of her biological reproductive function, any emotional conflicts in these areas will give rise to intrapsychic conflicts manifesting themselves by symptoms, the most frequent of which are depression, sense of worthlessness, and guilt.

Pregnancy has been compared to other critical periods called "developmental crises" by Erickson (5) and by Bibring (6). As this term implies, pregnancy revives psychic conflicts of earlier developmental phases. By doing so, it precipitates emotional upheaval yet also represents the opportunity for new, more mature psychological resolutions. Pregnancy, therefore, could also be an important catalyst for further emotional growth. The concept of reactivation of earlier unresolved conflicts by pregnancy is significant and we wish to illustrate this by clinical examples. Because pregnancy revives memories and feelings from her own experiences with her mother, a woman who suffered maternal deprivation, physical or emotional abandonment, or an unsatisfactory relationship with a parent early in life may experience depression precipitated by her pregnancy. She may feel anger and envy toward the unborn child, because she feels so needy herself (7). The clinical picture may be one of anxiety, depression, or ambivalence about continuation of the pregnancy. She may remain unaware of the causes of her depression and conse-

quently may not be able to resolve it without treatment. A woman who felt lonely and unloved may instead want a child very much in order to feel loved forever. Such a woman will feel very happy during pregnancy. Emotional difficulties are very likely to arise later, especially in allowing the child to separate and become interested in others (separation-individuation phase) (8).

Pregnancy may, at times, be an unconscious means of avoiding loneliness, emptiness, or a way to put off confronting other life tasks such as school or career that the woman may feel she is inadequate to achieve and is afraid to tackle. The emotional difficulties may remain relatively silent and may not lead to outwardly discernible symptomatology.

The incidence of severe postpartum psychosis or depression is estimated to be 1–2/1000 births (9, 10). But many more women may benefit significantly from psychiatric help, therefore, the question of referral for psychiatric evaluation is an important one. For many women, the obstetrician may be the only person in a position to observe increasing emotional difficulties that may result in psychological decompensation during pregnancy (11). The obstetrician is in a unique position of being alerted from the beginning of pregnancy that a pregnant woman may be more likely to experience emotional difficulties. Table 26.1 summarizes the risk factors suggested as signal areas for the obstetrician to pay greater attention to and to consider a psychiatric evaluation (12).

With the progressive emancipation of women, our society is altering its views and expectations of female behavior. Leafing through Mother Goose nursery rhymes, we find: "What are little girls made of?"

What are little girls made of?
Sugar and Spice and All that's nice,
And that's what little girls are made of, made of
                    Benet, 1943, p. 16 (13)

Sleeping Beauty, Gretel in Hansel and Gretel, and Cinderella were all passive, helpless, relatively mindless and dependent female figures who depended emotionally and physically on male figures. The men were free to think, make decisions, and move about. These

Table 26.1.   Psychological Risk Factors as Indication for Psychiatric Evaluation

1. Previous history of psychiatric treatment
2. A past history of emotional/behaviorial difficulties at other critical maturational stages, such as puberty, or after leaving home
3. A history of early maternal deprivation or loss
4. Conflicts about sexual identity
5. Conflicts about role as a mother, concerns about adequacy as a mother, or ability to care for a child
6. Severe marital or other family difficulties
7. Past emotional difficulties with pregnancy, delivery, or abortion
8. Major individual or family medical problems or deaths
9. Familial or congenital diseases
10. Unmarried state
11. History of prolonged infertility, stillbirths, or previous adoption
12. Previous birth of a defective child or the possibility of defective birth with this pregnancy
13. Extremes in age range (under 17, over 40)

1. Higher education
2. Work outside the home
3. Sport and physical activity
4. The arts

One psychological dimension of women's growing involvement is its relative newness. There are fewer female role models compared with male role models. Traditionally, these were masculine areas. The reactions to women's growing participation have been, at times, negative. This negative reaction can become internalized, producing anxiety, guilt, depression, and undermining women's self-esteem and their sense of entitlement to pursue their potential.

The very fact of the newness and of the emergent quality of female participation against a background of historical exclusion may add to a sense of impatience, urgency, and anger in some women; anger at having to wait or to postpone any longer their personal aspirations. In the area of exercise in pregnancy, this may cause frustration at having to consider any limits to physical activity during pregnancy. Some women may feel particularly sensitive to limits and caution especially when these are suggested by male experts, seeing them as excessively restrictive or authoritarian toward women. Men and women alike must be aware of just how old myths and stereotypical notions affect us all. By doing so, we will not only be more helpful to our patients but also be more scientific as we approach our data. Pregnancy faces women with a difficult task: having to reconcile personal goals with the exigencies of pregnancy, childbirth, breast-feeding, and caring for the young.

The task is especially difficult for the woman professional athlete who invests considerable amounts of time, energy, and emotional commitment to her sport. The timetable for childbearing has its biologically inherent limits. These limits are irrevocable. The same can be said about the timetable for optimal athletic performance.

Individual solutions will vary and different women will feel differently about what is important for them at a given time in their lives. Some compromise is inevitable, as is

and other nursery rhymes and fairy tales sung and read to generations of little boys and girls are but a few examples of the socially transmitted values and expectations for what feminine behavior was to be. The words and the metaphors they conjure up are remembered all one's life. Our cultures, religions, and political institutions were shaped by these ideas and in turn, shaped, institutionalized, reified, and legislated them for generations.

There has been an enormous change. Our society does not so readily frown upon women who wish to exercise their minds and their bodies. Although women have exercised their bodies for generations, at times very strenuously, it was for the most part over domestic chores or for the benefit of their families. The essential difference between these physical activities and the ones we address here is that inherently we are dealing with activities carried out primarily as expression of women's wish to pursue personal goals rather than to serve others.

Women now turn more freely to areas other than domestic activities, areas that have been mostly reserved for men throughout centuries:

probably true of most things in life. Counseling may be helpful for some women.

We have seen some women approach exercise as a means to prevent the weight gain associated with pregnancy. Others hope it will shorten labor or eliminate pain in labor. At times, we see women who seem to want to have a baby without feeling or looking pregnant. In our experience, women who abhor the temporary bodily changes accompanying pregnancy are usually women who do not feel good about themselves or who have difficulty accepting their femaleness with emotional maturity (15). Although we feel it is certainly a healthy human desire to look and feel attractive, the point at which one becomes so extremely governed by this concern to the exclusion of all others, to where one sacrifices one's own needs and health, as well as neglecting the welfare of the developing fetus, represents unresolved emotional problems.

Being physically active and exercising, not out of fear but with enjoyment, contributes to a sense of well-being, self-confidence, and greater emotional and physical resilience. Although exercise may not shorten labor or eliminate pain, the increased stamina is certainly beneficial. It lessens the anxiety of the anticipated labor, which, in turn, improves pain tolerance.

The improved muscular strength may be especially beneficial in preventing back pain, may help in feeling agile, nimble, and may facilitate carrying the added weight and changing center of gravity.

There is no question that the improved stamina, resilience, physical well-being, and greater self-reliance will better prepare a woman to the real challenges, both physical and emotional, inherent in pregnancy, childbirth, and rearing of the young.

REFERENCES

1. Dishman RK, Landy FJ. Psychological factors and prolonged exercise. In: Lamb DR, Murray R, eds. Perspectives in exercise science and sports medicine: prolonged exercise, Vol 1. 1988; p. 281–356.
2. Greist JH, Klein MH, Eischens RR, Faris JT. Running out of depression. Phys Sports Med 1978; 6:49–50.
3. Morgan WP. Affective beneficence of vigorous physical activity. Paper presented at the NIMH Workshop on Coping with Mental Stress: The potential and limits of exercise intervention. Bethesda, MD, April 1984.
4. Varrassi G, et al. Effects of physical activity or maternal plasma β-endorphin levels and perception of labor pain. Am J Obstet Gynecol 1989; 160:707–712.
5. Erickson E: Identity and the life cycle. New York: W.W. Norton & Co., 1959.
6. Bibring G. Some consideration of the psychological process in pregnancy. Psychoanalytic Study of the Child 1959; 14:113.
7. Spitz R. The first year of life. A psychoanalytic study of normal and deviant development of object relations. New York: International University Press Inc., 1981.
8. Mahler M. The psychological birth of the human infant. New York: Basic Books, Inc.
9. Pugh TE, Jerath BK, Schmidt WM, et al: Rates of mental disease related to childbearing. N Engl J Med 1963; 268:1224.
10. Gitlin M, Pasnau R. Psychiatric syndromes linked to reproductive function in women: A review of current knowledge. Am J Psychol 1989; 146:11.
11. Parks J. Emotional reactions to pregnancy. Am J Obstet Gynecol 1951; 62:2339.
12. Nadelson C. "Normal" and "special" aspects of pregnancy: A psychological approach. In: Notman MT, Nadelson CC, eds. The woman patient—medical and psychological interfaces. New York: Plenum Press, 1979.
13. Benet WR. Mother goose: a comprehensive collection of the rhymes. New York: Heritage Press, 1943.
14. Stoller R. Primary femeninity. In: Blum HP, ed. Female psychology. New York: International University Press, 1977.
15. Winnicott DW, ed. The maturational processes and the facilitating environment. New York: International Universities Press, 1965.

27

Legal Aspects of Exercise Prescription and Pregnancy

Elizabeth Gallup

Little is written in the sports medicine or cardiology literature regarding exercise and pregnancy. This is in sharp contrast to exercise testing and prescribing in general. Therefore, the legal aspects of exercise prescribing and testing in the pregnant patient must be extrapolated from case law arising from the exercise prescription and testing in the non-pregnant state. This, however, is how new principles of law are commonly derived. Certainly, keeping in stride with the current liability crisis, the legal basis of liability will be tested in the court in the not too distant future.

BASIS OF LIABILITY

Negligence is usually the legal basis for suits involving the exercise prescriptionist tester, regardless of whether that person is a physician, physical therapist, or fitness tester. To be found negligent, the practitioner must meet the four elements of negligence; duty, breach, causation, and damages. The act of prescribing or testing of a patient engenders the obligation of a duty to prescribe or test in a non-negligent manner. If the duty is breached and that breach causes the patient harm (damages), then there is negligence. For negligence, all four elements must be met. A duty must be owed the patient, it must be breached, and that breach must actually cause that patient harm or injury. Without all four elements, negligence cannot be found.

The duty that inures to the practitioner is the duty of meeting the standard of care. But what is this standard? There are no specific standards for either exercise testing or exercise prescription in the pregnant patient. The standard will be extrapolated from standards already determined for exercise prescribing and testing in the nonpregnant state. Incor-porated into these standards will be the special considerations that pregnancy generates. The general standard for negligence is that of the minimally competent practitioner in the field. What this means is that if the practitioner is a physician, the standard to which the physician is held is the minimally competent physician. It is the standard of what the minimally competent physician would do in the same or similar circumstances. The minimally competent physician is not the same as the average physician, which is actually a higher standard. In the case of an exercise physiologist, physical therapist, and so forth, the standard would be what a minimally competent exercise physiologist or physical therapist would do in the same or similar circumstances.

EXERCISE TESTING AND PREGNANCY

Both the American College of Sports Medicine and the American College of Cardiology have published guidelines for exercise testing. Neither of these documents mention testing in the pregnant state (1, 2). These programs differ markedly on the degree of physician supervision required during the exercise test. These differences highlight some of the controversial aspects of exercise testing and prescription. The American College of Cardiology Guidelines (ACC), which were developed with the American Heart Association (AHA), require the actual on-site presence of the physician and ultimate control by the physician of the exercise test. The ACSM guidelines, on the other hand, call for shared control between the physician and other exercise personnel. This degree of shared responsibility is dependent on the expertise of the exercise personnel and any special considerations generated by the patient. In general, if the patient is healthy (pregnancy is not defined as an unhealthy state), then consideration is given to the patient's risk factors for cardiovascular disease and the patient's age. If the patient has no coronary artery disease or risk factors and is below the age of 35 years, then it could be argued that the patient would be a low-risk candidate for exercises testing and prescription (3). Low risk is defined from the viewpoint of risk or cardiovascular disease. If, in fact, the patient is considered low risk, then argument could follow that the patient's exercise test could be carried out by a nonphysician. However, if an untoward result were to occur as a result of the test and litigation were to follow, you can be sure that the plaintiff's attorney would argue that the ACC guidelines that require physician-administered tests should have been followed (4).

It is notable that some states require that a physician be readily available during the administration of an exercise test (5). Readily available has been interpreted to mean anything from in the same room to in the same building. In any case, to conduct an exercise test on a pregnant patient without a physician available in the immediate area would probably be found to be substandard and, thus, open to liability. Because of this, it is recommended that pregnancy be considered an increased risk and that physicians should administer exercises tests.

There is no documentation in the medical literature that physicians are required for safe exercise testing in pregnancy. However, legal precedence sometimes prescribes medical guidelines and this is an example of such. Certainly nurses and exercise physiologists who have special training in the administration, interpretation, and complications of exercise testing can perform such testing in a safe manner. As exercise testing in healthy patients becomes more and more available and the demand increases, then perhaps a different standard than physician-administered testing for pregnant patients will emerge.

EXERCISE PRESCRIPTION AND PREGNANCY

Guidelines for exercise in pregnancy should reflect the increased risk of exercising in the pregnant state (see Appendix A). Careful consideration must be given to patient selection. When selecting the patient for exercise prescription, it is imperative to be aware not only of the contraindications to exercise and exercise prescription in the nonpregnant state, but also of the contraindications and special risks associated with exercise and pregnancy. If a patient is improperly selected and an injury occurs to either the patient or the fetus, a claim of negligence and malpractice is very likely to arise.

Exercise programs designed for the pregnant patient, like programs for the nonpregnant patient, will usually be done at home or in some other unsupervised place. Therefore, specific tailoring of the prescription must occur for such areas. It is not enough to say "start a walking program or jogging program." Give specific recommendations. The prescription for exercise should be much like that of a medical prescription for a drug. It should be clear and specific, and preferably in writing. The prescription must be understandable by the patient and not contraindicated for the patient. The prescription must be capable of being carried out by the patient in an unsupervised setting and risks and side effects of the prescription must be explained to the patient (6).

If exercise is prescribed, it is necessary to determine the safety of the locale at which the exercise will occur. Factors that enter into this are environmental conditions such as extremes of temperature, humidity, sun, wind, pollen, pollution, ice, and other. If environmental extremes are likely to occur, the patient must be warned of these possibilities and given specific advice to minimize the risks imposed thereof, which include not exercising. Sometimes advice about environmental concerns may seem like stating the obvious but liability has been found for failure to warn about obvious environmental conditions. Keep in mind:

1. Is the area appropriate for the activity?
2. Is the area relatively safe and free from latent defects and danger?
3. Is the area free of rapid and changing environmental conditions?

4. Is the area relatively safe from criminal activity?
5. Is the area populated?
6. Is the area close to emergency facilities? and
7. Is the area close to phones (6, p. 93)?

It is also essential to continue following the patient after the initiation of the exercise program. With the pregnant patient, this is usually not difficult because follow-up visits are routinely scheduled throughout the pregnancy. Remember to ask the patient how she is adjusting to the routine. Does she feel better or is she excessively fatigued? Has she lost weight? Ask the patient if she is following the specific instructions and warnings given or if she has modified the program. If she has modified anything, make a note of this in the chart because if a complication arises later it could have been caused by her modification and the documentation will be an important defense to her claim.

IMPORTANCE OF DOCUMENTATION

In all areas of negligence, the most important element of a defense to a claim is that of adequate documentation. From a defense attorney's standpoint, it is impossible to over-document. The more you document, the more evidence there is that the standard of care was met. Document that the patient was screened for all the contraindications and relative contraindications to exercise testing and prescription in pregnancy. Document that the benefits and risks of exercise were discussed with the patient, document whether or not the patient followed the prescription. Document, document, document!

INFORMED CONSENT

Documentation is especially significant in the area of informed consent. There must be documentation that specific information regarding the risks of exercise testing and prescription were given and that the patient consented to the test or prescription after being informed. This is especially true in the area of exercise testing. There have been court cases that found that, even though the chances for a stroke are remote, failure to warn a patient that a stroke is a possibility is necessary, and, absent such a disclosure, the pa-

tient would not have taken the test. The finding emphasizes the importance of informing the patient of all known risks of exercise testing.

Obviously, it is impossible to disclose all the risks inherent in exercise but it is possible to disclose known risks that are easily identifiable in the literature and are enumerated elsewhere in this text. As discussed, in addition to the risks of testing and prescription in the nonpregnant state, the patient must be informed of the special risks that pregnancy carries to both the mother and the fetus. If the patient decides to undergo the test or carry out the prescription and suffers an untoward result as a complication and the possibility of this complication had been disclosed to her, then this will afford some degree of protection from liability.

There are many forms available that enumerate the risks of prescription and testing of exercise; however, these documents in and of themselves do not guarantee protection against liability. They are used as evidence that the risks were, in fact, disclosed to the patient. These forms usually do not include the special considerations that must be disclosed to the pregnant patient and by no means should these forms take the place of discussion between the patient and physician or exercise tester/prescriber. The informed consent document should be clear and concise and written in language easy for the lay person to understand. The document should not contain a "no suit" clause where the patient waives the right to sue. Such a clause confuses the issue of informed consent with an exculpatory release, two very different issues.

PROSPECTIVE RELEASES

Release documents are contracts. The contract is between the health care provider and the patient and is an agreement not to sue. In an exculpatory waiver, the patient effectively relinquishes her right to sue. The issue of the legality of exculpatory waivers has many ramifications. In many states, exculpatory waivers have been found to be against public policy and, thus, not valid. Courts have held that the services offered by physicians are of such public import and are of such great personal necessity that a party who holds himself or herself out as willing to perform essential services pursuant to state regulations cannot, in the interest of greater public good, exculpate the provider from liability due to his or her own negligence. These courts have held that the release is a shield behind which the practitioner should not be allowed to hide (7).

Recently, some states have allowed exculpatory waivers but the language is very specific as to how these waivers must be worded and in what instances they can be used. Usually these are limited to experimental medical procedures or waivers used in nonmedical settings, such as fitness centers. When allowed for use in fitness centers, the waiver is only for the use of the center and not the actual exercise prescription generated by an employee of the center. Where the waiver has been allowed, there was evidence that the patient indeed understood the language of the waiver, was not under the influence of alcohol or drugs when he or she signed the waiver, had read the waiver, and signed it with the intent to give it legal effect (7, p. 90).

ASSUMPTION OF RISK

Exercise in and of itself implies some risk. In the past, implied assumption of risk has precluded liability for an untoward result. An example of this would be a voluntary participation by a football player in the sport of football, which is known to have a high injury rate. By participating, there is an implication that the player knew and assumed the risk of injury. More and more courts are doing away with implied assumption of risk but are allowing express assumption of risk (8).

Express assumption of risk involves the use of a document. This document, like the document involving informed consent and exculpatory releases, should be written only after appropriate legal consultation is obtained. In general, the forms should require review by the exercise prescriber/tester and the patient of the risks of the exercise prescribed. The document should also contain checkpoints where the patient can initial that she understood the legal meaning of the document as well as the contents of the document itself.

NONPHYSICIAN EXERCISE PRESCRIBER, TESTER, AND/OR SUPERVISOR

There is interest by many different people in the adult fitness boom. There has been rapid growth of fitness centers catering to the adult population that wants to "get in shape." This population includes the pregnant patient. Such fitness facilities are also found in the corporate world. These facilities often undertake exercise testing and prescribing and it is rare that a physician is connected, much less on-site at such facilities. The question then arises regarding the liability of such fitness centers and those persons who are employed as exercise specialists there.

Many different types of individuals may be lumped under the title of exercise specialist or fitness instructors. These include exercise physiologists, nurses, athletic trainers, physical therapists, physical education majors, and those individuals whose training is limited to a multiple week course on fitness instruction. Of course, the degree of responsibility to the exercise program by such individuals should be circumscribed by their training. It must be remembered though, that pregnancy in and of itself may limit exercise prescription and testing to those individuals with extensive training, such as physicians with special expertise in the area. Again, as discussed previously, careful consideration to exercise testing should be given and, for the pregnant patient, we recommend that a physician either administer the test or be immediately available during the administration of the exercise test.

If fitness instructors are used at facilities to supervise prescribed exercise, these instructors should be certified. There are many certification programs available and with the certification programs come standards. In addition to ascertaining certification and recertification of fitness instructors, administrators of fitness facilities should ensure that all personnel at the facility are certified in cardiopulmonary resuscitation and that an individual certified in advanced cardiac life support is always on-site and readily available. The administrator should also ensure maintenance of proper and adequate liability insurance.

LIABILITY INSURANCE

Accompanying the boom of the fitness industry is a corresponding boom in fitness industry insurance. Physicians are already too well aware of the liability crisis currently in progress and its associated effect on the cost and availability of liability insurance. Liability insurance should be acquired for exercise prescribing or testing employees of facility. The type and amount of insurance is influenced by such considerations as the type of client served (the pregnant patient would place the insured at a higher risk), the size of the facility, and the responsibilities of the insured, i.e., an individual who assists the physician in exercise testing versus the individual who administers the test him- or herself.

Many times, insurance companies recognize certification in fitness instruction in the form of reduced premiums. It follows that this recognition may be presumptive evidence of competency of the certified individual, which further underscores the evolution of something akin to "standard of care" in an area similar to exercise prescription and testing.

DEVELOPMENTS IN LEGISLATION

Many states have put forth proposals for regulating the exercise professional. Such legislative initiatives will vary from state to state but commonly include fitness center staff requirements, CPR training for all employees, and procedures governing approval of fitness centers by the states (9). The legislative proposals in isolated states foretell the future where such regulations will be nationwide.

SUMMARY

Exercise testing and prescribing for the pregnant patient bring to mind added liability considerations. This is because the pregnant patient brings with her not only the risks of exercising and exacerbation of cardiovascular disease, but also the added risks of pregnancy. In addition, the risks of exercising in pregnancy include the risk imposed on fetal development. The exercise prescriber and tester must carefully consider the issues of proper, well-delineated instructions, informed consent, and assumption of risk. The importance of adequate documentation cannot be overstressed.

REFERENCES

1. American College of Sports Medicine. Guidelines for exercise testing and prescription. Philadelphia: Lea & Febiger, 1986.
2. American College of Cardiology/American Heart Association. Guidelines for exercise testing: a report of the ACC/AHA task force on assessment of cardiovascular procedures (Subcommittee on exercise testing). J Am Coll Cardiol 1986; 8:725–738.
3. Rochmis P, Blackburn H. Exercise tests: a survey of procedures, safety and litigation experience in approximately 170,000 tests. JAMA 1971; 217:1061–1066.
4. Herbert D. Trends, physician must be present for administration of graded exercise tests. Exercise Standards Malpractice Reporter 1987; 1:75.
5. Statement of the North Carolina Board of Medical Examiners. June, 1987.
6. Herbert D. Selected liability considerations of prescribed but unsupervised cardiac rehabilitation activities. Exercise Standards Malpractice Reporter 1988; 2:89–94.
7. Herbert D. The use of prospective releases containing exculpatory language in exercise and fitness programs. Exercise Standards Malpractice Reporter 1986; 1:75–78 and 1986; 1:89–90.
8. Herbert D. Express assumption of risk. Exercise Standards Malpractice Reporter 1987; 1:91–94.
9. Herbert D. Legislative proposal for regulating exercise professionals becomes law. Exercise Standards Malpractice Reporter 1989; 3:13–14.

28

Exercise Guidelines for Pregnancy

Raul Artal Mittelmark, Robert A. Wiswell, Barbara L. Drinkwater, and
Wendy E. St. Jones-Repovich

Daily exercise has become a way of life for many women and physicians are frequently asked to provide specific advice. Women who become pregnant want to learn all they can about how they can remain active during their pregnancy, how much exercise is safe for them and their fetus, what are the benefits and risks of continued activity, how pregnancy will affect their sports performance, and how exercise may affect their pregnancy. Previous chapters in this book have addressed the physiological changes of pregnancy and how exercise may magnify the effects of these changes on both the woman and her fetus. This chapter will attempt to build on that background in offering guidelines for exercise during pregnancy for the recreational athlete. The motivation for continuing an exercise program for these women is often quite different from that of the professional or elite athlete. Women who are exercising primarily for fun and fitness are more likely to accept the modifications that pregnancy will place on their exercise programs. Some of these suggested guidelines are based on the theoretical effects intense exercise might have on the woman and the fetus; others are based on observations of how the physical changes during the latter months of pregnancy actually limit athletic performance.

The motivations for continuing to exercise during pregnancy may be complex (Chapter 26). However, those most frequently expressed revolve around the belief that maternal exercise will benefit the fetus as well as the mother. In fact, there is no evidence that the fetus benefits; on the contrary, there are potential risks to the fetus as noted in previous chapters. The woman may benefit both psychologically and physically by retaining some portion of her prepregnancy fitness. However, there is no truth to the myth that fit women deliver easier and quicker. Fitness does not affect the duration of labor although perception of pain may be lessened.

As demonstrated by Blair et al. (1), the health benefits of exercise can be obtained at exercise intensities considerably lower than those recommended (2) for increasing aerobic power.

Because attempts to limit a woman's physical activity during pregnancy can be interpreted as patronizing and anachronistic, the physician's advice should recognize the importance of exercise to the general well-being of the woman while emphasizing the potential long-term health benefits and relatively lower risk to the fetus of light to moderate exercise intensities.

Of all the subgroups in the general population of healthy adults, pregnant women are the only ones who have no exercise standards derived from large studies. At present, recommendations for pregnant and postpartum women are based on limited knowledge acquired in the exercise laboratory and on clinical observations and experience. Many specific programs for exercise in pregnancy can be found that have based their routines on this limited information alone. Past reviews of many highly specific programs revealed medical content that was, in many cases, inappropriate, inaccurate, or incomplete (3). Some of these programs imply that exercise may affect and shorten labor and delivery while others use motivational techniques such as suggesting that lack of fitness may make labor and delivery more difficult to tolerate. Some of these programs capitalize on the public image of one celebrity or another and, although the authors of these programs may be well intentioned, none of these programs has been properly researched, if at all.

There is no organization that presently regulates exercise programs in pregnancy, but it is the opinion of these authors that such a forum should be created to regulate these programs, monitor qualifications for instructors, and maintain guidelines and standards as they become available. Ideally, a multidisciplinary medical advisory committee should recommend the appropriate exercise programs and update the criteria for medical clearance for the participants. Such a committee should be multidisciplinary and include obstetricians, exercise physiologists, and sports medicine experts. The American College of Obstetricians and Gynecologists (ACOG) in its attempt to aid obstetricians has published guidelines for exercise in pregnancy and postpartum (Appendix); they have also created a collection of home exercise video programs that were carefully designed and considered medically safe. These guidelines and programs are for the pregnant recreational athlete and the general population, and they are periodically reviewed and updated as necessary.

By and large, pregnant women who engage in exercise programs are healthy but very few are aware of the anatomical and physiological changes of pregnancy that might predispose them to injuries. In addition, the short- and long-term effects of maternal exercise on the fetus should always be considered. It is logical to believe that with proper guidelines pregnant women can maintain a reasonable level of cardiorespiratory fitness, body composition, and muscular strength and endurance. In this chapter we will address the commonly asked questions: What types of exercise are safe in pregnancy? What are the potential risks? How much exercise? Who may exercise?

OBSTETRICAL AND MEDICAL SCREENING

Although the American College of Sports Medicine guidelines indicate that if an individual is asymptomatic, less than 35 years of age, has no evidence or history of cardiovas-

cular disease, has no risk factors for coronary heart disease, and has had a medical evaluation during the previous year, no medical clearance is necessary before an increase in physical activity level, these guidelines do not apply to pregnant women. All pregnant women should obtain an obstetrical and medical examination early in gestation and before engaging in exercise programs.

Guidelines for exercise should be safe and consider the normal physiological responses of the pregnant woman to various types of activity.

CONTRAINDICATIONS

The absolute and relative contraindications to exercise in pregnancy are listed in Table 28.1. Before approving an exercise program, a careful history of the cardiovascular, pulmonary, metabolic, and musculoskeletal systems should be taken.

Physicians will have to individualize exercise programs for women with relative contraindications. Some of these individuals may

Table 28.1. Contraindications to Exercise in Pregnancy

Absolute contraindications
1. Active myocardial disease
2. Congestive heart failure
3. Rheumatic heart disease (Class II and above)
4. Thrombophlebitis
5. Recent pulmonary embolism
6. Acute infectious disease
7. At risk for premature labor, incompetent cervix, multiple gestations
8. Uterine bleeding, ruptured membranes
9. Intrauterine growth retardation or macrosomia
10. Severe isoimmunization
11. Severe hypertensive disease
12. No prenatal care
13. Suspected fetal distress

Relative contraindications (patients may be engaged in medically supervised programs)
1. Essential hypertension
2. Anemia or other blood disorders
3. Thyroid disease
4. Diabetes mellitus
5. Breech presentations in the last trimester
6. Excessive obesity or extreme underweight
7. History of sedentary life-style

Additional contraindications should be left for the physician to evaluate

---

actually benefit from a medically supervised exercise program (e.g., diabetic patients).

The following symptoms and signs should signal the patient to stop exercise and contact her physician: *(a)* pain of any kind; *(b)* uterine contractions (at 15-min intervals or more frequent); *(c)* vaginal bleeding, leaking amniotic fluid; *(d)* dizziness, faintness; *(e)* shortness of breath; *(f)* palpitations, tachycardia; *(g)* persistent nausea and vomiting; *(h)* back pain; *(i)* pubic or hip pain; *(j)* difficulty in walking; *(k)* generalized edema; *(l)* numbness in any part of the body; *(m)* visual disturbances; and *(n)* decreased fetal activity. Patients should be educated to recognize and be alert to these signs and symptoms.

Exercise testing in pregnancy is investigational only, but could be utilized in the future to test cardiac functions and placental reserve capacity (4). Exercise testing provides a unique opportunity to test all body functional reserves, exposing conditions that otherwise would not have been uncovered. If exercise testing is undertaken in pregnancy, every effort should be made to test the fetus electronically before and after the procedure. A reactive fetal heart rate pattern with no obvious signs for fetal distress should be reassuring. In addition, monitoring the frequency of fetal movements is a useful but crude tool for self fetal monitoring of individuals engaged in exercise programs.

Based on our observations, maximal exercise capacity will decline in the recreational athlete by approximately 20–25% in the second and third trimester of pregnancy; conversely, the professional or elite athlete can maintain her $\dot{V}_{O_2max}$ (L/min) at prepregnancy levels.

EXERCISE GUIDELINES FOR THE GENERAL POPULATION IN PREGNANCY

Guidelines for the general population differ from those given to the highly trained or professional athlete. The risks are similar and the precautions taken should be similar, nevertheless, a professional or elite athlete may exercise more intensly if she is under the close supervision of a physician and thor-

Table 28.2.   Risks of Exercise in Pregnancy

Maternal risks
1. Increased risk of musculoskeletal injuries
2. Cardiovascular complications
   a. Supine hypotension
   b. Aortocaval syndrome, arrhythmias
   c. Heart failure
3. Spontaneous abortion
4. Premature labor
5. Hypoglycemia

Fetal risks
1. Fetal distress
2. Intrauterine growth retardation
3. Fetal malformations
4. Prematurity

Neonatal risks
1. Decreased adipose tissue
2. Hypothermia

oughly instructed in how to recognize symptoms of impending problems.

The creation of exercise programs for pregnant women should specify the intensity, duration, frequency, and the type of activity. Safety for both mother and fetus should be a primary concern. Table 28.2 lists a few of the potential risks for exercise in pregnancy.

Although some of the listed risks may be theoretical, caution should be exercised to prevent potential complications. To minimize the risks, the intensity, duration, and frequency of exercise routines utilized during pregnancy should be altered, especially in the general population whose supervision could be logistically difficult. Under unsupervised conditions, the intensity of the exercise should be reduced by approximately 25%, maximum maternal heart rate should not exceed 140 bpm, and the periods of strenuous activities should be limited to 15–20 min interspersed with low-intensity exercise and rest periods. We believe that moderating activity in this way can significantly reduce the incidence for the previously listed risks.

Determining exercise intensity is essential for the purpose of exercise prescription. Intensity of exercise is usually expressed in terms of the demand on the cardiovascular system as a percentage of maximal heart rate, percentage of heart rate reserve, or in METs. The relationship between $\dot{V}_{O_2}$, METs, and

Table 28.3. Intensity of Exercise

	% V_{O_2max}	METs	% HR max
Light	15–30	1.2–2.7	40–50
Moderate	31–50	2.8–4.3	51–65
Heavy	51–68	4.4–5.9	66–80
Very heavy	69–85	6.0–7.5	81–90
Unduly heavy	86+	7.6+	90+

heart rates for the average woman are listed in Table 28.3. Determining $\dot{V}_{O_2max}$ or HR max may not be practical for the clinician, an alternative guideline to determine exercise intensity is the degree of respiratory distress. If the woman can converse with ease while she is exercising, she will be exercising at a light to moderate exercise intensity.

With the publication of guidelines by ACOG in 1985 (Appendix), concern was expressed that setting maximum heart rate at 140 bpm was too low to achieve cardiovascular fitness. The obvious questions are: (a) How much should the pregnant woman exercise to derive cardiovascular benefits? (b) Why not above 140 bpm? One fact that is emerging is that the linear relationship between $\dot{V}_{O_2}$ and heart rate established for nonpregnant women differs during pregnancy (Fig. 28.1). This rela-

tionship is most probably altered also by age and gestational age. These changes and the wide variation in heart rate responses to strenuous exercise in pregnancy have been among the major reasons for recommending that maternal heart rate should not exceed 140 bpm.

One other concern is the potential hemodynamic changes during sustained tachycardia in pregnancy. Normally during pregnancy, the heart rate increases 10–15%. Transient sinus tachycardia is not infrequent and of no clinical significance in pregnancy; conversely, paroxysmal supraventricular tachycardia (140–240 bpm) is quite rare with an incidence of less than 1%. The main concern during strenuous exercise is that, in the presence of unrecognized organic disease, atrial tachycardia along with a rapid ventricular rate can precipitate heart failure. Because most pregnant women are not medically supervised while exercising, a prudent approach is recommended.

In view of these concerns, it is our opinion that pregnant women can derive health benefits from regular exercise at a light-moderate intensity (Table 28.3).

Special consideration must be given to

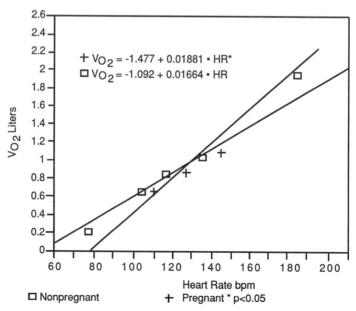

Figure 28.1. Correlation between oxygen consumption (V_{O_2}) and heart rate (HR) during exercise to predict V_{O_2} from submaximal HR. (Adapted from Wiswell RA, Artal R, Romem Y, Kammula R, Dorey F. Hormonal and metabolic response to exercise in pregnancy. Med Sci Sports Exerc 1985; 17:206.)

Table 28.4. Potential Mechanisms Leading to Injuries During Exercise in Pregnancy[a]

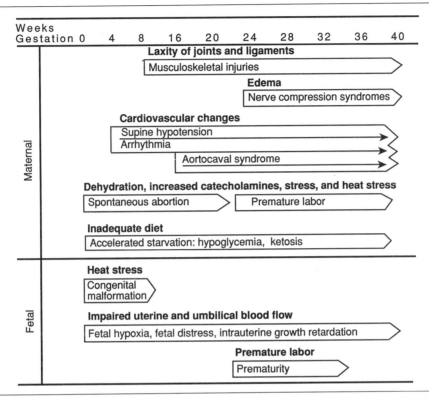

[a]The top of each box lists the etiology for potential injuries included in each box. The spacing of the boxes reflects the gestational age during which the injury is most likely to occur.

changes that occur in the first, second, and third trimesters of pregnancy and could result in injury (Table 28.4). To recapitulate, nausea, vomiting, and tachycardia can affect the ability to engage in exercise activities through pregnancy. The progressive anatomical and physiological changes of the second and third trimesters that affect activity are: change in center of gravity, increased connective tissue laxity with resulting joint instability, lordosis and kyphosis, edema potentially resulting in nerve compression syndrome, increase in blood volume, tachycardia, hyperventilation, and reductions in cardiac reserve and residual lung capacity.

The goal should be to maintain physical fitness within the physiological limitation of pregnancy. Exercise programs in pregnancy should also be directed toward muscle strengthening to minimize the risk of joint and ligament injuries and toward correcting postural changes that could result in lower back pain. Strain and fatigue should be avoided, and exercise periods should be interspersed with rest and relaxation.

A clear distinction must be made between the scope of exercise programs available in pregnancy:

1. Childbirth preparatory programs
2. Recreational and sports activities
3. Exercise prescription in pregnancy
4. Postpartum exercise

Childbirth Preparatory Programs

Currently, obstetricians and their patients include physical activity as a regular and acceptable part of the prenatal period. Childbirth preparatory education emphasizes the learning of relaxation techniques that could aid coping with the pain of labor and delivery. Through the years, many theories evolved on what type of exercise is good or even essential for the mother and/or the baby and whether the exercises did, in fact, ease the actual pregnancy or facilitate labor, birth, and the postpartum return of fitness. Unfortunately, early and many current prescriptions often have no scientific basis.

Around the turn of the century, obstetricians noted that the lower, working class mothers in England had easier labors and it was decided that this was due to their physical activity. Thus, in several of the early antenatal books, "gentle exercises" such as croquet were recommended (5, 6). These thoughts continued to affect prenatal preparation until the 1950s when controlled research found no significant differences in the length of labor or the incidence of complications between women who exercised and women who did not (7, 8).

Earlier exercise prescription emphasized mobility or flexibility exercise and avoided those exercises that stimulated the cardiovascular system. This was based on the accepted assumption that the maintenance of good posture during pregnancy and then labor was important. An exercise that was often recommended as beneficial was the squat. Because it was known that primitive people squatted during labor, squatting was suggested to be the natural way to an easy labor. While these prescriptions were being put forth, concurrent research demonstrated that the squat exercise did not, in fact, change the dimensions of the pelvis (9), nor was there distension or separation of the pubic symphysis during the actual labor (10). Even though the literature does not support the contention that squatting exercise has a significant anatomical effect, there are still two proposed benefits of proper squatting with the back straight. One is good balance, which keeps strain off the lower back when lifting. The other is the prevention of heartburn later in pregnancy when bending over too far can cause regurgitation (11). A more recent prospective controlled trial of 427 primipara compared the outcome of labor in women randomly allocated to squatting (218) or conventional semirecumbent (209) management in labor. The squatting group had relatively fewer forceps deliveries (9% vs. 16%) and shorter second stages (median length, 31 vs. 45 min) than the semirecumbent group

(12). As pointed out in the literature, to maintain a squatting position, the body weight has to be supported by way of hyperflexed hips and knees on flatly positioned feet, with stretched achilles tendons and dorsiflexed ankles. Due to the changes in joints and ligaments that occur in some pregnant women, those exercises may become impractical. Gardosi et al. (12) recommend supported squatting position during labor with the aid of a specially designed birth cushion. Some women may find this information advantageous and elect to conduct preparatory squatting exercises or utilize it in labor only.

Pelvic floor exercises (the Kegel or elevator exercises) are overrated by the lay literature; they were originally prescribed to increase the elasticity and tonicity of the perineum and to prevent tears during labor. However, there has been no scientific evidence to support this and, in fact, once an episiotomy is performed the activity of these muscles are completely abolished. In modern obstetrics, the standard of practice is to perform an episiotomy during the delivery stage rather than to overstretch the perineum and cause lacerations. The suggested benefit of pelvic floor exercises is for the postpartum period when they may help the muscles return to their prepregnancy condition (11, 13) and, viewed from this perspective, these exercises may offer some advantage.

Since the increased fitness awareness of the 1960s, there has been a shift in emphasis from calisthenics toward sports or aerobic exercises (jogging, swimming, bicycling, or aerobics). These activities could be done independently or in conjunction with prenatal education.

Many proposed but not proven benefits of exercise for the pregnant woman have been suggested. These include shorter labor, fewer complications during pregnancy, faster recovery from labor and delivery, prevention of varicose veins, thrombosis, and leg cramps, and improved mental outlook of the patients (11, 13–16).

With the popularity of "natural childbirth," mothers and fathers are increasingly encouraged to attend classes to learn how to prepare for labor and delivery. Undoubtedly, these classes fulfill an important educational role and have a major psychological impact on both parents and may increase the fetal-maternal-paternal bonds. In general, classes include a section on the anatomy, physiology, and psychology of labor and birth. These classes include instruction in relaxation and breathing techniques to be utilized in labor and delivery. As stated earlier, there is no scientific evidence that any of these exercises results in shorter labors, easier labors, less complications, or benefit to the baby (11); these exercises do, however, help some pregnant women to cope with the pain of labor. Proper toning exercises that are used may have some benefit in pregnancy in maintaining proper posture and preventing lower back pain and, after the birth, facilitate recovery. Some of the stretching routines, though, may have to be modified to prevent injuries.

The exercises are generally divided into areas of the body, first emphasizing the upper body, next the legs, and finally, the stomach area. They combine yoga, dance, and calisthenic routines. There are no standard exercises employed in these programs and many instructors may be unqualified (17–19). Moderation and individualization should be advised and there is no reason not to modify such activities if they are too difficult to perform as originally described; i.e., a sit-up from the semirecumbent position is a good exercise for the abdomen, but as the abdomen begins protruding, perhaps a sit-back, where the mother begins in the up position and slowly lies down in the semirecumbent position, could be easier to perform. Supine exercises should not be performed in pregnancy under any circumstances. This is to avoid the high incidence of orthostatic hypotension and the aortocaval compression syndrome. It is very important to remember that there is already major stress on the lower back in pregnancy because of the extra weight in the stomach area, so all exercises that require the mother to be on her back need to be done in a semirecumbent or, preferably sitting, position with the legs bent and the knees up. If unable to mobilize both legs, exercise may include one leg at a time in something like a leg-lift exercise routine.

Consistency is the most important part of any exercise program; if the individual is not willing to exercise regularly, she would probably be better to significantly reduce the intensity of her exercise routine. By doing so, she will prevent injuries associated with sporadic exertion. Pregnancy is an ideal time for behavior modification and the introduction of sedentary individuals to principles of an active life-style is warranted for its long-term effects.

Recreational and Sports Activities

This section will examine the types of activities that can be performed by pregnant women who want to remain active throughout their pregnancy. Table 28.5 lists the most popular activities for girls and active women in the general nonpregnant population. Such activities have an unknown incidence of injuries. The number of untreated or self-treated injuries is most likely considerably greater than the treated injuries. Whether or not the risk of strains and sprains in pregnant women is significantly greater than in the general population is not known. Nevertheless, it should be obvious that there is an orthopedic risk associated with some of these activities and continuance during pregnancy may increase that risk. Exercise programs should be modified during the pregnancy to allow for the physical and mental changes taking place and then resumed after delivery to facilitate recovery to prepregnancy conditions (20).

We recommend that pregnant women engaged in fitness programs be examined pe-

Table 28.5. The 10 Most Popular Activities for High School Girls and Active Women

High School Girls	Active Women
1. Basketball	1. Walking
2. Track and field	2. Jogging/running
3. Volleyball	3. Calisthentics/aerobics
4. Softball (fast pitch)	4. Weight lifting
5. Tennis	5. Softball/baseball
6. Cross country	6. Bicycling
7. Soccer	7. Swimming
8. Swimming/diving	8. Volleyball
9. Field hockey	9. Racquet sports
10. Softball (slow pitch)	10. Basketball

riodically to assess the effect of their exercise program on the developing fetus and have their programs readjusted to their level of tolerance or discontinued if necessary.

Each activity should begin with a 10- to 15-min warm-up period and end with a 10- to 15-min cool-down period. During exercise, maternal HR should not exceed 140 bpm. The cardiorespiratory changes as well as changes in the ligaments and joints require special care be taken to exercise safely (see Chapters 5, 11, 15, and 16). Exercise stretching should be avoided in pregnancy.

CARDIORESPIRATORY ENDURANCE ACTIVITIES

Jogging

Many women have found jogging to be an excellent form of exercise and want to continue for as long as possible into the pregnancy. This activity is not one that should be initiated after the pregnancy has begun. For those who continue their jogging programs, special precautions should be taken during the first trimester if certain common complications occur, e.g., nausea, vomiting, or poor weight gain. Ketosis and hypoglycemia are more likely to occur during prolonged strenuous exercise in pregnancy. Because of nausea, vomiting, and/or the feeling of fatigue that is prevalent in pregnancy, women may be unable to run any long distances. In pregnancy, we advise the recreational athlete to reduce mileage to no more than 2 miles per day. This is a precautionary step intended to prevent injuries from either hyperthermia or dehydration.

In published longitudinal studies of exercise throughout pregnancy, women averaged from 1.5–2.5 miles per day with no apparent deleterious effects (21, 22). During the second and third trimesters, increased body weight may make running more difficult. During this period, other factors, such as lower limb edema, varicose veins, or joint laxity, may also affect performance. Furthermore, coordination of the gross motor movements may be impaired as a result of the joint laxity, suggesting that pregnant women need to be especially alert to their running path (13) (see Chapter 11).

In the studies where jogging distances were

reported by the subjects rather than assigned by the investigator, there was a voluntary reduction from 2.5 miles per day on an average during the first trimester to approximately 1.75 miles per day in the second, and decreased to 1 mile per day in the third trimester (22). In the study by Hauth and Gilstrap (21), the subjects continued at 1.5 miles per day throughout. These distances were all well tolerated by the mothers and by their fetuses. These studies and others are, in part, the basis for the ACOG distance recommendation. Because pregnant women are running to maintain fitness rather than training for competition, the shorter distances should suffice. During the first trimester, if subjects would like to exceed 2 miles per day, such activity could be coordinated with the obstetrician to allow closer obstetrical follow-up.

Should pregnant women be unable to jog, they could engage in a brisk walking program. Such a program could include a 4- to 6-mile walk depending on terrain and climate conditions. This could be a reasonable alternative to a jogging program; the same precautions should be taken to avoid hyperthermia and dehydration.

1. Do not begin a jogging program while pregnant, the risk for musculoskeletal injuries is increased.
2. Reduce mileage to less than 2 miles per day.
3. If temperature and/or humidity is high, do not exercise (see Chapter 23). Adverse conditions may cause fetal loss.
4. Special attention should be given to terrain and running surface due to connective tissue changes associated with pregnancy.
5. Wear running shoes with proper support.

"Aerobics" Programs

In the last 5–10 years, women who wanted to get the benefit of the aerobic workout associated with jogging but did not like running by themselves searched for another way to exercise. This spawned, in part, the aerobics enthusiasm. Aerobics combined dance with an aerobic workout allowing women to work out in groups using a form of exercise they enjoyed and thus kept them exercising long enough to improve their aerobic capacity. The number of women who wanted to continue an aerobic activity during their pregnancy has led to a proliferation of aerobic classes specifically for pregnant women. Unfortunately, many of these programs are conducted by unqualified exercise leaders who are unaware of the basic physiology of pregnancy and have no formal training in physical education. Because aerobics is a weight bearing exercise, the same concerns that are associated with jogging should be considered by the mother during the progress of her pregnancy (heat stress, potential joint and ligament injuries, and unrecognized fetal distress). If necessary, these programs should be modified. We recommend closer obstetrical follow-up for these women to determine how they and their fetuses are responding to the program. We strongly believe that such programs should be supervised by a certified exercise leader qualified also to conduct programs for pregnant women. Exercise leaders should be required to maintain a record of injuries, and to modify programs to lower the incidence of injuries.

1. Programs should have a scientific basis.
2. Specific exercises that should be avoided include overextension and exercises performed on the back.
3. Avoid hard surfaces when exercising. Limit repetitious movements to 10.
4. Warm-up and cool down gradually.

Bicycling

There are several aerobic exercises that do not involve weight bearing—bicycling is one of them.

Bicycling is not without risk; with a stationary bicycle heat dissipation may become a problem, and exercising out of doors in traffic and smog may have unknown negative effects on both mother and fetus. Bicycling may strain the lower back in the aerodynamic position while riding a 10-speed, as the weight of the stomach accentuates the lordosis. This can be reduced by using a more upright position and/or exercising to strengthen the abdominal wall. Also, the extra weight and especially its distribution could make the woman less stable and more prone to falls. Cycling on a stationary bicycle (with

a fan) could provide a reasonable alternative to all those who wish to continue this type of exercise.

1. The program can be started during pregnancy.
2. A stationary bicycle is preferable to standard cycling due to weight and balance changes during pregnancy.
3. Bicycling may cause low back stress.
4. Bicycling should be avoided out of doors during high temperatures and high pollution levels.

Swimming

Swimming is another nonweight bearing aerobic exercise. Many consider swimming to be the most adequate aerobic exercise for the pregnant woman (23) (also see Chapter 24). We tend to agree because the changing body composition makes the mother more buoyant and, therefore, swimming is easier. However, with a change in weight distribution during the second and third trimesters, breathing may be more difficult. Lap swimming is one means of maintaining aerobic capacity. Also, as long as the temperature of the water is not too high (above 85–90°F), thermoregulation is not a problem being in a swimming pool (24). Water calisthenics and walking-in-water programs can augment swimming as an aquatic activity.

Throughout the pregnancy, the mother may be able to maintain a given distance but take longer to complete it (23).

1. Respiratory changes may make swimming difficult in late pregnancy.
2. Calisthenic exercise in water is encouraged for maintenance of strength and flexibility.
3. Swimming in water that is either too cold or too hot should be avoided.
4. Jacuzzi temperatures above 38.5°C should be avoided.

Scuba Diving

Based on the available information, it is presently recommended that women who are or may become pregnant not dive (20, 25, 26). The risks of diving during pregnancy are not warranted considering its potential effects. Both experimental and case reports indicate that the fetus may be at greater risk than the diving mother. The potential effects consist of decompression sickness, hyperoxia, hypoxia, hypercapnia, and asphyxia. There are insufficient data to establish safe diving tables for the pregnant woman and her fetus. The Undersea Medical Society (26) recommends that pregnant women who choose to dive against medical advice be informed that the potential risk to the fetus apparently increases as the no-decompression limits are approached, as the oxygen tension of the inspired gas increases, and perhaps also as a function of other factors that remain to be identified.

MUSCULAR STRENGTH AND ENDURANCE ACTIVITIES

Weight Lifting

For many years, weight lifting was not recommended for women in general; for pregnant women it was unheard of. As more and more health clubs began opening, weight lifting became a complementary exercise for whatever form of aerobic exercise was being undertaken. Because women who become pregnant do not want to give up any part of their routine, they need to know how to lift weights safely. As weight machines are used frequently rather than free weights, the fear of damage to the baby by dropping a weight is alleviated. This is not to say that free weights cannot be used, but rather that "spotting" is more necessary to avoid injury at this time. The fetus is well protected by the maternal anatomical structures, but there is evidence that blunt trauma to the abdomen could damage the uterus or cause placental abruptio (20). The only available weight training program in print is the Nautilus program, "Making Mama Fit: The Ultimate Game Plan" (27). Although a scientific basis for the program is claimed, none is cited. Such programs may place pregnant women at high risk for spinal and disc injuries facilitated by the relaxation of joints and ligaments in pregnancy. Any program that works the entire body, promoting toning and flexibility, can be recommended only within certain limits. One possible problem that could arise for the inexperienced weight lifter is transient hypertension caused by the Valsalva maneuver, which causes a significant decrease in venous return to the heart, an increase in arterial pressure, and increased work for the heart. The decreased cardiac output blood flow to the brain may cause orthostatic hypotension. It may also cause decreased perfusion of the uterus. Breathing properly, i.e., exhaling during a lift, will keep this from happening. Low weights and moderate repetitions should make up the program to maintain flexibility while toning the muscles. Using very light weights (2–5 kg) as the pregnancy progresses is recommended to prevent injuries to joints and ligaments (13). Exercises should not be performed while in the supine position. Heavy weight lifting or high resistance activities should be limited or avoided in pregnancy and done only under strict prescription and supervision.

1. Training with light weights can be cautiously continued throughout pregnancy.
2. Heavy resistance on weight machines should be avoided.
3. The use of heavy free weights should be avoided.
4. Proper breathing is necessary to avoid the Valsalva maneuver.

Recreational and Sports Activities

All sporting events include some inherent danger to the participants. When a pregnant woman desires to engage in such activities, she must be advised and consider these dangers and decide whether she can modify her activities accordingly or whether she may elect to avoid the activity altogether. Contact sports such as basketball are better avoided not just for fear of potential trauma to the abdomen from falling, but also because of the unpredictability of the opponent's movements. Volleyball, gymnastics, and horseback riding follow closely on the list of potentially dangerous sports (13, 20).

Racquet sports such as tennis, racquetball, and squash are considered, within certain limits, fairly safe sports. The intensity should be reduced as the pregnancy progresses to prevent injuries due to impaired coordination secondary to the new weight distribution and change in center of gravity. Especially in racquetball and squash, heat stress should be considered because they are played in a confined area with little air circulation (20). In addition, overstretching could be traumatic to joints and ligaments, thus it is preferable that this activity be limited to women with well-toned and well-developed muscles who exercise regularly.

Water sports such as water skiing also should be engaged in with caution.

Two sporting activities that can be safely continued throughout the pregnancy with little inherent danger are golf and slow-pitch softball. The golf swing may have to be modified, but the walk around the golf course could provide a nice diversion from the usual walk around the neighborhood for the woman who is using walking as her form of exercise. Slow-pitch softball, if the game is not too competitive, can also be continued throughout the pregnancy. The pregnant woman should be advised that her balance is compromised by additional weight and not to take unnecessary risks (13, 20). Actions such as sliding into bases and blocking bases should be avoided.

Winter activities can also be enjoyed if care is taken to protect against the cold. The function of the cardiopulmonary system is altered by pregnancy, and exercise in the cold can put an additional strain on it. Exposure to extreme cold must be avoided. If the pregnant woman is skiing (either downhill or cross-country) or skating, she is probably already expert in an activity that could be inherently dangerous to an unskilled person. These sports should not be taken up by a novice during pregnancy. For the competent athlete, these activities should not be undertaken competitively during pregnancy; i.e., fatigue and strain should be avoided. Because of the possibility of injuries caused by poor balance during pregnancy, downhill skiing and skating should be given up sooner than cross-country skiing (20). For the mother who lives in a climate where snow and cold weather are common for much of the winter, cross-country skiing can be a very good activity for maintaining cardiovascular fitness. Such activities should be interspersed with frequent periods of rest and adequate hydration. Cross-country skiing stresses the cardiovascular system to a higher degree than either of the other activities because all the large muscle groups are being used and, therefore, cross-country skiing at a moderate pace will promote a higher fitness level.

The muscle and joint injuries associated with sports activities may be avoided if a woman is skilled and in good physical condition (28).

NONSTRENUOUS RELAXATION ACTIVITIES

Yoga

Yoga has experienced a popularity with pregnant women for two reasons: first is the relaxation effect that many women seek during their pregnancy, and second is the desire to maintain muscle tone and flexibility throughout the 9 months (29, 30). These are both good reasons, and as long as yoga is accompanied by some form of aerobic work, it can be an adequate form of workout. Yoga postures may have to be modified as the pregnancy progresses, i.e., using chairs, or pillows, or another person for better balance or posture. Yoga can be done alone or in a class, depending on the expertise of the mothers but as with every form of exercise, consistency is the most important component of the program. Supine and prolonged standing exercises should be eliminated because they may induce the aortocaval syndrome or hypotension. The yoga plan and exercises that include extreme stretching should be eliminated as well.

Exercise Prescription in Pregnancy

Exercise is being routinely prescribed for various clinical conditions in the nonpregnant woman, but has not been offered to pregnant women in the past because of the fear that the potential maternal benefits could be offset by potential fetal risks. Exercise prescription requires a thorough knowledge of exercise physiology and recognition of potential risks associated with exercise during pregnancy. As emphasized numerous times throughout this text, such risks are amplified in pregnancy by normal anatomic and physiological changes in pregnancy.

EXERCISE FOR PREGNANT DIABETICS

One significant step was recently taken in utilizing exercise as an adjunct or alternative therapeutic modality for the control of blood glucose levels for pregnant diabetics. Recent acquired information has made it possible to initiate such investigational programs in the type II pregnant diabetic (31–33). Comparative physiological studies between weight bearing and nonweight bearing exercise in pregnancy may indicate a preferential utilization of carbohydrates during nonweight bearing exercises in pregnancy (34).

The risks of low-intensity exercise during pregnancy in previously sedentary individuals (as many diabetics are) are minimal and predominantly include soft tissue musculoskeletal injuries; thus, nonweight bearing exercises may be more suitable (i.e., bicycle, arm exercise). The risks to the fetus are remote in these types of exercise.

However, individuals at risk for premature labor as some diabetics may be could have labor precipitated by physical activity even at the lowest intensity. These individuals should not be enrolled in exercise programs.

A previously published clinical protocol (35) appears to be particularly suited for the type II diabetic (Fig. 28.2). Patients entering such a program are initially screened and examined to rule out intercurrent medical or obstetrical complications. Then they undergo a symptom-limited $\dot{V}_{O_2max}$ bicycle ergometer test to determine the individual's work capacity. The patient is then instructed to follow the following program: before each meal (breakfast, lunch, and dinner), the patient rests for 30 min, during which time she monitors fetal activity and records the movements (this provision is included to allow a crude evaluation and home monitoring of the fetus' well-being after 26 weeks' gestation). The patient is in-

structed to skip the next exercise session if the fetus did not move during the 30-min preexercise period or to notify the physician if the fetus has moved less than 10 times in 24 hr. Thereafter, she checks her own blood glucose with a home blood glucose monitoring device. If the blood glucose is <60 mg/dl, or >250 mg/dl, or if ketonuria is present, she is to skip the exercise session and notify the physician. In the absence of the previously stated conditions, the patient will consume her prescribed meal and then exercise on a stationary cycle ergometer at 50% of her predetermined maximum aerobic capacity. Immediately after the exercise, the patient will again check her blood glucose, rest for 30 minutes, and count fetal movements. The patient should be aware of uterine activity and if uterine contractions should become regular and/or occur at intervals of 15 min or less, she should consult her obstetrician. The subjects sign an informed consent and are informed of potential complications. They are also required to keep accurate records of their blood glucose determinations, food intake, fetal movements, and certainly, their own physical activities. Beginning after approximately 32 weeks' gestation, fetal heart rate monitoring (nonstress testing) is conducted weekly. Further fetal testing is done as indicated. Preliminary available information indicates that exercise could be safely utilized by the pregnant diabetic, provided that appropriate steps were taken to avoid complications. A program of adequate frequency and intensity specifically tailored for the pregnant diabetic patient could improve insulin sensitivity and attain normoglycemia.

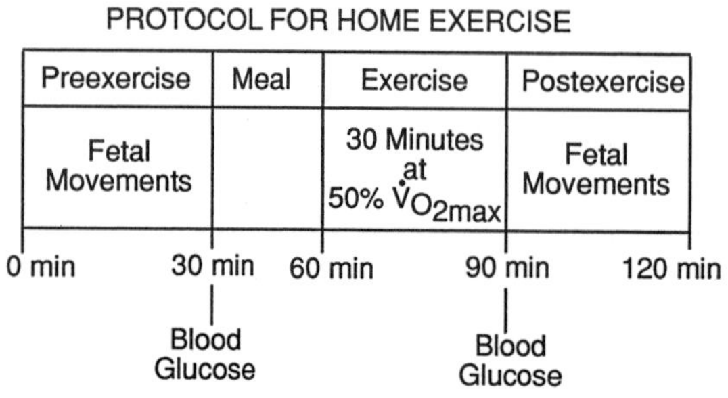

PROTOCOL FOR HOME EXERCISE

Preexercise	Meal	Exercise	Postexercise
Fetal Movements		30 Minutes at 50% $\dot{V}_{O_2max}$	Fetal Movements

0 min	30 min	60 min	90 min	120 min
	Blood Glucose		Blood Glucose	

Figure 28.2.   Protocol for home exercise.

Postpartum Exercise

With the process of delivery the continuous anatomic and functional changes of pregnancy start the slow process of reversal that traditionally is thought to take 6 weeks. From the athlete's perspective, recovery from pregnancy labor and delivery is to overcome a detraining period. The process of regaining complete physical fitness is a gradual one that includes restorative processes complicated, in part, by the persistent changes associated with pregnancy.

To recapitulate the anatomic changes that occur in the postpartum period: the uterus involutes to its prepregnancy size in 6 weeks. The lochia discharge gradually diminishes within 3–6 weeks. The abdominal wall remains soft and flabby for weeks and only gradual training will return it to its prepregnancy shape. The changes in the urinary tract take at least 8 weeks to reverse. The episiotomy and vaginal lacerations heal quickly within 1–2 weeks and the perineum appears completely recovered by 6 weeks. Most of the hormonal pregnancy-related changes reverse to prepregnancy levels within 30 days. Although the serum concentrations of relaxin produced by the corpus luteum of pregnancy decline to normal within 3–7 days postpartum, its anatomic effects may persist as long as 12 weeks. Physical recovery from any medical condition is a gradual process that varies from one individual to another. If the woman had a vaginal delivery, she could engage in some form of physical activity the day after her delivery, i.e., brief walk through the hospital ward. In the case of cesarean section, meaningful physical activities cannot be resumed as long as pain persists. For women who breast-feed, the dietary intake has to be increased by 600 cal. It also appears that the quality of the milk may differ after exercise, thus, it may be advisable to breast-feed immediately before engaging in physical activities rather than after.

The same general principles applied for any detrained population can be utilized by women recovering from delivery.

POSTPARTUM EXERCISE

1. Gradual but regular exercise (at least three times per week), correct anemia before engaging in moderately strenuous activities;
2. Ballistic movements, extreme stretching, heavy weight lifting, and weight resistance machines should be avoided for 12 weeks or longer if joint laxity persists;
3. Target heart rates and limits should be established in consultation with a physician;
4. Liquids should be taken liberally, caloric intake should be balanced and adequate.

SUMMARY

The guidelines outlined in this chapter are in compliance with those issued by ACOG (Appendix) and are for the general population. They are the product of a comprehensive overview of the available scientific literature and its interpretation by these authors. An attempt was made to separate "empirical" advice from "common sense" advice. Sports activities and exercise in pregnancy are by and large recreational, thus whenever the potential consequences of one or more activities is not known, medical practice dictates a prudent approach by erring on the safe side. We also recognize that fetal complications and injury are more difficult to identify than maternal side effects or injury. Guidelines should be viewed strictly as guidelines; as more pertinent information becomes available, they can be easily modified. In the interim, these guidelines reflect the consensus opinion about preventing injuries to both mother and fetus while engaging in activities that have not been shown to improve pregnancy outcomes for the mother or fetus. Adopting modified and individualized exercise programs is certainly a prudent approach and, as proven in the general non-pregnant population, such programs can also promote health benefits.

REFERENCES

1. Blair SN, Chandler JY, Ellisor DB, Langley J. Improving physical fitness by exercise training programs. South Med J 1980; 73:1594–1596.
2. American College of Sports Medicine. Guidelines for exercise testing and prescription, 3rd ed. Philadelphia: Lea & Febiger, 1986.
3. ACOG. Home exercise programs—Exercise during pregnancy and the postnatal period. Washington, DC: ACOG, 1985.
4. Brotanek V, Surean G. Exercise test as a physiological form of antepartum test. Int J Gynaecol Obstet 1985; 23:327–333.
5. Johnstone RW. A textbook of midwifery. London: Adams, Charles & Black, 1913; p. 101.
6. Haultan WFT, Fahmy ECF. Antenatal care. Edinburgh: Livingston, 1929, p. 13.
7. Burnett C. Value of antenatal exercise. J Obstet Gynaecol Br Emp 1956; 63:40.
8. Roberts H, Wooton IDP, Kane KM, Burnett WE. The value of antenatal preparation. J Obstet Gynaecol Br Emp 1953; 60:404.
9. Young J. Relaxation of pelvic joints in pregnancy. J Obstet Gynaecol Br Emp 1940; 47:49.
10. Heyman J, Lundquist A. The symphysis pubis in

pregnancy and parturition. Acta Obstet Gynaecol Scand 1932; 12:191.

11. Blankfield A. Is exercise necessary for the obstetric patient. Med J Austral 1967; 1:163–165.

12. Gardosi J, Hutson N, Lynch BC. Randomized, controlled trial of squatting in the second stage of labour. Lancet 1989; 2:74–77.

13. Danforth DN. Pregnancy and labor from the vantage point of the physical therapist. Am J Phys Med 1967; 46:653–658.

14. Jarrett II JC, Spellacy WN. Jogging during pregnancy: an improved outcome? Obstet Gynecol 1983; 61:705–709.

15. Pomerance JJ, Gluck L, Lynch VA. Physical fitness in pregnancy: its effect on pregnancy outcome. Am J Obstet Gynecol 1974; 119:867–876.

16. Speroff L. Can exercise cause problems in pregnancy and menstruation? Contemp OB/GYN 1980; 16:57–63.

17. Simkin D. The complete pregnancy exercise program. New York: New American Library, Mosby Times Mirror, 1980.

18. Harris NF. Controlled childbirth. Palm Springs, CA: Harris Industries, 1976.

19. Bing E. Six practical lessons for an easier childbirth. New York: Grosset & Dunlap, 1978.

20. Bullard JA. Exercise and pregnancy. Can Fam Physic 1981; 27:977–982.

21. Hauth JO, Gilstrap LC, Widmer K. Fetal heart rate reactivity before and after maternal jogging during the third trimester. Am J Obstet Gynecol 1982; 142:545–547.

22. Jarrett JC, Spellacy WN. Jogging during pregnancy: an improved outcome? Obstet Gynecol 1983; 61:705–709.

23. Katz J. Swimming through your pregnancy, the perfect exercise for pregnant women. New York: Dolphin Books, Doubleday, 1983; p. 1–159.

24. St. John W. Body composition of female college age swimmers. Master's thesis, University of Cincinnati, 1978, p. 15.

25. Kizer KW. Women and diving. Phys Sports Med 1981; 9:84–92.

26. Fife WP. Effects of diving on pregnancy. Undersea Med Soc 36, 1980.

27. Hall DC, Geinl GK. Making mama fit: the ultimate game. New York: Leisure Press, 1982, p. 177–192.

28. Astrand PO, Rodahl K. Textbook of work physiology, ed 2. New York: McGraw-Hill, 1977.

29. Thompson J. Healthy pregnancy the yoga way. New York: Dolphin Books, Doubleday, 1977.

30. Leboyer F. Inner beauty inner light yoga for pregnant women. New York: Bolzoi Book, Alfred A. Knopf, 1978.

31. Artal R, Wiswell R, Romem Y. Hormonal responses to exercise in diabetic and nondiabetic pregnant patients. Diabetes 1985; 39:78–80.

32. Jovanovic L, Durak EP, Peterson CM. Randomized trial of diet versus diet plus cardiovascular conditioning on glucose levels in gestational diabetes. Am J Obstet Gynecol 1989; 161:415–419.

33. Summary and Recommendations of the Second International Workshop—Conference on Gestational Diabetes Mellitus. Therapeutic strategies. Diabetes 1985; 34:125.

34. Artal LR, Masaki DI, Khodiguian N, Romem Y, Rutherford SE, Wiswell RA. Exercise prescription in pregnancy: weight-bearing versus non-weight-bearing exercise. AM J Obstet Gynecol 1989; 161:1464–1469.

35. Artal R, Masaki D. Exercise in gestational diabetes. Prac Diabet 1989; 8:7–14.

ACOG Guidelines: Exercise During Pregnancy and the Postnatal Period

The American College of Obstetricians and Gynecologists (ACOG) is the national specialty society that represents the 29,000 practicing obstetricians and gynecologists in the United States and Canada. It is dedicated to maintain and improve the quality of health care for women through the development of physician self-assessment programs and a wide variety of other educational programs for its members and their patients. The College also sets practice parameters, develops quality assurance guidelines, and maintains active government relations, professional liability, and public information departments.

The ACOG is organized using an elected Executive Board supported by an extensive Commission and Standing Committee structure with additional support from subcommittees and task forces. The College is located in Washington, DC and employs a staff of 175 people.

Fulfillment of its continuing medical education responsibilities to its membership and playing its role in the continuum of education for the obstetrician and gynecologist is one of the College's major responsibilities. In that context, it produces many publications of an educational nature to assist its members to become familiar with current knowledge and technology. The College does not do the original medical research, but rather develops consensus documents through the work of committees and task forces composed of its members who have both special expertise and practice experience. These documents are intended to be educational aids to present recognized methods and techniques of clinical practice for consideration by obstetrician-gynecologists for incorporation into their practices. Variations of practice taking into account the needs of the individual patient, resources, and limitations unique to the institution or type of practice may be appropriate.

The educational bulletin "Exercise During Pregnancy and the Postnatal Period" is an example of one of these ACOG publications. It was originally published in May, 1985 following deliberations of an educational task force of eight content experts. It describes the physiological changes that occur during pregnancy that relate to exercise and it suggests how to develop an exercise prescription for pregnant women. It also lists risk factors during pregnancy. Recent review by the same group indicates that new scientific knowledge has not shown any need to change these recommendations and that these guidelines for exercise during pregnancy are still pertinent.

—Harrison C. Visscher, MD
Director of Education
The American College
of Obstetricians and Gynecologists

With increasing frequency, women are turning to their physicians for advice about exercise during pregnancy and the postpartum period. Although regular exercise would appear to be beneficial to women at these times, the unique physical and physiological conditions that exist during pregnancy and the postpartum period create special risks that do not affect nonpregnant women.

The societal pressures to exercise today and the competitive spirit that challenges some women to place performance goals above safety indicate the need for a scientific approach to recommendations for exercise. Furthermore, the changing nature of exercise opportunities presents some additional concerns.

The number and type of exercise programs available now to pregnant and postpartum women have increased dramatically. Some of these programs were designed by nonprofessionals who lack the scientific background to appreciate potential problems and take steps to minimize their occurrence. A recent review of several exercise programs being marketed to pregnant and postpartum patients revealed medical content that was often inappropriate, inaccurate, or incomplete.

Exercise standards for pregnant women, one of the major subgroups in the general population, have not been set. At present, recommendations for pregnant and postpartum patients are based largely on intuition and "common sense." Little research has been done on the effects of exercise during pregnancy and the postpartum period, and ethical considerations make it almost impossible to define limits of safety.

It is noteworthy that no evidence exists to support the popular notion that regular exercise will improve the outcome of pregnancy. Those studies that have been done reveal no change in the length or quality of labor and no reduction in the number of maternal or fetal complications. There is some evidence that increased occupational activity and heavy endurance exercise will shorten the length of gestation and result in lower infant birth weights. The significance of this finding can only be speculated upon.

Guidelines for exercise during pregnancy and the postpartum period should be based on consideration of the physiological changes that take place at these times. When establishing an exercise program for patients, physicians should advise them of limitations, contraindications, warning signs, and any special concerns.

It should be noted that recommendations designed for a general cross-section of the population may not be appropriate for a particular patient. A physically fit pregnant patient may tolerate a more strenuous program, whereas an unfit, overweight individual with a sedentary life-style should restrict activities to those that are less vigorous.

CHANGES DURING PREGNANCY THAT AFFECT EXERCISE

Maternal Considerations

CONNECTIVE TISSUE

Under the influence of hormones such as estrogen, progesterone, and elastin, the ground substance and connective tissue become softer and more easily stretched. This results in connective tissue laxity and joint instability, rendering joints more susceptible to injury.

As pregnancy progresses, the enlarging uterus and breasts produce changes in the body's center of gravity. There is increased lordosis during pregnancy and increased strain on the sacroiliac and hip joints. This causes additional strain on the back and creates balance problems, increasing the risk of falls, especially during exercise. Back and hip pain are considerably more common.

Other problems of particular concern at this time include nerve compression syndromes such as carpal tunnel syndrome and, more rarely, separation of the symphysis pubis.

CARDIOVASCULAR RESPONSE

During normal pregnancy, maternal blood volume increases by about 30% and sometimes more, and heart rate and cardiac output are significantly elevated at rest. Hematocrit levels are lower during pregnancy, but the tendency toward hemoconcentration increases during exercise. When pregnant women exercise vigorously, it is common to observe a rise in the hematocrit of 10 percentage points within 15 min. These cardiovascular and hemodynamic changes persist for approximately 4 weeks after delivery and remain a significant factor during postpartum exercise.

These changes significantly reduce the cardiac reserve during increased physical activity. They must be taken into consideration in establishing the intensity level of exercise during pregnancy and the postpartum period and in determining safe target heart rates. Heart rate is utilized as an approximate index of aerobic fitness, although a better way to evaluate fitness is to measure the amount of oxygen used during exercise. In general, target heart rates for pregnant and postpartum women should be set approximately 25–30% lower than would be appropriate at other times.

The major hemodynamic response to exercise is redistribution of blood flow, away from the splanchnic organs and toward the working muscles. During exercise, the blood flow to the brain and heart remain unchanged. Animal studies suggest that at least 50% of uterine blood flow must be redistributed before it will affect the fetus, but there is no human research to corroborate or refute this.

It should be noted that even more variability in cardiovascular response to exercise exists during pregnancy and the postpartum period than at other times. Pregnant and postpartum women who exercise should be advised to measure heart rates during activity and given limits to follow. The physician should be especially concerned with women whose oxygen-carrying capacity is compromised by anemia and with women who are extremely sedentary or obese. The response of these patients to even mild exercise is significantly abnormal.

After the fourth month of pregnancy, the enlarging uterus is capable of interfering with venous return by compression of the vena cava. This can cause supine hypotensive syndrome, affecting cardiac output and interfering with uterine circulation, and it has been implicated as a cause of placental abruption.

RESPIRATORY RESPONSE TO EXERCISE IN PREGNANCY

Near the end of pregnancy, the enlarging uterus displaces the diaphragm upward, reducing the height of the pleural cavities by as much as 4 cm and, in some women, creating discomfort and a feeling of dyspnea. However, pulmonary function is not impaired at rest in pregnancy, as there is concomitant lateral expansion of the rib cage and increased tidal volume. The increased tidal volume results in increased ventilation at rest. The increased oxygen requirements of normal pregnancy are easily met.

This hyperventilation increases with mild exercise during pregnancy, but does not increase proportionately with moderate and severe exercise in comparison with nonpregnant women. During mild levels of activity, the expected increases in oxygen consumption occur. However, during high-intensity exercise, the increase is less than expected, suggesting that pregnant women are unable to maintain high levels of aerobic activity. This also indicates a decrease in pulmonary reserve and an inability to compensate effectively for anaerobic exercise. This respiratory inefficiency increases the risk of lactic acidosis if high-intensity exercise is maintained for long periods.

NUTRITIONAL CHANGES

Approximately 300 extra calories are required each day to meet the metabolic needs of pregnancy. Very active women need even more. These women should be encouraged to eat enough to supply the additional energy requirements of exercise during pregnancy. The use of exercise to promote weight reduction should be discouraged during pregnancy.

The risk of dehydration during exercise is increased in pregnant women. Dehydration can increase the core temperature to dangerous levels. Because of this, patients should be advised to drink liquids before and after exercise and, if necessary, to interrupt activity to replenish fluids.

On an average, women who do not breastfeed will have gained about 6 lb when their weight stabilizes postpartum. With repeated pregnancies, the accumulation of excess weight can reach medically significant levels. To correct this tendency, weight control through exercise and dietary measures is appropriate after each pregnancy.

METABOLIC RESPONSE

Temperature Control

Vigorous physical activity for sustained periods of time increases the body core temperature. In nonpregnant women, 30–60 min of strenuous exercise can increase the core temperature to 39°C. Strenuous exercise for 15 min will usually not increase the temperature over 38°C. Data are not available for pregnant women, but the basal body temperature is higher during pregnancy and it must be assumed that the same temperature response to exercise will occur.

Evidence from animal studies indicates that increased temperatures may be capable of inducing neural tube defects. No prospective studies have been done in humans; however, sporadic reports suggest that the same problem might occur. The problem of hyperthermia is of special concern during pregnancy because the fetus has no mechanisms (such as perspiration or respiration) through which excess heat can be dissipated. Pregnant women should be cautioned not to exercise when they are febrile or in hot, humid weather (when their own mechanisms for heat dissipation are compromised).

Endocrine Factors

During pregnancy, fasting blood glucose levels and glucose levels in general are lower than in nonpregnant women. Since pregnant women utilize carbohydrates at a greater rate during exercise, hypoglycemia may occur under conditions of prolonged or strenuous exercise.

Epinephrine and norepinephrine levels increase significantly during physical activity. Epinephrine tends to inhibit uterine muscle activity, while norepinephrine increases the frequency and amplitude of contractions. The increased levels of norepinephrine have the potential for precipitating premature labor in a susceptible individual. Women at risk for premature labor should avoid vigorous exercise.

FETAL RESPONSE TO MATERNAL EXERCISE

There is a close correlation between the level of sympathetic activity in the mother and the extent of fetal movements and breathing. The fetal heart rate almost always rises after maternal exercise. During exercise, however, the fetal heart rate may occasionally decrease. Fetal bradycardia has been reported in association with vigorous maternal exercise, but the actual incidence and significance is unknown. It is possible that this represents brief periods of fetal asphyxia.

DEVELOPING AN EXERCISE PRESCRIPTION

The safety of the mother and infant is the primary concern in any exercise program prescribed in conjunction with pregnancy. The potential for maternal and fetal injury is significant because of the musculoskeletal and cardiovascular changes at this time. Although the risk of fetal injury is probably small, there are insufficient scientific data to support this belief. Therefore, exercise recommendations must err on the conservative side.

The goal of exercise during pregnancy and the postpartum period should be to maintain the highest level of fitness consistent with maximum safety. Given this constraint, it is not possible to maintain cardiovascular fitness at optimum levels, nor to achieve the level of strength-training that would be reasonable in the nonpregnant state, at least as far as our knowledge at present is concerned.

In the postpartum period, fetal safety is no longer a concern. However, persistent musculoskeletal and cardiovascular changes continue to present potential problems for the woman. In addition to the concern about injuries, certain exercise routines create significant discomfort for postpartum women. This condition is further altered by the fact that women are likely to have been especially inactive immediately prior to their postpartum exercise, and regular activity is made more difficult by the responsibility of caring for a newborn child.

The *ACOG Pregnancy and Postnatal Exercise Programs* were designed for a broad section of the population. They incorporate restrictions and modifications made necessary by the physiological changes of pregnancy and the postpartum period and by a primary concern for safety. Based on their previous level of activity, some women may be able to tolerate more strenuous exercise, whereas others may need to restrict activities to those that are less vigorous such as walking.

The ideal exercise program will offer women a variety of options, including walking, swimming, stationary cycling, and modified forms of dancing or calisthenics. There is an extremely wide spectrum of ability and need to exercise in pregnancy and the postpartum period. There is also great variability in the way different pregnant women will respond to the same activity (more so than in the nonpregnant state).

Thus, no single exercise or exercise program will be able to meet the needs of all women. It is incumbent on the physician to assess the abilities and needs of the individual patient and assist her in constructing a program for her particular situation. The need for communication between physician and patient cannot be overemphasized. The patient who is alert to the potential hazards of exercise, aware of the warning signs, and in touch with her physician is less likely to suffer problems as a result of exercising during pregnancy or the postpartum period.

It is also important to remind the patient that exercise is but one activity out of many that make up a healthy life-style. Pregnant women should be made aware, also, of the importance of good nutrition and avoidance of the use of tobacco products, alcohol, and unnecessary drugs.

Exercise Guidelines

The following guidelines are based on the unique physical and physiological conditions that exist during pregnancy and the postpartum period. They outline general criteria for safety to provide direction to patients in the development of home exercise programs.

PREGNANCY AND POSTPARTUM

1. Regular exercise (at least three times per week) is preferable to intermittent activity. Competitive activities should be discouraged.
2. Vigorous exercise should not be performed in hot, humid weather or during a period of febrile illness.
3. Ballistic movements (jerky, bouncy motions) should be avoided. Exercise should be done on a wooden floor or a tightly carpeted surface to reduce shock and provide a sure footing.
4. Deep flexion or extension of joints should be avoided because of connective tissue laxity. Activities that require jumping, jarring motions or rapid changes in direction should be avoided because of joint instability.
5. Vigorous exercise should be preceded by a 5-minute period of muscle warm-up. This can be accomplished by slow walking or stationary cycling with low resistance.
6. Vigorous exercise should be followed by a period of gradually declining activity that includes gentle stationary stretching. Because connective tissue laxity increases the risk of joint injury, stretches should not be taken to the point of maximum resistance.
7. Heart rate should be measured at times of peak activity. Target heart rates and limits established in consultation with the physician should not be exceeded (see Table A.1 for recommended postpartum heart rate limits).

Table A.1. Heart Rate Guidelines for Postpartum Exercise

Age	Beats per Minute	
	Limit[a]	Maximum
20	150	200
25	146	195
30	142	190
35	138	185
40	135	180
45	131	175

[a]Each figure represents 75% of the maximum heart rate that would be predicted for the corresponding age group. Under proper medical supervision, more strenuous activity and higher heart rates may be appropriate.

8. Care should be taken to rise gradually from the floor to avoid orthostatic hypotension. Some form of activity involving the legs should be continued for a brief period.
9. Liquids should be taken liberally before and after exercise to prevent dehydration. If necessary, activity should be interrupted to replenish fluids.
10. Women who have led sedentary life-styles should begin with physical activity of very low intensity and advance activity levels very gradually.
11. Activity should be stopped and the physician consulted if any unusual symptoms appear.

PREGNANCY ONLY

1. Maternal heart rate should not exceed 140 bpm.
2. Strenuous activities should not exceed 15 min in duration.
3. No exercise should be performed in the supine position after the fourth month of gestation is completed.
4. Exercises that employ the Valsalva maneuver should be avoided.
5. Caloric intake should be adequate to meet not only the extra energy needs of pregnancy, but also of the exercise performed.
6. Maternal core temperature should not exceed 38°C.

Special Exercises for Pregnancy and the Postpartum Period

EXERCISES FOR THE BACK

The back is subjected to significant stress during pregnancy and the postpartum pe-

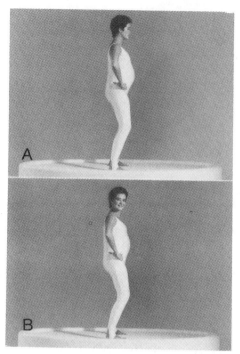

Figure A.1. Pelvic tilt. *A,* The patient is instructed to stand with her feet shoulder-width apart. The knees are bent slightly. *B,* The muscles of the buttocks and abdomen are contracted and the pelvis is gently thrust forward, rotating the pubic bone upward. This position is held for 10 sec and then released.

riod. Many traditional back strengthening exercises are not recommended during pregnancy because they require the supine position or the Valsalva maneuver. One exercise that can be done throughout pregnancy, however, is the "pelvic tilt," which strengthens abdominal musculature and reduces the lower lumbar lordosis. The exercise is performed in the following manner, as illustrated in Figure A.1.

The pelvic tilt can also be performed while lying or sitting down. Pregnant women should be encouraged to perform this maneuver as many times as possible throughout the day.

After delivery, back pain and injury remain a significant problem, because of the repeated bending, lifting, and carrying associated with child-rearing. At this time, a full program of strengthening and stretching exercises for the abdomen, back, and legs can be incorporated into the patient's daily program. The pelvic tilt should still be continued.

EXERCISES FOR THE PELVIC MUSCLES (KEGEL'S EXERCISES)

The physical and hormonal changes of pregnancy cause relaxation of the pelvic supporting tissues. Vaginal delivery stretches these tissues even further. Most women are not troubled by these changes, but some will complain of discomfort or of stress incontinence. Others may be concerned about looseness of the vagina during intercourse.

Exercise will not alter major anatomic defects. However, in patients with mild pelvic relaxation, the regular use of Kegel's exercises may be all that is necessary to provide symptomatic relief in the postpartum period. Symptomatic patients should be taught how to perform these exercises and encouraged to use them.

RISK FACTORS DURING PREGNANCY

Relative Contraindications

The physician will need to evaluate each patient individually with respect to an exercise program. The following conditions may contraindicate vigorous physical activity during pregnancy.

- Hypertension
- Anemia or other blood disorders
- Thyroid disease
- Diabetes
- Cardiac arrhythmia or palpitations
- History of precipitous labor
- History of intrauterine growth retardation
- History of bleeding during present pregnancy
- Breech presentation in the last trimester
- Excessive obesity
- Extreme underweight
- History of extremely sedentary lifestyle
- History of three or more spontaneous abortions
- Ruptured membranes
- Premature labor
- Diagnosed multiple gestation
- Incompetent cervix
- Bleeding or a diagnosis of placenta previa
- Diagnosed cardiac disease

Absolute Contraindications

The following conditions are considered contraindications to vigorous exercise during pregnancy.

The physician must be aware that complications arising during pregnancy may contraindicate vigorous activity in a woman who was previously able to exercise without restriction.

WARNING SIGNS AND SYMPTOMS

Most pregnant women and postpartum women who exercise will be doing so without supervision or with inadequate supervision. Physicians must develop and approve exercise programs with this constraint in mind and must prepare patients to recognize warning signs and symptoms that would alert them to problems. Patients should be encouraged to discuss all exercise-related questions with the physician.

The following symptoms and signs should signal the patient to stop exercise and contact her physician.

- Pain
- Bleeding
- Dizziness
- Shortness of breath
- Palpitations
- Faintness
- Tachycardia
- Back pain
- Pubic pain
- Difficulty walking

SUMMARY

There are inherent benefits to exercise: it maintains muscle tone, strength, and endurance; protects against back pain; and is felt to have a positive effect on energy level, mood, and self-image. These benefits can be appreciated during pregnancy and the postpartum period if precautions are taken in consideration of women's special needs at these times. An individualized, closely monitored exercise program can help promote fitness and, at the same time, ensure the safety of women during pregnancy and the postpartum period.

This document was developed under the direction of the Division of Education of the American College of Obstetricians and Gynecologists. The College wishes to thank Raul Artal, MD, FACOG, for his assistance in its preparation. It sets forth current information and opinions on subjects related to women's health. It does not dictate an exclusive course of treatment or procedure to be followed and should not be construed as excluding other acceptable methods of practice. Variations taking into account the needs of the individual patient, resources, and limitations unique to a type of practice may be appropriate.

From the American College of Obstetricians and Gynecologists. Exercise during pregnancy and the postnatal period. ACOG Home Exercise Programs. Washington, DC: ACOG, 1985.

BIBLIOGRAPHY

American College of Obstetrics and Gynecology: Pregnancy, work and disability. (Technical Bulletin No. 58). Washington, DC, ACOG, 1980.

Artal R, Wiswell R: Maternal Exercise. Baltimore, Williams and Wilkins, 1985

Artal R, Platt LD, Sperling M, et al: Maternal exercise: Cardiovascular and metabolic responses in normal pregnancy. Am J Obstet Gynecol 140:123, 1981

Artal R, Romem Y, Paul RH, Wiswell R: Fetal bradycardia induced by maternal exercise. Lancett II 258–269, 1984

Blankfeld A: Is exercise necessary for the obstetric patient? Med J Aust 1:163–165, 1967

Bruser M: Sporting activities during pregnancy. Obstet Gynecol 32:721, 1968

Collings CA, Curet LB, Mullin JP: Maternal and fetal responses to a maternal aerobic exercise program. Am J Obstet Gynecol 145:702, 1983

Dressendorfer RH, Goodlin RC: Fetal heart rate responses to maternal exercise testing. Phys Sports Med 8:91–96, 1980

Erkkola R: The influence of physical training during pregnancy on physical work capacity and circulatory parameters. Scand J Clin Lab Invest 36:747, 1976

Hauth JC, Gilstrap LC, Widmer K: Fetal heart rate reactivity before and after maternal jogging during the third trimester. Am J Obstet Gynecol 142:545, 1982

Longo LD et al: To what extent does maternal exercise affect fetal oxygenation and uterine blood flow? Fed Proc 37:905, 1978

Lotgering FK, Gilbert RD, Longo LD: Exercise responses in pregnant sheep: Oxygen consumption, uterine blood flow and blood volume. J Appl Physiol 55:834, 1983

Lotgering FK, Gilbert RD, Longo LD: Maternal and fetal responses to exercise during pregnancy. Physiological Reviews 65:1, 1985

Naeye RL, Peters EC: Working during pregnancy: Effects on the fetus. Pediatrics 69:724, 1982

Pernoll ML, Metcalfe J, et al: Ventilation during rest and exercise in pregnancy and postpartum. Resp Physiol 25:295, 1975

Platt LD, Artal R, et al: Maternal exercise: Fetal responses. Am J Obstet Gynecol 147:487, 1983

Pomerance J, et al: Physical fitness in pregnancy: Its effect on pregnancy outcome. Am J Obstet Gynecol 119:867, 1974

Ueland K, Navy MJ, Metcalfe J: Cardiorespiratory responses to pregnancy and exercise in normal women and patients with heart disease. Am J Obstet Gynecol 115:4, 1973

Index

Page numbers in *italics* denote figures; those followed by "t" denote tables.